Major Sponsors
supporting the European Vascular Course

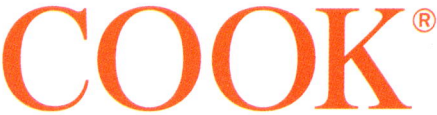

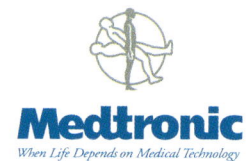

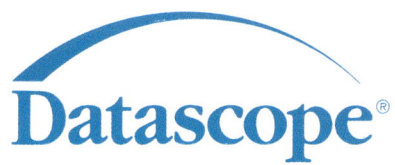

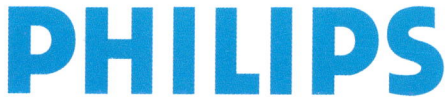

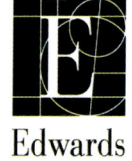

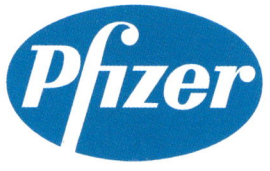

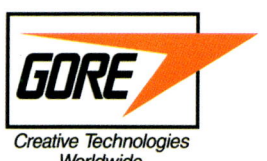

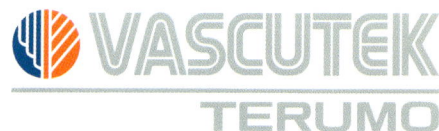

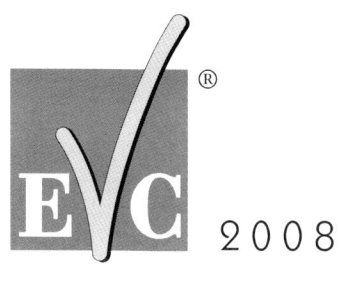

2008

ENDOVASCULAR AORTIC REPAIR: THE STATE OF THE ART

Endovascular Aortic Repair: the State of the Art

Edited by

Alain Branchereau, MD
University Hospital, Marseille, France

&

Michael Jacobs, MD
University Hospital, Maastricht, The Netherlands
University Hospital, Aachen, Germany

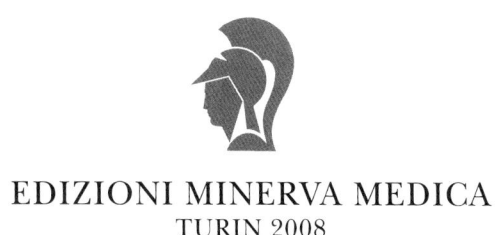

EDIZIONI MINERVA MEDICA
TURIN 2008

ISBN 10: 88-7711-604-8
ISBN 13: 978-88-7711-604-8

© 2008 – Edizioni Minerva Medica S.p.A. – Corso Bramante 83/85 – 10126 Torino (Italy)
www.minervamedica.it - E-mail: minervamedica@minervamedica.it

All rights reserved. No part of this publication may by reproduced, stored in a retrieval system, or transmitted in any form or by any means.

LIST OF CONTRIBUTORS

Chapter 1

Albert CLARÁ, Eduard MATEOS,
Francesc VIDAL-BARRAQUER
> Vascular Surgery Department
> Hospital del Mar
> Paseo Maritimo 25-29
> 08003 Barcelona, Spain

and

Begoña ROMÁN
> Theoretical and Practical Philosophy Department
> Universitat de Barcelona
> Montalegre 6
> 08001 Barcelona, Spain

Chapter 2

Andrea Maria DIRRIGL, Hermann BERGER,
Alexander ZIMMERMANN, Christian REEPS,
Andreas KÜHNL, Heiko WENDORFF,
Hans-Henning ECKSTEIN
> Department of Vascular Surgery,
> Department of Interventional Radiology
> Klinikum Rechts der Isar
> Technical University of Munich
> Ismaninger Strasse 22
> 81675 Munich, Germany

Chapter 3

Nabil CHAKFE, Olivier CRETON, Fabien THAVEAU,
Yannick GEORG, Jean-Georges KRETZ
> Department of Vascular Surgery
> Les Hôpitaux Universitaires de Strasbourg
> 1, place de l'Hôpital
> B.P. 426
> 67091 Strasbourg Cedex, France

and

Andrei IVANENKO, Daniel MATHIEU,
Bernard DURAND
> Laboratoire de Physique et Mécanique Textile
> ENSISA
> Mulhouse, France

Chapter 4

Gianbattista PARLANI, Paola DE RANGO,
Fabio VERZINI, Giuseppe PANUCCIO,
Gustavo IACONO, Piergiorgio CAO
> Department of Vascular and Endovascular Surgery
> University of Perugia
> Ospedale S. Maria della Misericordia
> Loc. S. Andrea delle Fratte
> 06156 Perugia, Italy

Chapter 5

Pierre ALRIC, Ludovic CANAUD, Frédéric JOYEUX,
Pascal BRANCHEREAU, Charles MARTY-ANE,
Jean-Philippe BERTHET
> Service de Chirurgie Thoracique et Vasculaire
> CHRU de Montpellier
> Hôpital Arnaud de Villeneuve
> 371 Avenue du Doyen Gaston Giraud
> 34295 Montpellier Cedex 05, France

Chapter 6

Aysel CAN, Giovanni TORSELLO, Thomas UMSCHEID
> Department of Vascular Surgery
> St. Franziskus Hospital
> Hohenzollernring 72
> 48145 Münster, Germany

Chapter 7

Martin MALINA, Tim RESCH, Björn SONESSON
> Vascular Center Malmö-Lund
> Department of Vascular Disease and Endovascular Center
> Malmö University Hospital
> 20502 Malmö, Sweden

Chapter 8

Geoffrey GILLING-SMITH
> Regional Vascular Unit
> Royal Liverpool University Hospital
> Prescot Street
> Liverpool L7 8XP, England

Chapter 9

Andrew ENGLAND
> Division of Medical Imaging & Radiotherapy
> University of Liverpool
> Liverpool, England

and

Richard McWILLIAMS
> Department of Radiology
> Royal Liverpool and Broadgreen University Hospitals
> Prescot Street
> Liverpool L7 8XP, England

Chapter 10

Roberto CHIESA, Germano MELISSANO,
Luca BERTOGLIO,
Massimiliano Maria MARROCCO-TRISCHITTA,
Efrem CIVILINI, Yamume TSHOMBA,
Fabio Massimo CALLIARI, Enrico Maria MARONE,
Giliola CALORI
    "Vita-Salute" University, Scientific Institute H. San Raffaele
    Department of Vascular Surgery
    IRCCS H. San Raffaele
    Via Olgettina, 60
    20132 Milan, Italy

Chapter 11

Timothy CHUTER
    Division of Vacular Surgery
    UCSF
    400 Parnassus Ave., A-581
    San Francisco, CA 94143, USA

Chapter 12

Stéphan HAULON, Richard AZZAOUI,
Elixène jEAN-BAPTISTE, Tommaso DONATI,
Piervito D'ELIA, Sébastien AMIOT,
Jonathan SOBOCINSKI, Mohamad KOUSSA
    Chirurgie Vasculaire
    Hôpital Cardiologique
    CHRU de Lille
    Boulevard du Professeur Jules Leclerq
    59037 Lille Cedex, France

Chapter 13

Tara MASTRACCI, Roy GREENBERG, Coletta VIDMAR
    Endovasular Research
    Department of Vascular Surgery
    Cleveland Clinic
    9500 Euclid Avenue
    Cleveland, OH 44195, USA

Chapter 14

Andrew CHOONG, Nicholas CHESHIRE
    Section of Vascular Surgery
    Department of Biosurgery and Surgical Technology
    Imperial College London
    Regional Vascular Unit, St Mary's Hospital
    Mary Stanford Wing,
    Praed Street, Paddington
    London W2 1NY, England

Chapter 15

Christos KARKOS, Zoran RANČIĆ, Murat AKSOY,
Alexei SVETLIKOV, Yuriy SPIRIN
    Department of Vascular Surgery
    Clinical Center Niš
    Bul. Dr. Zorana Đinđića 48
    18000 Niš, Serbia

Chapter 16

Pierre-Edouard MAGNAN, Nabil SEDKI,
Michel BARTOLI, Alain BRANCHEREAU
    Faculté de Médicine de Marseille
    Université de la Méditerranée
    Assistance Publique Hôpitaux de Marseille
    Hôpital la Timone
    Service de Chirurgie Vasculaire
    13385 Marseille Cedex 05, France

Chapter 17

Meryl DAVIS, Peter TAYLOR
    Guy's and St. Thomas' NHS Foundation Trust
    St. Thomas' Hospital
    Lambeth Palace Road
    London SE1 7EH, England

Chapter 18

Geert Willem SCHURINK,
Tanja LETTINGA VAN DE POLL, Thomas KOEPPEL,
Stephan LANGER, Gottfried MOMMERTZ,
Michiel de HAAN, Michael JACOBS
    European Vascular Center Aachen-Maastricht
    Department of Vascular Surgery
    University Hospital Maastricht
    P.O. Box 5800
    6202 AZ Maastricht, the Netherlands

Chapter 19

Jan BRUNKWALL, Vladimir MATOUSSEVITCH,
Michael GAWENDA
    Department of Vascular and Endovascular Surgery
    University Clinics
    University of Cologne
    Kerpener Strasse 62
    50931 Cologne, Germany

Chapter 20

Matt THOMPSON, David SAYER, Ian LOFTUS,
Rob MORGAN
    St. George's Vascular Institute
    4th Floor St. James Wing
    St. George's Hospital
    London SW17 0QT, England

Chapter 21

Stephan LANGER, Gottfried MOMMERTZ, Thomas
KOEPPEL, Geert Willem SCHURINK, Michael JACOBS
    European Vascular Center Aachen-Maastricht
    Klinik für Gefaesschirurgie
    Universitätsklinikum Aachen
    Pauwelsstrasse 30
    52074 Aachen, Deutschland

Chapter 22
Clark ZEEBREGTS, Eric VERHOEVEN,
Ignace TIELLIU, Wendy BOS, Ted PRINS,
Roy DE JONG, Jan VAN DEN DUNGEN
  Department of Surgery
  University Medical Center Groningen
  P.O. Box 30 001
  9700 RB Groningen, the Netherlands

Chapter 23
Zoran RANČIĆ, Dieter MAYER, Christian SCHMID,
Mario LACHAT
  Clinic for Cardiovascular Surgery
  University Hospital Zürich

and

Thomas PFAMMATTER
  Institute for Diagnostic and Interventional Radiology
  University Hospital Zürich
  Ramistrasse 100
  8091 Zürich, Switzerland

Chapter 24
David BECKETT, Steven THOMAS,
Syed Tansheet MUSTAFA, Mathew KADUTHODIL
  Sheffield Vascular Institute
  Northern General Hospital
  Herries Road
  Sheffield S5 7AU, England

FOREWORD

Aortic pathology comprises an extensive range of diseases, which can be located along the entire length, from the ascending aorta to the iliac bifurcation. Apart from aneurysms, pathology includes acute and chronic dissection, inflammatory and ulcerating disease, atherosclerotic degeneration, connective tissue abnormalities, traumatic rupture, fistula with surrounding organs like lung, esophagus, bowel and veins. Involvement of side branches with subsequent organ dysfunction like the brain, spinal cord, intestines, kidneys and extremities further determine the complexity of diagnosis and therapy of aortic diseases.

Since the Egyptian, Indian and Greco-Roman times, the history of aortic interventions has known a wide spectrum of exotic procedures. From the 16th to the mid-19th century surgical treatment included cauterization of aneurysms and introduction of foreign bodies. From the 19th century ligation, resection, wiring and wrapping without repair were introduced and gradually evolved to the current techniques of open repair of thoracic and abdominal aortic pathology during the last 50 years of the 20th century. Following, the spectacular idea of endovascular solutions was introduced only two decades ago and we all had the privilege to witness a tremendous development of technology and devices. At present, treatment of aortic diseases is primarily dictated by endovascular measures, requiring that all of us working in this field are familiar with the available endovascular technology, strategy planning and practical handling.

The subject of the 2008 European Vascular Course is Endovascular Aortic Repair: the State of the Art, *and the aim is to gather the latest and most updated knowledge on this theme. The experts in the field have covered the entire spectrum of endovascular aortic repair addressing training and educational matters, characteristics of stent-graft material, assessment and sizing, solving intraprocedural problems and handling postoperative complications. The challenging development of side branch technology is extensively presented including aortic arch and thoraco-abdominal pathology. Furthermore, false and infected aneurysms as well as traumatic injuries are included and treatment of acute and chronic dissections broadly discussed. Finally, surveillance and short-time morbidity-mortality of abdominal and thoracic endografting are defined and detailed.*

Since the number of vascular meetings addressing endovascular aortic repair is overwhelming, it would be justified to ask why the European Vascular Course selected this topic in 2008. Apart from covering the entire spectrum and offering the latest update, the answer to the question is this high standard textbook which comprises the most recent experiences, reviews of the literature, tips and tricks, dangers and pitfalls, drawings and illustrations: a reference book for the vascular interventionalist.

We are greatly indebted to our invited authors for their significant contribution. Our new publisher Minerva Medica has realized an immense challenge and we are grateful to Mrs Eugenia Battaglio and Mrs Cecilia Ponsat who accomplished the editing and production of the English and French textbook. We thank Dr Nabil Sedki and our secretaries Mrs Annie Barral and Mrs Claire Meertens for their assistance in preparing this book.

The appearance of this work is only possible with the continuous support of our major sponsors to whom we express our sincere gratitude.

Maastricht, Aachen - Marseille, 2008

Michael Jacobs - Alain Branchereau

CONTENTS

List of Contributors VII

Foreword XI

1 Transgressing the Boundaries: the Hermeneutics of Endovascular Aortic Repair's Enthusiasm
Albert Clará, Eduard Mateos Begoña Román, Francesc Vidal-Barraquer 1

2 How to Learn Endovascular Aortic Procedures - Theoretical and Practical Education
Andrea Maria Dirrigl, Hermann Berger Alexander Zimmermann, Christian Reeps, Andreas Kühnl, Heiko Wendorff Hans-Henning Eckstein 9

3 Characteristics of Aortic Stent Grafts Including Durability and Fatigue Testing
Nabil Chakfe, Olivier Creton Andrei Ivanenko, Fabien Thaveau Daniel Mathieu, Yannick Georg Jean-Georges Kretz, Bernard Durand 23

4 Different Types of Infrarenal (Modular, Unibody, Aorto-Uni-Iliac) and Thoracic Endografts: Advantages and Drawbacks
Gianbattista Parlani, Paola De Rango Fabio Verzini, Giuseppe Panuccio Gustavo Iacono, Piergiorgio Cao 35

5 Preoperative Assessment for Descending Thoracic Aortic Endografting
Pierre Alric, Ludovic Canaud, Frederic Joyeux Pascal Branchereau, Charles Marty-Ane Jean-Philippe Berthet 51

6 The Arterial Approaches for Endovascular Aortic Grafting
Aysel Can, Giovanni Torsello Thomas Umscheid 57

7 Management of Intra-Procedural Problems
Martin Malina, Tim Resch Björn Sonesson 63

8 EVAR and TEVAR: Endoleaks and Endotension
Geoffrey Gilling-Smith 75

9 Migration and Dislocation of Aortic Devices During Follow-Up
Andrew England, Richard McWilliams 83

10 The Risk of Spinal Cord Ischemia During Thoracic and Abdominal Aortic Endografting
Roberto Chiesa, Germano Melissano Luca Bertoglio Massimiliano Maria Marrocco-Trischitta Efrem Civilini, Yamume Tshomba Fabio Massimo Calliari Enrico Maria Marone, Giliola Calori 95

11 Endovascular Repair of Aortic Arch Aneurysms
Timothy Chuter 107

12 Branched and Fenestrated Endografts: Technology, Planning Process and Implantation Technique
Stéphan Haulon, Richard Azzaoui
Elixène Jean-Baptiste, Tommaso Donati
Piervito D'Elia, Sébastien Amiot
Jonathan Sobocinski, Mohamad Koussa 115

13 Fenestrated and Branched Endografts: Current Results
Tara Mastracci, Roy Greenberg
Coletta Vidmar 123

14 Debranching Procedures for Thoraco-abdominal Aortic Aneurysms
Andrew Choong, Nicholas Cheshire 133

15 Endovascular Repair of Ruptured Abdominal Aortic Aneurysms
Christos Karkos, Zoran Rancic
Murat Aksoy, Alexei Svetlikov
Yuriy Spirin 141

16 Endovascular Treatment of Anastomotic False Aneurysms of the Abdominal Aorta
Pierre-Edouard Magnan, Nabil Sedki
Michel Bartoli, Alain Branchereau 155

17 Endovascular Treatment of Infected Aortic Aneurysms
Meryl Davis, Peter Taylor 167

18 Endovascular Treatment of Traumatic Aortic Ruptures
Geert Willem Schurink
Tanja Lettinga Van De Poll, Thomas Koeppel,
Stephan Langer, Gottfried Mommertz
Michiel De Haan, Michael Jacobs 181

19 Endovascular Treatment of Acute Thoracic Aortic Dissection
Jan Brunkwall, Vladimir Matoussevitch
Michael Gawenda 191

20 Endovascular Treatment of Chronic Dissecting Aneurysms
Matt Thompson, David Sayer, Ian Loftus
Rob Morgan 195

21 Damage Repair after Thoracic EVAR
Stephan Langer, Gottfried Mommertz
Thomas Koeppel, Geert Willem Schurink
Michael Jacobs 207

22 Surveillance after EVAR: Indications, Cost and Modalities
Clark Zeebregts, Eric Verhoeven, Ignace Tielliu,
Wendy Bos, Ted Prins, Roy De Jong
Jan Van Den Dungen 221

23 Short-Term Morbidity and Mortality of AAA Endografting
Zoran Rancic, Dieter Mayer, Christian Schmid
Thomas Pfammatter, Mario Lachat 229

24 Short-Term Mortality and Morbidity in TAA Endografting
David Beckett, Steven Thomas
Syed Tansheet Mustafa
Mathew Kaduthodil 243

# 1

TRANSGRESSING THE BOUNDARIES: THE HERMENEUTICS OF ENDOVASCULAR AORTIC REPAIR'S ENTHUSIASM

ALBERT CLARÁ, EDUARD MATEOS, BEGOÑA ROMÁN
FRANCESC VIDAL-BARRAQUER

An atmosphere of optimism and enthusiasm has surrounded the development of endovascular aortic repair over the last decade. Seen from outside our profession, such collective fever in pursuing innovation and change could only be understood on the basis of a clinical need or a radical improvement of previous results. Neither one nor the other seem to have been the case at least for the most frequent of aortic aneurysms. Opposite to what might happen in other greyer areas of our specialty, conventional open repair of abdominal aortic aneurysms was at the beginning of the 90s in its golden age. Short time before important series had accredited better than ever-immediate results together with a well-established long-term durability. At the opposite end, endovascular aortic repair has never been able to accomplish a radical improvement of previous results. After fifteen years (!), several generations of devices and three clinical trials, EVAR's objective success can be summarized in an initial mortality advantage for patients with large abdominal aortic aneurysms who are also fit for open repair.

The paradigm shift in the repair of aortic aneurysms that is taking place within our specialty needs thus to be re-interpreted from another perspective. This point of view must go, of course, beyond the self-evident competition among (or within) specialties or the economic factor. Commercial profit may appear as a necessary requisite for such a complex technological innovation to succeed but it is clearly not a sufficient one. Innovation and development in surgery emerge from inside the profession and if results or need do not appear to be the keystones, our hermeneutical approach must be aimed to disclose uncovered causes. Transgressing the boundaries of accepted ways of perceiving how innovation succeeds within surgery thus appears a requisite for our enterprise. To this task the present essay is addressed.

A decade of scientific enthusiasm for aortic aneurysms

THE FACTS

With little doubt aortic aneurysms have become the focus of a surprising enthusiasm within the public arena of vascular specialists over the last decade. As a result a plethora of worldwide initiatives such as conferences, symposia, meetings, workshops, courses and other postgraduate activities have been organized around this topic during this period. Medline citations have not remained beyond this enthusiasm either. Over the period 1980-2005 Pubmed citations for human studies have increased from 170 674 to 441 493, which mean a lineal 2.58-fold increase. Within the same period *aortic aneurysm* (Mesh term) citations for human subjects have raised from 395 to 1 347, which mean a 3.41-fold increase. Surprisingly this differential ratio has become only apparent since 1993 (Fig. 1), soon after the seminal contribution by Parodi et al. in November 1991.

ASSOCIATION WITH EVAR's EMERGENCE

From a theoretical point of view the scientific enthusiasm for aortic aneurysms seen over the last decade might have several explanations. Most of them, however, can be straightforwardly rejected. Aortic aneurysm is neither a new disease, such as AIDS or antiphospholipid syndrome, nor has re-emerged from a "glorious" past, such as tuberculosis. Diagnostic tools for aortic aneurysms have improved over the years but clearly not to an extent greater than that observed for many other diseases. To end no major discoveries regarding etiology, natural history or conventional open repair have emerged over the last years. With this background in mind, there is no other reason for such above-mentioned enthusiasm than the development of endovascular repair techniques for both abdominal (AAA) and thoracic aortic aneurysms and dissections (TAA/D).

A NAÏVE INTERPRETATION

From a naïve perspective it might be thought that the enthusiasm for endovascular aortic repair has obeyed to a radical change in the perspective of results as might have happened 50 years ago when conventional open repair (OR) arose. Surprisingly, however, for a long period of almost 15 years the possibility that endovascular aortic repair (EVAR) could become superior in hard endpoints to open surgery for AAA repair has been extremely uncertain.

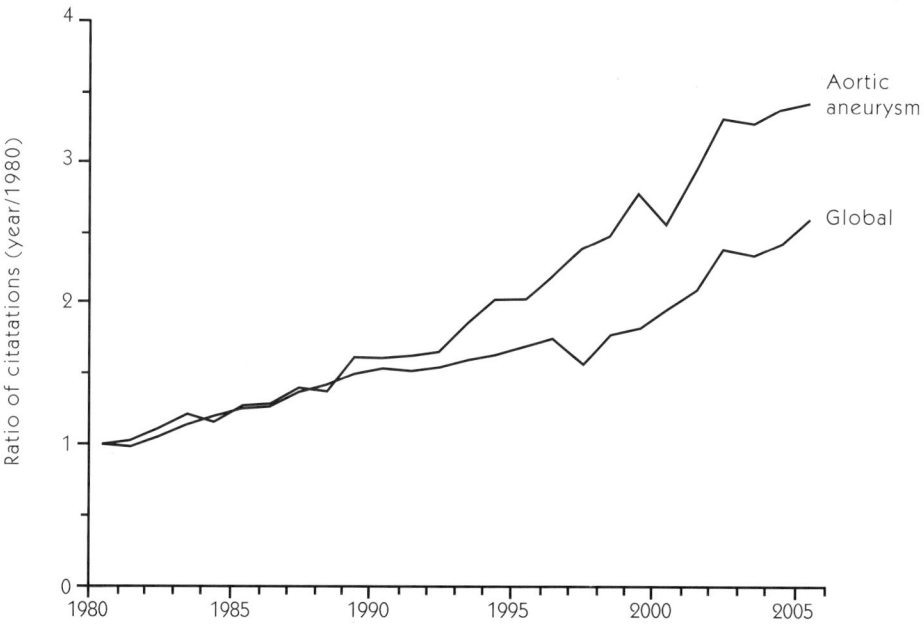

FIG. 1 Growth in the number of Pubmed citations (referred to 1980's citations) considered globally or under the Mesh term "aortic aneurysm" over the period 1980 - 2005.

In deed, prior to the publication of DREAM and EVAR trials in 2005, our knowledge about EVAR results, brilliantly summarized by Rutherford [1], was the following: 1) EVAR advantaged OR by reducing cardiac and pulmonary morbidity, hospital length stay and transfusion requirements; 2) no significant difference was observed in 30-day operative mortality; 3) late survival after EVAR was not better, and more often worse than that after OR, possibly due to the frequent need for reintervention in EVAR; and 4) new complications, such as endoleaks, endotension or rupture, and other problems, such as surveillance or higher overall costs, all specific to EVAR, were of great concern.

The scenario for TAA/D has been quite different. Although level I evidence is yet to arrive, EVAR has been regarded with great expectation from the beginning. Without doubt behind this it is the risky and highly demanding nature of thoracic open procedures to which EVAR easily compares better. Nevertheless, the above-mentioned enthusiasm for EVAR cannot be sustained on the basis of TAA/D. After all TAA/D continue to be much less frequent than AAA together with the fact that few vascular surgical teams continue to be involved in their management on a regular basis. Dear reader, the reasons for the vascular surgeons' enthusiasm towards EVAR over the last decade must be found elsewhere but not precisely in need or results. To this task of interpretation of our more recent past, hermeneutics in a broad sense, will be devoted the rest of the essay.

A hermeneutical approach to EVAR'S enthusiasm

Not until the nineteenth century was it possible plausibly to claim, as Friedrich Nietzsche did, that "everything is interpretation". Nonetheless, the interpretive arts are ancient. The origin of the term "hermeneutics" is Greek—hermeneia, or interpretation—probably after Hermes, who made human sense of the sometimes obscure utterances of the gods. While for many centuries hermeneutics has been centered in the interpretation of biblical texts, contemporaneous hermeneutics applies to the human world in all its manifestations, which resemble a text that requires reading. Hermeneutics consists in a dialectic of comprehending and explaining. However, within the scientific arena this task requires external reference points to avoid excessive ideological, social or economic distortions in the interpretation. These external reference points can be found in our issue at hands in accepted models explaining how communities respond to innovation or empirical data.

STANDARD MODELS EXPLAINING HOW COMMUNITIES RESPOND TO INNOVATION

Surgery, as one of the oldest technical fields, builds upon continuous innovation. The history of surgery is paved with a plethora of innovations enabling unprecedented benefits. While many fail in their purposes after a brief period of time, some of them succeed. Social researchers have long developed models to explain how communities respond to discontinuous innovations. These models may help us in our first hermeneutical approach to EVAR's enthusiasm. With this purpose in mind two recent models adapted to technological markets will be regarded from the perspective of EVAR's paradigm shift and the vascular surgeons' community.

The Rogers/Moore's technology adoption cycle model

Definition of the model. On the basis of the model of Everett Rogers, later adapted by Geoffrey Moore [2] to technological markets, when a marketplace is faced with the opportunity to switch to a new product or service that requires the end users to dramatically change their past behavior, members segregate according to their level of risk aversion.

The model adapted to EVAR innovation. The early market consists of the *technology innovators*. Among them, for example, all those working since the mid 80s in the transfemoral placement of intraluminal prosthesis in the aorta of dogs or sheeps, with one eye in the previous success of open surgical sutureless intraluminal grafts for aortic aneurysms and dissections [3], and the other in the evolving technology of balloon-expandable and nitinol stents. The names of most of them, such as A. Belko from Providence VA Medical Center, A. H. Cragg from University of Minnesota Hospitals or D. Mirich from the University of Texas M.D. Anderson Cancer Center remain still today quite unfamiliar to us.

The *visionaries* (early adopters) are in deed the true revolutionaries. They are the first to exploit the new capabilities to achieve a competitive advantage in the marketplace. Their names (Parodi, May, Veith, Moore, among others) are often associated with the paradigm shift. At this moment of the cycle, however, the early market means no other thing that journal papers or meeting abstracts but little penetration into the marketplace.

The people that determine the success of a discontinuous innovation, in our case EVAR, are not the innovators or the visionaries; success depends on the bulk of potential consumers, in our case the majority of vascular surgeons. Success depends on acceptance by the *pragmatists* (early majority), that is, those who adopt innovation only after favorable evidence emerges, and the *conservatives* (late majority), that is, those sceptical and demanding surgeons who accept innovation when it is simplified and commoditized to the point where it just works.

Discussion. Moore's model gives us some insight about the emergence of EVAR yet fails to justify the enthusiasm that has surrounded it over the last decade. Level I evidence has not been available until 2005 and the procedure is still far away to be commoditized to the desires of many conservative surgeons. The massive adoption of EVAR among vascular teams has preceded the usual requirements for a discontinuous innovation to succeed according to Moore's model.

The Christensen's Disruptive Innovation Model

Definition of the model. According to C. M. Christensen [4] a disruptive innovation is a technology that brings a much more affordable product or service that is much simpler to use into a market. It frequently allows the emergence of a whole new population of consumers, whereas historically, the ability to access was limited to people who had a lot of money or a lot of skill.

The model adapted to EVAR innovation. Disruptive innovations usually start as low segment differentiated products. Taking EVAR as our case of study this low segment might comprise high-risk patients with anatomically suitable AAA. Marginal players, for example new surgical teams or those other without a highly renowned experience in aortic surgery, might occupy this segment and started growing rapidly, solving initial quality problems while retaining its advantages.

Market leaders, namely renowned aortic surgical teams in our case, no matter how visionary, were forced to ignore the opportunity because 1) their results in open repair were good enough, 2) their definition of high risk patient was very restrictive, and 3) the disruptive product was not yet good enough for its mainstream customers. They did sustaining innovation by improving the existing techniques (open repair) and it was precisely their ability to do this what became their disability to do a disruption. Marginal players went through a learning curve, solved their quality problems and suddenly started threatening market leaders in its main markets.

Empirical data supporting the model. Central to Christensen's model is the prediction, almost by definition, that disruption depends on marginal players rather than on market leaders. This hypothesis can be indirectly tested by analyzing the degree of open surgical expertise of EVAR's early adopters as it can be inferred from their previous published experience in AAA open repair.

With this purpose in mind we conducted a search on PubMed (January 1992 to December 1996) looking for the first institutional EVAR clinical series including at least 10 patients. Whenever one group had published more than one case series within that period only the first of them was chosen for the analysis. New searches on Pubmed were then performed over the first, second, third and last authors of each series looking for previous (before 1992) published research (basic, clinical or otherwise) on abdominal aortic aneurysms.

The literature search yielded 2 229 citations, of which 14 published clinical series on EVAR fulfilled our eligibility criteria. New searches on Pubmed related to the first, second, third and last authors (n=37 surgeons) revealed that 5 (13.5%) had been at least first authors of a clinical series on AAA, 4 (10.8%) had been at least first authors of a case report or other type of citation, 7 (18.9%) had been simply coauthors of others' citations and 21 (56.8%) had no previous published research on AAA at all. Seen from an institutional perspective, and taking again only in consideration the first three authors and the last one, only 3 (21.4%) EVAR early series had one author (2 first authors and 1 third author) with relevant (at least 3 AAA clinical series as first author or coauthor) previous published research on AAA.

Christensen's prediction thus fits EVAR paradigm shift by showing that very few of those EVAR early-adopter surgeons had accredited aortic open surgical expertise as it can be inferred from their previous published experience in AAA open repair.

Discussion. Although Christensen's model may explain certain scientific characteristics of EVAR's early adopters, it fails to predict adequately EVAR's success since it is unclear to what extent disruption has brought a much more affordable product or service that is much simpler to use into a market. Abdominal EVAR is only simpler than open repair in selected cases and by no means is it a cheaper therapeutic option. Thoracic EVAR probably fits better Christensen's model yet its media-tic success has emerged later together with the fact that TAA/D are still much more infrequent conditions. Thoracic EVAR, in short, does not appear to have been the sticking point of this technological disruption.

EVAR's Enthusiasm Understood from Inside

While some aspects of research in the broad field of innovation are directly applicable to surgery, many unique aspects of our craft and practice require specialized thought. As such, perhaps it is the surgeon's responsibility to describe and study innovation as it applies to our field. Surprisingly while innovation in surgery has a rich tradition, the field and study of surgical innovation is quite new. Riskin et al. [5], for instance, showed that over the last 10 years less than a dozen of peer-reviewed articles focusing on surgical innovation had been published.

The traditional approach to innovation in surgery

Innovation understood from inside forces us to ask ourselves why do certain procedures in vascular surgery become obsolete. Classically seven forces influencing obsolescence have been identified [6]. They include: 1) better understanding of pathogenesis; 2) improved materials and techniques; 3) less morbid and mortal approaches; 4) the ease to perform and teach a technique; 5) the encouragement or obstruction of colleagues; 6) durability of the procedure; and 7) cost. Some of them may apply to EVAR's paradigm shift, namely forces number two, three and four. It has to be noted, however, that they may apply now, once level I evidence has become available, yet not precisely over the last decade when enthusiasm was already present within the vascular public arena. Other forces, namely durability or cost, do not seem to apply to EVAR yet.

Interestingly durability has long been recognized as one of the most important features of success of a procedure. Many will easily remember how lack of durability has been the coup of grace for many vascular interventions. Few decades ago no vascular technique would have received such an indulgence as it has been tolerated to EVAR over the last years. May be our eyes are changing as postmodern society evolves. Three decades ago durability was important in life, from jobs to freezers. You paid more but you knew that your German washing machine was going to last. Now neither the same salesman can promise you durability. We live within a culture of use and throw away, a culture unconcerned by the long-term, a culture that of course permeates surgery.

Transgressing causes of innovation in surgery

Classical forces seem to add little to our understanding of the EVAR revolution. Our hermeneutical task from inside must include, perhaps, other less evident, or at least less publicited, reasons. They can be easily named as strategical forces and for each of them some evidence will be provided to support their role.

Aortic aneurysms are a market in expansion. The first and more obvious strategical cause is that aortic aneurysms are a market in expansion. Approximately 200 000 new cases are diagnosed each year in the United States. Ruptured AAA is responsible for approximately 15 000 deaths in this country, making it the 14th leading cause of death, similar in magnitude to emphysema, renal disease and homicide.

It is clear that our society is ageing. The impact of this is the certainty of more aneurysms, because abundant data exist to show that the prevalence and rupture risk increases sharply with advancing age. Besides ageing, other factors must be involved, because the incidence of small aneurysms has increased almost 30-fold. Certainly, better diagnosis and more frequent imaging studies are involved, but it appears there has probably been a true increase in prevalence as well.

It is certain that in coming years vascular surgeons are going to deal with more patients with AAA in their practice, many of whom will be elderly and high risk. Therefore, the possibility of a less invasive method of treatment, such as EVAR, that might reduce risk, improve recovery and extend the chance of successful repair to a greater number of patients may have tremendous appeal to vascular surgeons.

EVAR closed the endovascular circle. The immense majority of arterial diseases managed by vascular surgeons are occlusive or aneurysmal in nature. Any disruptive innovation aspiring to replace the good gold standard of open surgery was expected to provide at least a reasonable solution for both types of diseases. For many years, angioplasty, stenting and other related procedures have leaded the fight for arterial occlusive diseases from the endovascular side. It may be true that for many time their battle had been limited to iliac stenoses and some renal cases. However, any progress from these initial cases to the present scenario-where almost any stenotic or occlusive disease is open to endovascular (EV) repair-was not difficult to foresee. There was a commercial profit, competition among different specialists and even within the same specialty and a technological avant-garde coming from coronary interventionalists. In short, the evolution to our present EV technical capabilities in arterial occlusive diseases could be easily foreseen as a simple sustaining progress, unproblematic one.

Quite different was the EV approach to aneurysmal disease. Qualitatively it required a radical disruption. Of course there were precedents. Innovation never emerges from zero and the contribution of nitinol stents' development and open surgical sutureless grafts cannot be neglected. Yet a disruptive innovation was needed. Once it appeared the EV approach to arterial diseases became complete, the circle was closed. A therapeutic paradigm shift could then take place. Over the last half a century neither medical treatment nor laparoscopic surgery had been able to provide a solution for all the array of arterial disorders and for the first time an alternative to open surgery, seen as a whole, was theoretically possible. EVAR was not simply a new approach to AAA. EVAR closed the conceptual circle of EV capabilities and massively catalyzed the interest of vascular surgeons in EV techniques.

EVAR emerged precisely when open repair of AAA had begun a scientific decline. Some readers might wonder what would happen if a new technical approach to AAA, completely different of EVAR, would emerge today. Few probably would agree that such new technique would receive the enthusiasm accumulated by EVAR over the last decade. Although this belief may have several explanations there is at least one that may be significant and can be indirectly tested. Our question at hands is to what extent open repair had initiated a scientific decline prior or at the time of EVAR emergence. In other words, was there little left to say about open repair of AAA in vascular journals, meetings and courses at the late 80s or the beginning of 90s?

To answer this question we conducted a search on PubMed (January 1980 to December 1991) looking for citations on human research under the Mesh term "aortic aneurysm". We randomly chose 25% of each year's citations. We then identified for each selected citation the type of article (original article, case report, or other), main objective (basic/clinical, diagnosis, therapeutics), type of journal (surgical or not), mean journal's impact factor over the 90s decade and language.

The literature search yielded 1 532 citations of which 580 fulfilled the criteria of having AAA as their main issue. The 12-year period of study was then divided in four consecutive triennia (1980-1982, 1983-1985, 1986-1988, 1989-1991). AAA citations dealing with basic, epidemiological or clinical issues increased from 19.3% (1980-1982) to 46.1% (1989-1991), whereas citations dealing with diagnostic or open surgery issues decreased from 26.6% to 9.1% and from 54.1% to 44.8%, respectively, between the first and last triennia ($p<0.001$). This decline in open surgical citations was even greater when only original articles were considered (66% to 43.7%), whereas case report rates remained without significant change within the period of study.

At the end of the 12-year period AAA citations dealing with basic, epidemiological or clinical issues included more original articles (15.0% vs 45.1%) and less case reports (85.0% vs 36.6%) ($p=0.002$), more articles in English language (52.4% vs 81.7%, $p=0.01$) and published in more rated journals (14.2% vs 46.5%, $p=0.05$). These characteristics did not change significantly within the group of AAA citations dealing with open repair issues (technique, perioperative issues, results, short and long-term complications) with the exception of manuscripts's language with lesser English language articles at the end of the period (83.1% vs 63.8 %, $p=0.01$).

Although the number of citations had annually increased over the 12-year period, our results show a decline in the proportion of AAA citations dealing with open repair issues, especially in original articles, together with a shift to non-English language journals. AAA citations dealing with basic, epidemiologic or clinical issues showed the reverse of the coin, namely, more proportion of citations, original articles, manuscripts written in English language and published in more rated journals. With these results in mind it is not difficult to glimpse an adequate breeding ground for scientifically avid vascular surgeons to accept and promote a disruptive innovation in AAA therapeutics.

EVAR's Enthusiasm Promoted from Outside

Our hermeneutical framework would not be complete without a brief consideration to certain factors coming from outside clinical practice and how they may have influenced EVAR's enthusiasm over the last decade. These factors include commercial profit, esthetic motivations, technological influences and a change in the perception of the real.

Commercial profit

There is little to say about the influence of commercial profit on technology adoption that every average surgeon does not know beforehand. The price of an endovascular aortic graft is several times greater than that of a prosthetic graft for an open repair. For many, commercial profit is simply the keystone of EVAR's technological disruption. Market forecasts, for instance, are now assessing market size and growth potential of thoracic EVAR. They are aimed to busy executives in the medical device and venture capital industries. Based on current technology, published company and investment analysts and thought leaders they forecast the market to raise from US $ 70 million at 2006 to US $ 250 million, globally, by 2012. Furthermore it is expected that stent-grafts for AAA will represent a 1 billion dollar market in less than five years. With such background is there a need, someone may wonder, for additional reasons to explain EVAR's enthusiasm?

Truly without such a profit it is difficult to understand the scientific enthusiasm seen over the last decade, with the plethora of courses, meetings and other scientific activities that have taken place, many of them–if not all-direct or indirectly sponsored by industry. However, although all this may be true, the role of commercial profit does not go beyond a simple necessary but not sufficient cause. Commercial profit has been also behind many other technological innovations that have not succeeded over the past. All over the present chapter other factors have been analyzed as predisposing to a shift in AAA management. Some of them even appear as crucial as commercial profit, such as the status-quo of the visionaries or the scientific exhaustion of previous procedures. Seen altogether and with the addition of a profitable market the paradigm shift seems inevitable.

Esthetic forces: the fall of the paradigm "big surgeon, big incision"

In 1960 Jurgen Thorwald published *The Triumph of Surgery*, a fascinating and vivid account of the main features of the history of surgery during the 19th century and the first part of the XXth century. A similar enthusiasm emerged between the fifties and the seventies with the arousal of modern cardiac and vascular surgery. For some decades generations of vascular surgeons grew under a conception of surgery as an engaged way of life. For hundredths of vascular surgeons the idealization of both success and sacrifice became incarnated in the figures of the great popes of vascular surgery and their teams. Urban legends, reality and certain doses of esthetics for a very concrete understanding of a surgical way of life allowed a pseudo-heroical myth to grow. Great surgeons, big incisions, extremely complex cases, pseudo-orgasmic solutions, huge paraphernalia of instruments and devices, several cases done at a same time, daily surgical schedules almost incompatible with life, eternal on-call services, more the one hundredth hours per week of work time, in short, a referral of what any enthusiast in vascular surgery might expect to find in the heaven.

Yet at nineties together with the shift from reporting patency rates alone to include patient's quality of life in scientific papers, the question of surgeon's quality of life inconspicuously emerged as well. The "No pain" aphorism began to disappear from the notebook of new generations of surgeons in training as a consequence of a commoditized world, the length of the incision began to lose its "esthetic force" for society in general, political concern emerged around work hours per week and the great above-mentioned popes and their teams began to be seen as the result of a glorious past rather than living referrals. In short, a slow but gradual process of collectively eschewing previous values was taking place, while adopting attitudes toward the profession rooted in the reaction to the restrictions and limitations of the previous way of life. Within such postmodern setting any new procedure associated with promising features such as simplicity, rapidity and lesser post-procedural work-load was expected to be very welcomed.

Technological influences and the disappearance of the real

Surgery uses new technological opportunities as means for its "sacred" end. Yet at a same time technology uses surgical procedures as means for its autonomous and deterministic purposes. In his essay "The virtual surgeon: operating on the data in an age of medialization" Timothy Lenoir [7] suggests that we will soon reach a time when the ubiquity of computers and the prevalence of virtual interfaces for surgical applications will lead to surgical practices where the "real" is indistinguishable from the "virtual". According to Lenoir well before we enter the operating room of the future, it is clear that surgeons will be significantly influenced by medialization and postmodern distributed production.

Key to medialization will be the externalization of formerly internal mental processes in computer visualization, modelling, simulation and computer-generated virtual reality interfaces. All these new features will certainly affect the classical status of the surgeon. While some traditional background knowledge and skills will be retained, surgeons will require familiarity with new fields such as biophysics, computer graphics, animation, bio-robotics and mechanical and biomedical engineering.

It is obviously unrealistic to assume that surgeons will be able to assume expertise in all such complex fields. For that reason workload probably will be more distributed. Indeed central to post-modern distributed production it is to expect flat organizational structures and distributed teamwork, including software engineers, robotics experts and a host of others.

Nevertheless, beyond technological influences on how aortic patients are going to be treated in the future there appears to exist also a slow but steady tendency towards a disappearance of the real aortic aneurysm. For any vascular surgeon over 40 years old there is no other real AAA than that of a retro-peritoneal pulsatile mass surrounded by an annoying and bleeding fat tissue. For many present vascular surgeons in training the real AAA is becoming the clear, sharp, colored and 360°-visible CT reconstruction, in short, the hyperreal AAA.

Hyperreality is a means to characterize the way consciousness defines what is actually "real" in a world where a multitude of media can radically shape and filter the original event or experience being depicted. Hyperreal AAA obviously look better and serve best for present therapeutic purposes. Hyperreal AAA are more real than real. The metaphysical consequences of this shift are difficult to foresee but, whatever they are, it is a fact that hyperreality is permeating all our daily reality. Indeed wouldn't you be disappointed of seeing a real *Tyrannosaurus rex* in your Sunday's morning walk after having seen the more-real-than-real creatures of Steven Spielberg's *Jurassic Park*?

REFERENCES

1 Rutherford RB. Randomized EVAR trials and advent of level I evidence: A paradigm shift in management of large abdominal aortic aneurysms? *Semin Vasc Surg* 2006; 19: 69 - 74.

2 Moore GA. *Inside the Tornado: Marketing Strategies from Silicon Valley's Cutting Edge*. New York: HarperCollins Publishers; 1995, pp 1 - 244.

3 Lemole GM. Aortic replacement with sutureless intraluminal grafts. *Texas Heart Inst J* 1990; 17: 302 - 309.

4 Christensen, Clayton M. *The Innovator's Dilemma: When New Technologies Cause Great Firms to Fail*. Boston: Harvard Business School Press; 1997, pp 1 - 225.

5 Riskin DJ, Longaker MT, Gertner M et al. Innovation in surgery: an historical perspective. *Ann Surg* 2006; 244: 686 - 693.

6 Hallet JW. Presidential address: Back to the future of vascular surgery – Why certain procedures become obsolete. *J Vasc Surg* 1997; 25: 791 - 795.

7 Lenoir T. The virtual surgeon: operating on the data in an age of medialization. In Thurtle PH, Mitchell R, eds. *Semiotic Flesh: Information and the Human Body*. Seattle: University of Washington Press; 2002, pp 28 - 51.

HOW TO LEARN ENDOVASCULAR AORTIC PROCEDURES - THEORETICAL AND PRACTICAL EDUCATION

ANDREA MARIA DIRRIGL, HERMANN BERGER
ALEXANDER ZIMMERMANN, CHRISTIAN REEPS, ANDREAS KÜHNL
HEIKO WENDORFF, HANS-HENNING ECKSTEIN

The endovascular revolution in treating aortic aneurysms started with Volodos in 1988, Parodi in 1991 and Dake in 1994, respectively [1-4]. Meanwhile, results from large investigator-initiated prospective registries and randomized controlled trials constitute that endovascular aortic procedures have become standard procedures for properly selected patients with abdominal aortic aneurysms (AAA), thoracic aortic aneuryms (TAA) and traumatic thoracic aortic tears [5-14]. In addition, the combination of open and endovascular repair (hybrid procedures) and the introduction of fenestrated and side-branched endografts have further expanded the applicability of endovascular aortic repair (EVAR) to complex thoraco-abdominal aortic aneurysms and aneurysms of the aortic arch [15-18].

The wide variety of open and endovascular therapeutic options coupled with an increasing complexity of cases, reduction in working hours and patients' demands to be operated on by well-educated and experienced vascular surgeons leads to the question of how and where to train these procedures safely and effectively. Up to now, the sheer volume of exposure, rather than specifically designed curricula, is the hallmark of surgical training. Since opportunities for learning through work with "real" patients have diminished, interest in workshops and training curricula specifically designed to teach surgical skills has increased [19]. This is especially true for vascular patients. In order to achieve a high educational standard in a short period of time, endovascular training programs have been established by vascular scientific societies and by individual radiologists, cardiologists and vascular surgeons. This chapter aims to review current training recommendations for endovascular aortic procedures and to report experiences from the European vascular workshops in Pontresina, Switzerland. Additionally, the current developing endovascular curriculum of the German Society of Vascular Surgery will be introduced (www.gefaesschirurgie.de).

Methods

All published guidelines and recommendations on theoretical and practical endovascular training for aortic diseases were reviewed. In addition, MEDLINE was explored from 1991 to 2007 using the search terms "endovascular aortic procedure", combined with "learning", "workshop", "virtual reality" and "simulator training". Furthermore, reference lists of review articles and homepages from the European and North-American Vascular Societies were examined. The available information was analyzed for the end points: theoretical knowledge, basic endovascular skills for aortic procedures, the value of computer-generated virtual reality simulators and the benefits of simulator training on synthetic and animal models, including the experience of the European vascular workshops in Pontresina (Switzerland).

Theoretical requirements for endovascular aortic procedures

According to a multidisciplinary clinical competence statement, a minimal knowledge of vascular anatomy and vascular diseases is required to perform catheter-based interventions safely and effectively [20]. With respect to aortic diseases, it is necessary to have a thorough understanding of the following issues: aortic anatomy (Fig. 1), clinical manifestation and natural history of aortic diseases, the pros and cons of conservative, surgical and endovascular treatment options, invasive and non-invasive diagnostic tests, radiation protection and contrast agents (Table I).

Basic diagnostic, surgical and endovascular skills for aortic procedures

Since Duplex ultrasound is the diagnostic medium of choice for screening patients for AAAs, computed tomography (CT)-angiography is mandatory to assess aortic diseases in terms of the overall necessity to treat the condition, the different treatment options and the planning of endovascular procedure. The latter includes a distinct assessment of anatomical criteria with sufficient measurements of neck diameter, neck length, aneurysm diameter and length etc. Likewise, proximal and distal attachment zones, iliac tortuosity and/or calcifications, anatomical variations, (e.g. additional renal arteries) etc. have to be assessed (Table II, Figs. 2-4). Trainees should perform measurements by using a standardized form and comparing their results with the assessment from a senior colleague. Additional assessments by representatives or core labs from graft companies may be helpful in the setting of new types of endoprosthesis or a lack of personal experience with the specific device. In any case, the responsible surgeon should perform his/her own measurements and assessment for an endovascular procedure (Figs. 5-7).

Surgical skills for endovascular surgeons include the capability to obtain and repair access to the vascular system at the brachial, common femoral or common iliac artery levels and to perform standard extra-anatomic bypass procedures (left subclavian artery transposition, femoro-femoral bypass). Complex aortic aneurysms may be treated by hybrid procedures including technically demanding supra-aortic and/or visceral debranching procedures like transposition of the brachiocepha-

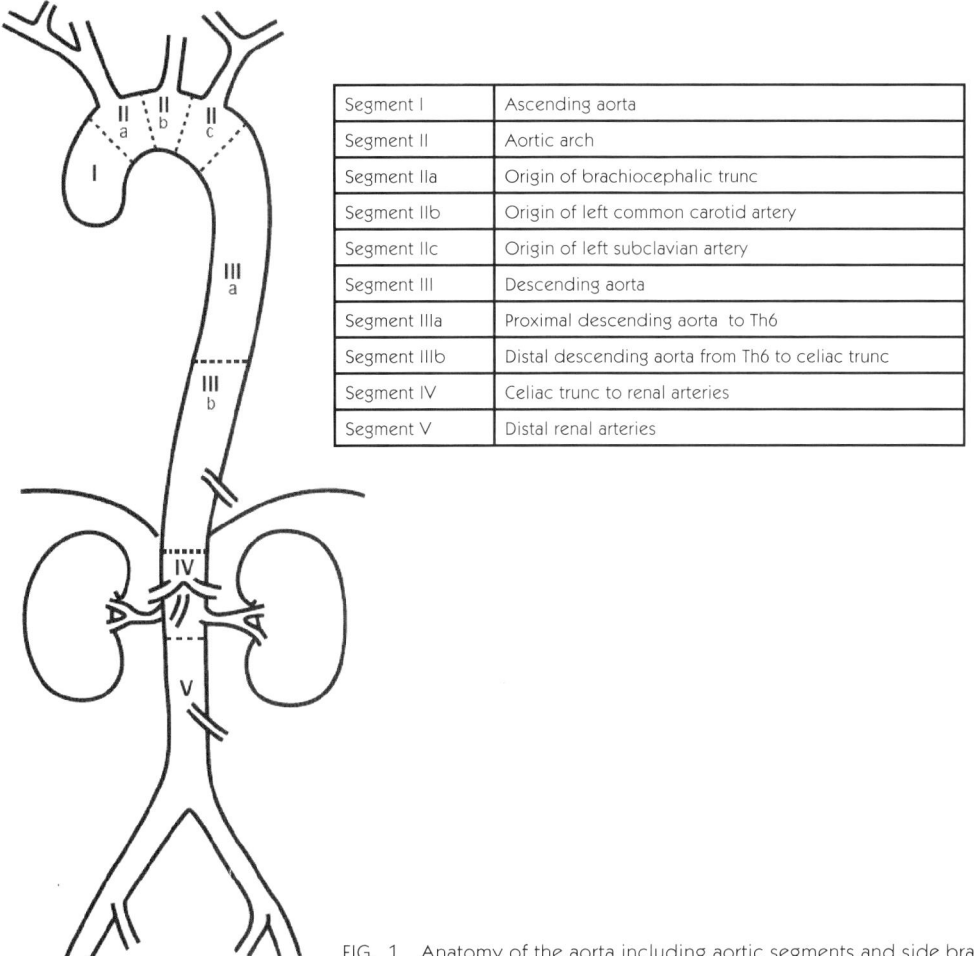

FIG. 1 Anatomy of the aorta including aortic segments and side branches.

Segment I	Ascending aorta
Segment II	Aortic arch
Segment IIa	Origin of brachiocephalic trunc
Segment IIb	Origin of left common carotid artery
Segment IIc	Origin of left subclavian artery
Segment III	Descending aorta
Segment IIIa	Proximal descending aorta to Th6
Segment IIIb	Distal descending aorta from Th6 to celiac trunc
Segment IV	Celiac trunc to renal arteries
Segment V	Distal renal arteries

Table I — MINIMAL THEORETICAL KNOWLEDGE REQUIRED FOR COMPETENCE IN AORTIC CATHETER-BASED INTERVENTIONS (MODIFIED FROM CREAGER 2004 [20])

- Anatomy of the aorta and its side-branches (Fig. 1)
- Incidence, prevalence and the role of ageing and atherosclerosis in aortic enlargement
- Clinical manifestation and natural history of aortic diseases below the diaphragm: AAA, aortic occlusive disease
- Clinical manifestation and natural history of aortic diseases above the diaphragm: thoracic and thoracoabdominal aortic aneurysms, acute and chronic aortic dissections, traumatic transsection, congenital aortic diseases (Ehlers-Danlos-Syndrome, Marfan-Syndrome), intramural hematoma and penetrating aortic ulcer
- Endovascular, surgical and conservative treatment options for aortic aneurysms (AAA, TAA, TAAA, arch aneurysms, including current classifications, Fig. 3), acute and chronic aortic dissections, aortic transsections and aortic occlusive disease.
- Indications, contraindications, accuracy and limitations of noninvasive and invasive diagnostic tests: duplex ultrasonography, CT-angiography, magnetic resonance angiography, catheter angiography
- Radiation physics, safety, and radiographic imaging equipment
- Advantages and potential complications of iodinated and noniodinated contrast agents

Table II	STANDARDS FOR THE ASSESSMENT AND MEASUREMENT OF ABDOMINAL AND THORACIC AORTIC ANEURYSMS (INCLUDING AORTIC DISSECTIONS)
Abdominal aortic aneurysm (AAA)	
Type of AAA and maximal diameter (mm)	EUROSTAR Classification Heidelberg (Allenberg) [21] classification (Fig. 5)
Shape of the aneurysm	Fusiform Saccular Others
Proximal AAA neck	Diameter (mm), at the level of the renal arteries and at the lower end of the proximal neck Length (mm) Angulation (degrees) Shape: tubular, cone, funnel, barrel, hourglass Circumferential thrombus (%) Circumferential calcification (%)
Distal aorta (mm)	Diameter (mm) Circumferential calcification (%)
Distance mesaurements ("center line")	Distance from renal arteries to aortic bifurcation Distance from aortic bifurcation to iliac bifurcation
Common and external iliac arteries (mm)	Diameter (mm): proximal, mid, distal Length (mm) Angulation (degrees) Calcification
Thoracic aortic aneurysm (TAA) and thoracic aortic dissection	
Etiology	Atherosclerotic Chronic Aortic Dissection Traumatic tear False aneurysm Penetreting aortic ulcer
Localization and diameter (mm)	Segment of the thoracic aorta Maximum diameter of aneurysm
Shape of the aneurysm	Fusiform Saccular Others
Proximal neck	Length (distance between TAA and left subclavian artery) Diameter of the proximal aorta
Distal neck	Length (distance between TAA and celiac trunk) Diameter of the distal aorta
Distance measurements ("center line")	Distance from left subclavian artery to celiac trunk
Aortic dissection	Site of entry and reentry Diameter of the true and the false lumen

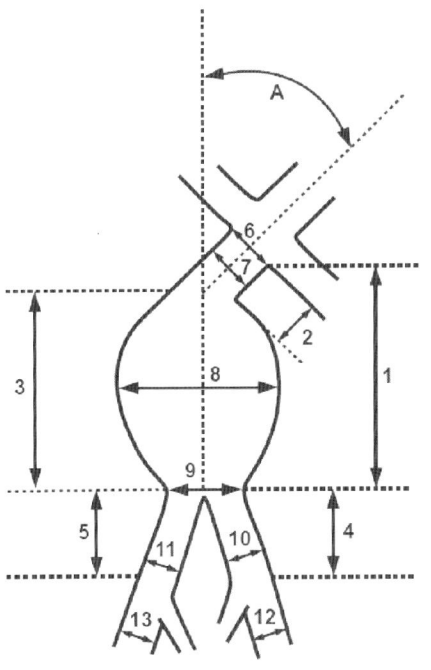

ANATOMICAL LOCATION		
A	Proximal aortic neck angle	°
1	Distance from renal arteries to bifurcation	mm
2	Aortic neck lenght	mm
3	Distance from proximal neck to bifurcation	mm
4	Lenght of left common iliac artery	mm
5	Lenght of right common iliac artery	mm
6	Aortic diameter at proximal implantation site	mm
7	Aortic diameter - 15 mm inferior to proximal implantation site	mm
8	Maximum outer aneurysm diameter	mm
9	Minimum diameter of distal neck	mm
10	Diameter of left common iliac artery	mm
11	Diameter of right common iliac artery	mm
12	Diameter of left external iliac artery	mm
13	Diameter of right external iliac artery	mm

FIG. 2   Measurement scheme for AAAs.

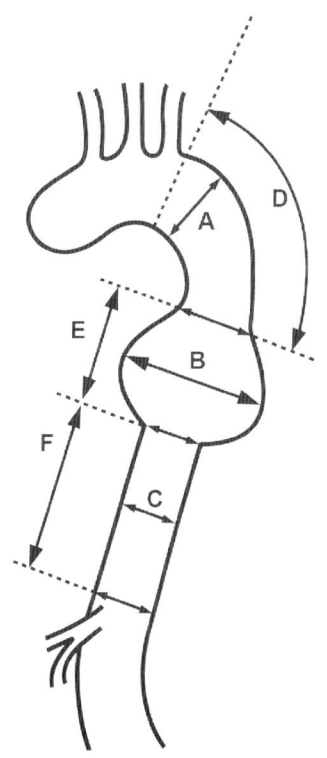

ANATOMICAL LOCATION		
A	Diameter of proximal neck	mm
B	Maximum aneurysm diameter	mm
C	Diameter of distal neck	mm
D	Proximal neck Distance from aneurysm to left subclavian artery	mm
E	Lengh of aneurysm segment	mm
F	Distal neck Distance from aneurysm to coeliac trunc	mm
D+E+F	Maximum possible lenght of aortic stent prothesis	mm

FIG. 3   Measurement scheme for TAAs.

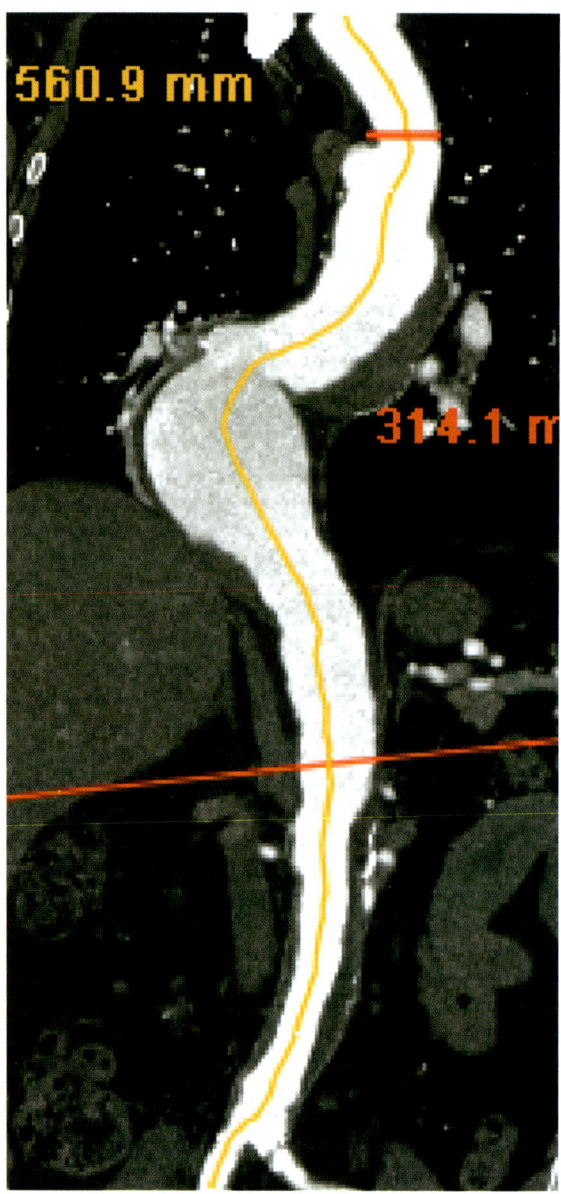

FIG. 4 3D-Reconstruction of a TAA based on CT-angiography. The center-line is assessed to measure the overall optimal length of the aortic endoprothesis (Image with friendly permission of Mr. Hendrik von Tengg-Koblik).

lic trunk, carotid-carotid bypass grafting and extra-anatomic bypasses to the renal arteries, the superficial mesenteric artery and the celiac trunk. These procedures are mostly performed by senior consultants and therefore should not be part of a vascular surgical training program. The same is true for immediate conversion procedures which always constitute an emergency situation (e.g. dislocated endoprosthesis, occlusion of important aortic side-branches, device not removable). Though the conversion rate from endovascular to open aortic repair has decreased significantly over the last years, aortic endovascular procedures should not be performed in a setting where no expertise in open aortic repair is immediately available.

Before starting endovascular aortic procedures, surgical residents have to be trained in using basic endovascular tools and techniques, including percutaneous and open puncture and sheath insertion techniques, the handling of different guide-

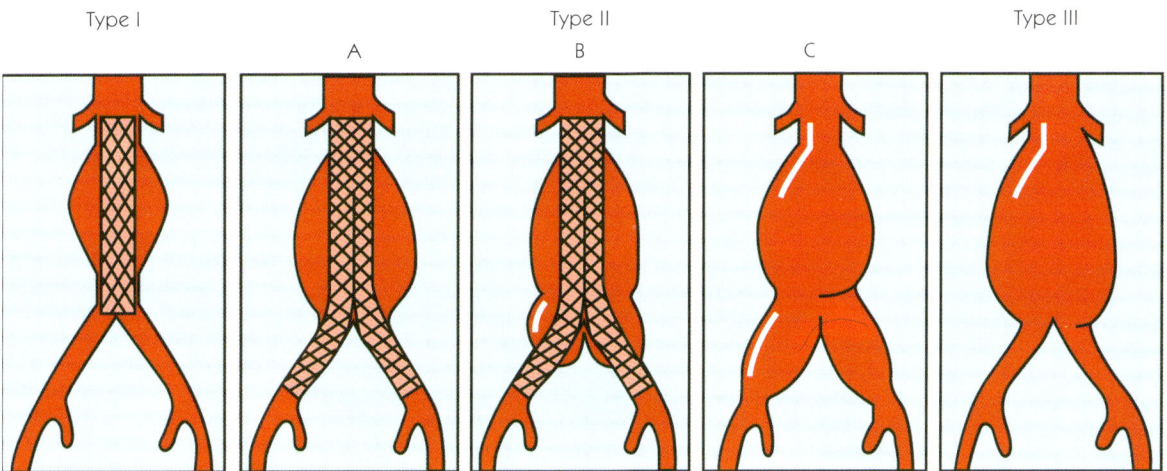

FIG. 5 Heidelberg (Allenberg)-Classification of AAAs [21]. Types I, IIA and IIB are suitable for EVAR, in type IIC both iliac bifurcations have to be covered, EVAR is only possible by use of a bifurcated iliac endograft. Type III is a juxtarenal AAA, EVAR would only be possible by use of a side-branched/fenestrated endograft.

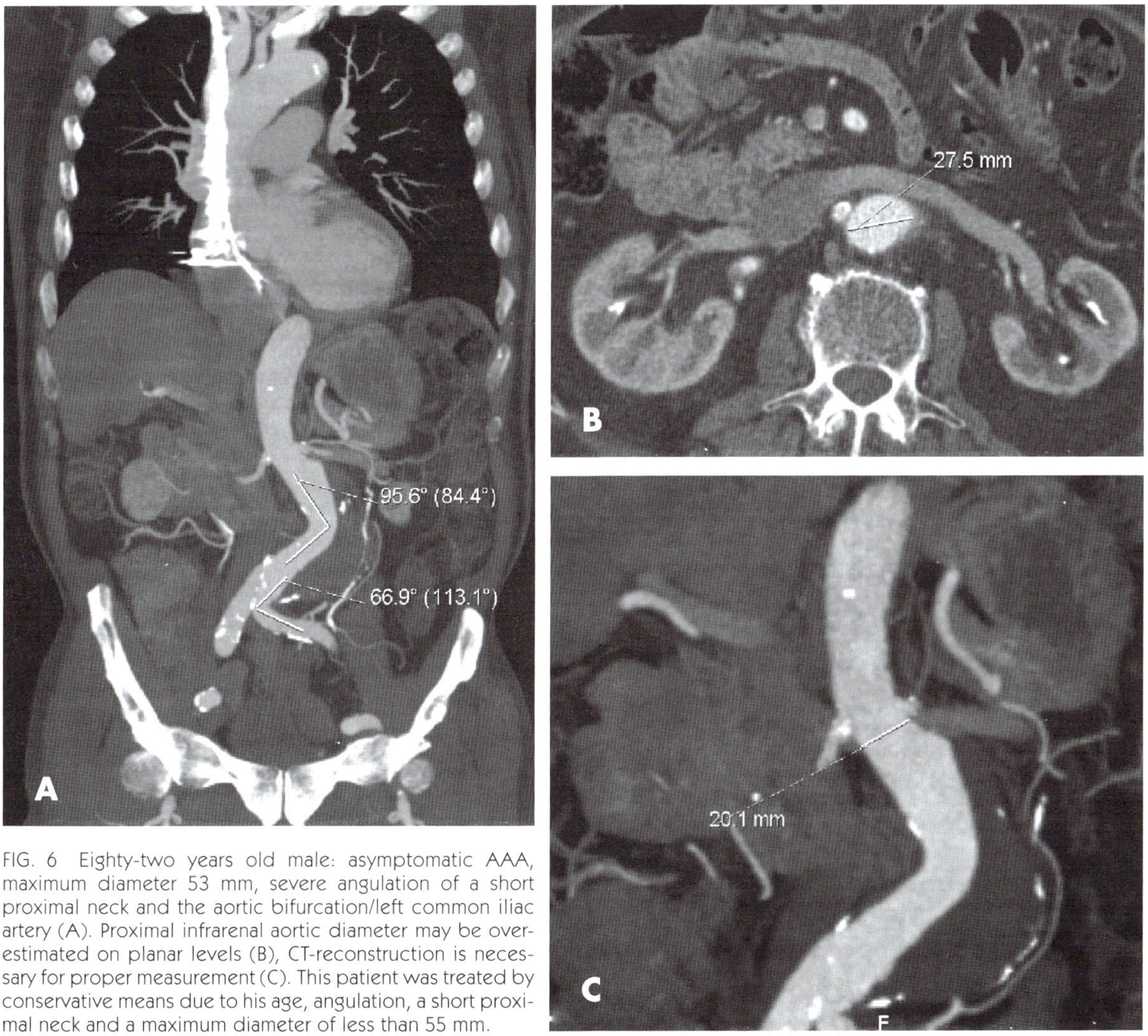

FIG. 6 Eighty-two years old male: asymptomatic AAA, maximum diameter 53 mm, severe angulation of a short proximal neck and the aortic bifurcation/left common iliac artery (A). Proximal infrarenal aortic diameter may be overestimated on planar levels (B), CT-reconstruction is necessary for proper measurement (C). This patient was treated by conservative means due to his age, angulation, a short proximal neck and a maximum diameter of less than 55 mm.

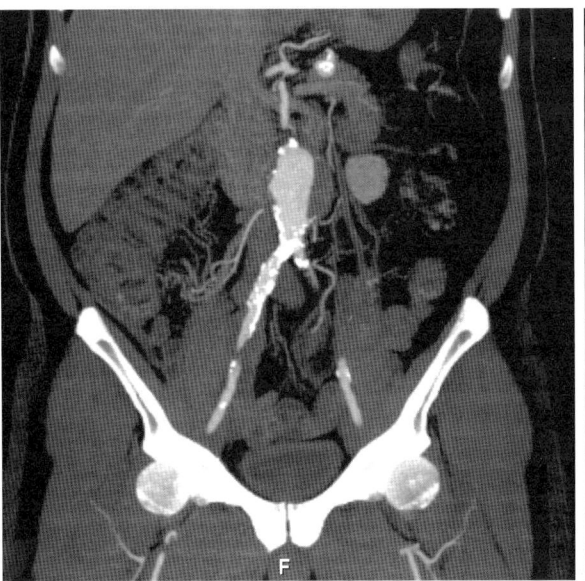 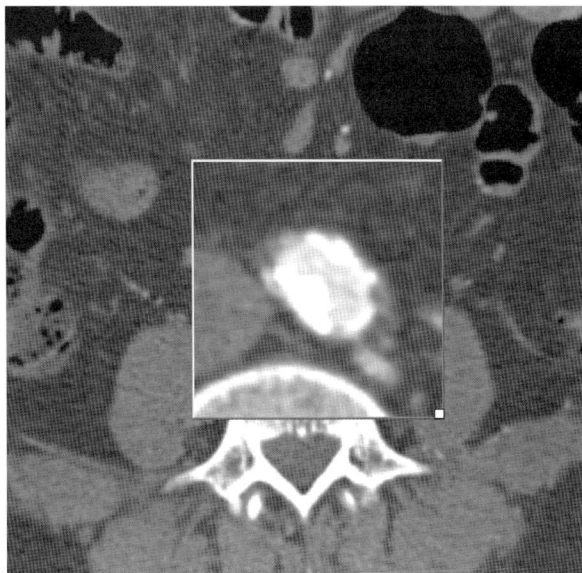

FIG. 7 Sixty-six years old male: AAA with a maximum diameter of 5.5 cm, severe calcification of the aortic bifurcation with a residual lumen of <10 mm. Open therapy preferred.

wires and angiography catheters and the use of balloon catheters, stents and endografts, respectively (Table III). It is also necessary to have personal experience with additional tools, like torque handles and snare guidewires and to be able to handle a mobile C-arm within the operating room or to work with a fixed stationary device including all means necessary for radiation protection. These basic skills and knowledge can be acquired by observations and direct learning from senior endovascular specialists, by hands-on-training in endovascular workshops and didactical workshops.

Virtual reality simulators

Over the last years, a handful of papers have been published reporting on virtual reality (VR) simulation in endovascular skills training (Table IV). There is good evidence that inexperienced interventionists' skills improve significantly through simulator performance on carotid stenting, renal and iliac interventions respectively [22-27]. In a randomized trial, the transfer from VR-acquired endovascular skills to the human model was demonstrated. Following didactical teaching, twenty general surgery residents were divided into two groups. The first group received two hours of VR simulation training on iliofemoral angioplasty before performing the procedure in the human model, whereas the second group had no VR-training. Compared with the control group, the simulator-trained group improved significantly using a procedure specific checklist and a global rating scale to assess performance [25].

The development of a VR aortic trainer is currently under evaluation by several companies (Mentice, Sweden and SimSuite, Medical Simulation Corporation, Denver, Colorado) and individual investigators [28], so the training effect of VR-simulation on EVAR has yet to be determined.

Simulator training on synthetic models - European vascular workshops (Pontresina, Switzerland)

The Pontresina Vascular Workshop was founded in 1991 by Jens Allenberg, Georg Hagmüller and Jon Largiader, who jointly aimed to propagate techniques and skills in vascular surgery (www.vascular-international.org). The following key issues were considered to be important: techniques should be trained by use of realistic models, the ratio between trainers and trainees should be low leading to a restricted number of participants, both beginners and experienced vascular surgeons should be addressed. Since 1991, more than 1 500 participants

Table III	BASIC EQUIPMENT AND TECHNIQUES FOR ENDOVASCULAR AORTIC SURGERY

- Puncture needles and puncture technique to gain access to the femoral and the iliac arteries and the aorta
- Introducer sheaths and insertion technique
- Guidewires (Teflon-coated, hydrophilic), different strengths, lengths, tips and diameters
- Angiography catheters (different lengths, end-hole, side-hole catheters, measuring catheters, flush angiography catheters, selective catheters)
- Angioplasty balloons (compliant, non-compliant)
- Stents (self-expandable, balloon-expandable, diameters, lengths, flexibility, axial movement after deployment, radiopacity)
- Endoluminal stentgrafts
- Additional tools: torque handles, snare guidewires
- Angio-Suite within the operating room with a mobile C-arm or a fixed stationary device including means for x-ray protection

Table IV	TRAINING TOOLS TO ACHIEVE COMPETENCE FOR ENDOVASCULAR AORTIC PROCEDURES (ADAPTED FROM NEEQUAYE [22])

	Advantages	*Disadvantages*	*Evidence in the literature*
Virtual Reality (VR)	- Standardized task - Multiple modules in various anatomical territories - Patient specific simulation possible - Endovascular tools re-usable - No x-ray	- Significant setup, transport and maintenance costs - Frequent breakdown - Technician required	- Significant improvement in simulator performance of novice interventionist and in-vivo performance for renal and iliac interventions - Currently no experiences for endovascular aortic procedures
Animal	- High degree of realism using live anesthetized animals - Full procedure simulation (including arteriotomy and closure)	- Single session use of animals and endovascular tools - Anesthesia required - Legal and ethical problems - Size and anatomical differences to human - High costs - X-ray	- Significant improvement in skills performance of novices using porcine training model
Synthetic models	- Standardized task - Full procedure simulation possible - Relatively easily transported - Basic models cheap - No x-ray - Simulation under dynamic flow conditions possible - Team training	- Endovascular tools (especially endografts) sometimes not re-usable - EVAR/TEVAR simulation expensive - Lacks validated assessment tool - Simulation of advanced tasks (renal, carotid interventions) demanding	- None

have been trained in three-day practical workshops, mostly in Switzerland but also in Italy, Germany, France and China. In addition, one-day-workshops were held at the annual meetings of the ESVS in Dublin, Istanbul and Helsinki.

Much effort was put into the development of a realistic leg model to practice bypass surgery and an abdominal model with pulsatile perfusion of inserted silicon AAAs for conventional surgical aortic procedures. Pandey et al. [29] examined the technical progress of 15 participants of the Pontresina workshop and was able to show that all end points (generic and procedural skills, aortic anastomotic techniques and time needed) improved significantly within 2.5 days.

Endovascular procedures are honed by a specifically designed pressurized and pulsatile model which enables the trainee to practice complete endovascular procedures, including the puncturing of the femoral artery, sheath and guidewire insertion and angiography without radiation. Iliac, renal and aortic interventions can be practiced with the use of different commercially available endografts for EVAR and TEVAR (Fig. 8). In 2008, the second generation of the Pontresina Endo-Trainer will be introduced. New features include compliant silicon models of AAA and TAAs and the option to perform angiography in different levels, which is obviously especially important for the thoracic aorta and the aortic arch (Fig. 9).

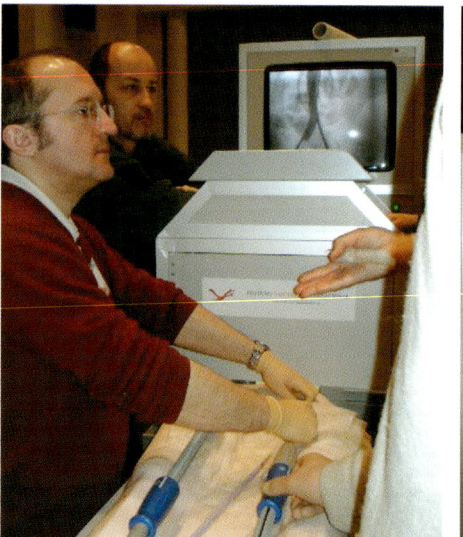
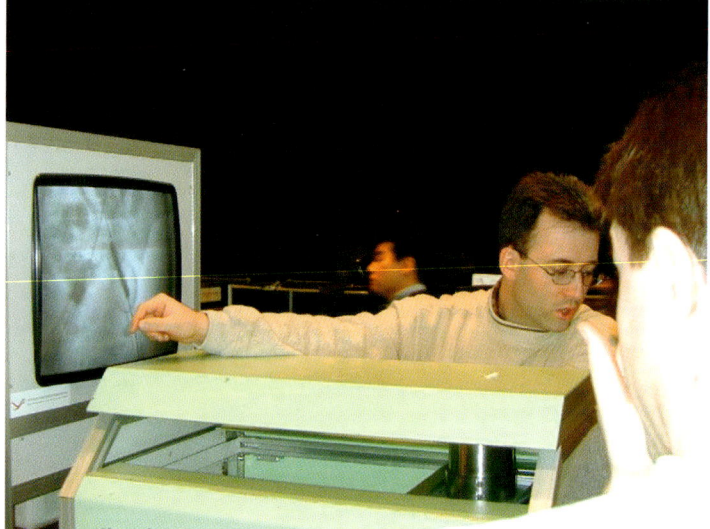

FIG. 8 Teaching and practicing EVAR with the Pontresina Endovascular Model (Pontresina Vascular Workshops).

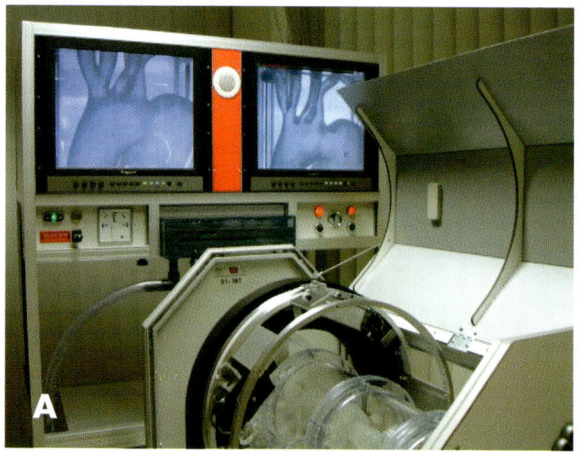
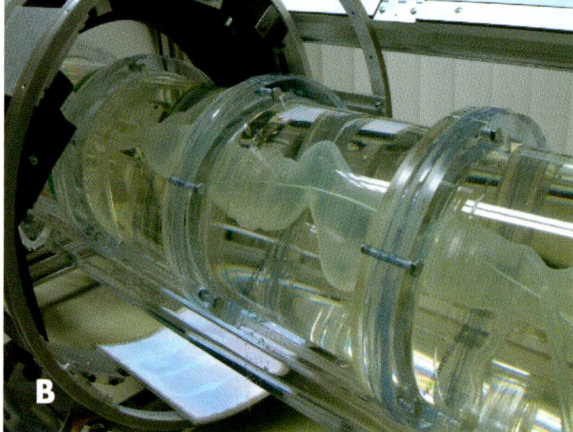

FIG. 9 Prototype of the second generation Pontresina Endovascular Model including better imaging on two screens (A) and pulsatile compliant silicon aortic segments (B), designed by Otmar Keel for Vascular International.

The endovascular curriculum of the German Society of Vascular Surgery

In 2007, the German Society of Vascular Surgery established an endovascular curriculum (Table V) to provide vascular surgeons with a detailed and structured training regimen for performing endovascular procedures [30]. The training program addresses surgical residents within their first two years (the so-called surgical common trunk, which is obligatory for all surgical specialties in Germany), vascular surgical residents and board certified vascular surgeons with a special interest in endovascular procedures. Workshops organized by individuals, clinical institutions or companies may apply for certification according to the course program by the German Society for Vascular Surgery. Following a series of advanced courses and at least three special courses, surgeons can apply for an individual degree as an *"endovascular specialist, certified by the German Society of Vascular Surgery"*. Applicants will have to provide evidence of at least 150 documented endovascular reconstructions with the following minimum numbers in various vascular territories: 50 supra-aortic (at least 30 carotid artery interventions), 10 thoracic, 15 visceral/renal, 20 shunt interventions and 30 distal interventions below the knee.

Current guidelines and recommendations

The implementation of endovascular curriculae in vascular surgery has only just begun. Only one

Table V — STRUCTURE OF THE ENDOVASCULAR CURRICULUM OF THE GERMAN SOCIETY OF VASCULAR SURGERY

	Topic/theory	Practice program
Basic endovascular skills for surgical residents in the first two years (common trunk trainees)		
4 hours	- Principles about radiation physics, safety, radiographic imaging equipment and complications of (non-)iodinated contrast agents - Guidewires, angiography catheters, stents and endografts	- Puncture technique - Insertion of guidewires and catheters - Catheter navigation - Balloon dilatation and stenting
Endovascular skills for vascular surgical residents and/or board-certified vascular surgeons		
Basic course (8 hours)	- Principles about radiation physics, safety, radiographic imaging equipment and complications of (non-)iodinated contrast agents - Sheaths, guidewires and angiography catheters - Stents and endografts - Occlusion systems - Management of complications	- Training on models in small groups: - Puncture technique - Insertion of guidewires and catheters - Balloon dilatation and stenting - Application of occlusion systems
Advanced courses for various vascular territories (8 hours each)	- Abdominal aorta - Iliac arteries - SFA	- Training on models in small groups - Live transmissions from the OR - Training within the OR/angiosuite - Proctering by experts
Special courses for vascular territories (8 hours each)	- Supra-aortic interventions including CAS - Thoracic aorta - Visceral and renal arteries - Shunt interventions - SFA, poplital and distal arteries	- Training on models in small groups - Live transmissions from the OR - Training within the OR/angiosuite - Proctering by experts

year ago, the Royal College of Surgeons and the Royal College of Radiology agreed to create the new specialty of endovascular specialists, however, a detailed and formal curriculum is still lacking. Due to widely different structures and traditions between and within the majority of western countries, the responsibilities for vascular patients and endovascular procedures differ widely between various disciplines. As a result, endovascular procedures are performed by interventional radiologists, neuroradiologists, cardiologists, angiologists and vascular surgeons, respectively.

Just recently, the Clinical Practice Counsil of the Society for Vascular Surgery (SVS) emphasized "that a fully trained vascular surgeon should be considered to be a vascular specialist who performs traditional open surgery, but who also perfoms endovascular interventions and is competent to treat vascular diseases with noninterventional and nonsurgical means". With respect to endovascular interventions, it was further stated that all vascular surgery residents currently are expected to have acquired sufficient training to perform vascular catheter-based intervention with a minimum number of endovascular procedures for training. These include 80 endovascular therapeutic procedures, 100 endovascular diagnostic procedures and 20 endovascular aortic aneurysm repairs (EVAR) [31]. It should be noted that, apart from these minimum numbers, the individual surgeon's learning curve shortens considerably while the institution's experience with EVAR increases [32].

For TEVAR, recent guidelines include full basic endovascular privileges with an experience of at least 25 EVARs, with 12 as the primary operator. The term "full basic endovascular privileges" means that the operator is fully qualified as defined by either American Heart Association guidelines or multispecialty guidelines [33,34]. Upon completion of their training, vascular residents performing TEVAR should be familiar with the peri-operative management of aortic surgical patients and are expected to have experience in performing adjunctive procedures for TEVARs, including iliac conduits, femoral artery exposures and repairs, and carotid-subclavian bypasses. The surgeon does not have to have pre-existing open thoracoabdominal privileges [31].

A recent multidisciplinary group recommended guidelines for certified vascular surgeons performing TEVAR. These include 10 TEVARS performed within the past two years and 10 continuing medical education hours devoted to TEVAR. The procedural numerical requirement may be reduced for surgeons with robust EVAR experience of at least 25 EVARs. The surgeon is not required to have pre-existing privileges for open thoracic or thoracoabdominal aneurysm repair. Similar to recent graduates of vascular residencies, certified surgeons already in practice performing TEVAR should be familiar with the peri-operative management of aortic surgical patients and are expected to have experience in performing adjunctive procedures for TEVAR [5]. This case volume for TEVAR, as recommended by the SVS, was supported by a recent study which showed that catheter-trained surgeons can achieve optimal results with thoracic lesions following 5 to 10 cases [5].

Conclusion

There is no doubt that endovascular aortic procedures are a key component of today's vascular surgeon's profile. Besides a minimal knowledge of aortic diseases, basic diagnostic, surgical and endovascular skills are a prerequisite before starting endovascular aortic procedures. Clinical competence in endovascular aortic repair can be achieved by the implementation of guidelines for vascular surgical training programs and the attendance of simulator training workshops. Since endovascular technology is rapidly improving, didactical workshops and simulator training on synthetic models may become a permanent assignment for vascular surgeons.

REFERENCES

1 Volodos NL, Karpovich IP, Shekhanin VE et al. A case of distant transfemoral endoprosthesis of the thoracic artery using a self-fixing synthetic prosthesis in traumatic aneurysm. *Grudn Khir* 1988; 6: 84-86.

2 Volodos NL, Karpovich IP, Troyan VI et al. Clinical experience of the use of self-fixing synthetic prostheses for remote endoprosthetics of the thoracic and the abdominal aorta and iliac arteries through the femoral artery and as intraoperative endoprosthesis for aorta reconstruction. *Vasa Suppl* 1991; 33: 93-95.

3 Parodi JC, Palmaz JC, Barone HD. Transfemoral intraluminal graft implantation for abdominal aortic aneurysms. *Ann Vasc Surg* 1991; 5: 491-499.

4   Dake MD, Miller DC, Semba CP et al. Transluminal placement of endovascular stent-grafts for the treatment of descending thoracic aortic aneurysms. *N Engl J Med* 1994; 331: 1729-1734.

5   Hodgson KJ, Matsumura JS, Ascher E et al. Clinical competence statement on thoracic endovascular aortic repair (TEVAR)–multispecialty consensus recommendations. A report of the SVS/SIR/SCAI/SVMB Writing Committee to develop a clinical competence standard for TEVAR. *J Vasc Surg* 2006; 43: 858-862.

6   Anonymous. Endovascular aneurysm repair and outcome in patients unfit for open repair of abdominal aortic aneurysm (EVAR trial 2): randomised controlled trial. *Lancet* 2005; 365: 2187-2192.

7   Anonymous. Endovascular aneurysm repair versus open repair in patients with abdominal aortic aneurysm (EVAR trial 1): randomised controlled trial. *Lancet* 2005; 365: 2179-2186.

8   Greenhalgh RM, Brown LC, Kwong GP et al. Comparison of endovascular aneurysm repair with open repair in patients with abdominal aortic aneurysm (EVAR trial 1), 30-day operative mortality results: randomised controlled trial. *Lancet* 2004; 364: 843-848.

9   Harris PL, Buth J. An update on the important findings from the EUROSTAR EVAR registry. *Vascular* 2004; 12: 33-38.

10 Blankensteijn JD, de Jong SE, Prinssen M et al. Two-year outcomes after conventional or endovascular repair of abdominal aortic aneurysms. *N Engl J Med* 2005; 352: 2398-2405.

11 Buth J, Harris PL, Hobo R et al. Neurologic complications associated with endovascular repair of thoracic aortic pathology: Incidence and risk factors. A study from the European Collaborators on Stent/Graft Techniques for Aortic Aneurysm Repair (EUROSTAR) Registry. *J Vasc Surg* 2007; 46: 1103-1111.

12 Leurs LJ, Harris PL, Buth J. Secondary interventions after elective endovascular repair of degenerative thoracic aortic aneurysms: results of the European collaborators registry (EUROSTAR). *J Vasc Interv Radiol* 2007; 18: 491-495.

13 Bown MJ, Fishwick G, Sayers RD et al. Repair of ruptured abdominal aortic aneurysms by endovascular techniques. *Adv Surg* 2007; 41: 63-80.

14 Franks SC, Sutton AJ, Bown MJ et al. Systematic review and meta-analysis of 12 years of endovascular abdominal aortic aneurysm repair. *Eur J Vasc Endovasc Surg* 2007; 33: 154-171.

15 Black SA, Wolfe JH, Clark M et al. Complex thoracoabdominal aortic aneurysms: endovascular exclusion with visceral revascularization. *J Vasc Surg* 2006; 43: 1081-1089.

16 Greenberg RK, West K, Pfaff K et al. Beyond the aortic bifurcation: branched endovascular grafts for thoracoabdominal and aortoiliac aneurysms. *J Vasc Surg* 2006; 43: 879-886.

17 Greenberg RK, Haddad F, Svensson L et al. Hybrid approaches to thoracic aortic aneurysms: the role of endovascular elephant trunk completion. *Circulation* 2005; 112: 2619-2626.

18 Moon MC, Morales JP, Greenberg RK. The aortic arch and ascending aorta: are they within the endovascular realm? *Semin Vasc Surg* 2007; 20: 97-107.

19 Reznick RK, MacRae H. Teaching surgical skills–changes in the wind. *N Engl J Med* 2006; 355: 2664-2669.

20 Creager MA, Goldstone J, Hirshfeld JW Jr et al. ACC/ACP/SCAI/SVMB/SVS clinical competence statement on vascular medicine and catheter-based peripheral vascular interventions: a report of the American College of Cardiology/American Heart Association/American College of Physician Task Force on Clinical Competence (ACC/ACP/SCAI/SVMB/SVS Writing Committee to develop a clinical competence statement on peripheral vascular disease). *J Am Coll Cardiol* 2004; 44: 941-957.

21 Schumacher H, Allenberg JR, Eckstein HH. Morphological classification of abdominal aortic aneurysm in selection of patients for endovascular grafting. *Br J Surg* 1996; 83:949-950.

22 Neequaye SK, Aggarwal R, Brightwell R et al. Identification of skills common to renal and iliac endovascular procedures performed on a virtual reality simulator. *Eur J Vasc Endovasc Surg* 2007; 33: 525-532.

23 Neequaye SK, Aggarwal R, Van Herzeele I et al. Endovascular skills training and assessment. *J Vasc Surg* 2007; 46: 1055-1064.

24 Dawson DL, Meyer J, Lee ES et al. Training with simulation improves residents' endovascular procedure skills. *J Vasc Surg* 2007; 45: 149-154.

25 Chaer RA, DeRubertis BG, Lin SC et al. Simulation improves resident performance in catheter-based intervention: results of a randomized, controlled study. *Ann Surg* 2006; 244: 343-352.

26 Aggarwal R, Black SA, Hance JR et al. Virtual reality simulation training can improve inexperienced surgeons' endovascular skills. *Eur J Vasc Endovasc Surg* 2006; 31: 588-593.

27 Berry M, Lystig T, Beard J et al. Porcine transfer study: virtual reality simulator training compared with porcine training in endovascular novices. *Cardiovasc Intervent Radiol* 2007; 30: 455-461.

28 Kunst E, Rodel S, Moll F et al. Towards a VR trainer for EVAR treatment. *Stud Health Technol Inform* 2006; 119: 279-281.

29 Pandey VA, Black SA, Lazaris AM et al. Do workshops improve the technical skill of vascular surgical trainees? *Eur J Vasc Endovasc Surg* 2005; 30: 441-447.

30 http://www.akademie-dgg.de/curriculum_endovasculaer.pdf. 2007. Ref Type: Generic.

31 Calligaro KD, Toursarkissian B, Clagett GP et al. Guidelines for hospital privileges in vascular and endovascular surgery: Recommendations of the Society for Vascular Surgery. *J Vasc Surg* 2008; 47: 1-5.

32 Forbes TL, DeRose G, Lawlor DK et al. The association between a surgeon's learning curve with endovascular aortic aneurysm repair and previous institutional experience. *Vasc Endovascular Surg* 2007; 41: 14-18.

33 Hirsch AT, Haskal ZJ, Hertzer NR et al. ACC/AHA Guidelines for the Management of Patients with Peripheral Arterial Disease (lower extremity, renal, mesenteric, and abdominal aortic): a collaborative report from the American Associations for Vascular Surgery/Society for Vascular Surgery, Society for Cardiovascular Angiography and Interventions, Society for Vascular Medicine and Biology, Society of Interventional Radiology, and the ACC/AHA Task Force on Practice Guidelines (writing committee to develop guidelines for the management of patients with peripheral arterial disease)–summary of recommendations. *J Vasc Interv Radiol* 2006; 17: 1383-1397.

34 White RA, Hodgson KJ, Ahn SS et al. Endovascular interventions training and credentialing for vascular surgeons. *J Vasc Surg* 1999; 29: 177-186.

3

CHARACTERISTICS OF AORTIC STENT GRAFTS INCLUDING DURABILITY AND FATIGUE TESTING

NABIL CHAKFE, OLIVIER CRETON, ANDREI IVANENKO
FABIEN THAVEAU, DANIEL MATHIEU, YANNICK GEORG
JEAN-GEORGES KRETZ, BERNARD DURAND

Endovascular treatment of abdominal aortic aneurysm (EVAR) undoubtedly represented one of the main developments in modern vascular surgery. The goal of this technique is to be less invasive than open surgery and then to allow the treatment of patients with a high surgical risk of morbidity and mortality, this risk being either related to the physiological status of the patient or to a specific morphology or pathology of the diseased aorta. The goal of EVAR is to eliminate the risk of aortic aneurysm rupture by excluding the aneurysmal sac. However, in order to develop this technique, it was necessary to create a specific device associating a membrane for the exclusion of the aneurysmal sac, and an attachment system for the anchorage of this membrane at the level of proximal and distal necks. This device needed to be flexible and deformable enough to allow an easy intra-vascular navigation from the site of arterial entrance to the diseased aortic area and to demonstrate a long-term stability in order to guarantee a durable efficiency of the treatment. Logically, the first generations of endoprostheses were constructed by using the biomaterials and structures that were available and accepted in clinical practice: vascular prostheses and stents. Consequently, the endoprosthesis was an hybrid structure associating deformable fibrous materials to low-deformable metallic materials.

Early experience

First clinical studies showed that the aneurysmal sac exclusion was not always achieved because of early or delayed arterial reinjections. The observation of these reinjections led to the concepts of endoleaks and endotension with a risk for the patient of aneurysmal expansion and rupture. The structural stability of the device was then considered as one of the major characteristics of the endoprosthesis to take into account in order to assume good long-term clinical results. Studies of explanted endoprostheses of the first generation showed early degradations characterized by dislocations of the stented structure and perforations of the membrane [1]. These degradations were observed either on the metallic structure, the stents, that showed corrosion phenomenons and ruptures, or on the membranes, that demonstrated opening of their structure and tears. These observations showed that it was necessary to better understand these degradation phenomenons in order to propose more durable generations of devices. The specific hybrid construction and the conditions of implantation of the endoprostheses represented biomechanic conditions that have not been studied before.

Basically, characteristics and factors influencing the stability and the durability of an endoprosthesis can be divided in two groups. The first group is represented by the biomechanical factors influencing the endoprosthesis mobility inside the aneurysmal sac, that we will call "macroscopic interactions". These factors of mobility can be considered as potentially responsible for migrations from the necks, for disconnections of modular devices, for direct interactions between the different materials of the endoprosthesis, and for the interactions between the endoprosthesis and its environment. The second group is represented by the biomechanical factors influencing the interactions between the different materials of the endoprosthesis, that we will call "microscopic factors". These factors characterized the knowledge about physical and chemical biomaterial interactions and about wearing and ageing phenomenons. Microscopic factors are partially related to macroscopic factors.

We propose a literature review on the updated knowledge about endoprostheses characteristics known as able to influence their stability, and on the different types of pre-clinical characterization proposed to predict their long-term behavior.

Behavior characteristics of the endoprostheses

CLINICAL DATA ABOUT ENDOPROSTHESES MIGRATION AND MOBILITY

Textile prostheses and stents were the main vascular devices available before the commercial introduction of endoprostheses. Since stents implanted for the treatment of occlusive vascular disease are stressed by the arterial wall on their entire length, they are not exposed to migration but can exceptionally present degradations or ruptures in areas of high arterial mobility. Textile prostheses performing a bypass are implanted in an extravascular environment since endoprostheses are placed inside the vessel. However, both devices are fixed at their extremities, by stents at the level of the necks for endoprostheses and by running sutures for textile prostheses. Biomechanically, this difference of fixation leads to, on one hand, a stable prosthesis-to-artery anastomosis related to the running suture, and on the other hand to an unstable endoprosthesis-to-artery fixation because of its potential mobility. In both cases, biomechanical stresses that will be applied to the devices are: the pulsatile flow, the angulations of the device, and the specificity of the adjacent anatomical structures. The impact of the stresses on the device can be influenced by different factors such as its own structure or its pre-stressed state.

Because of its endovascular placement, an aortic endoprosthesis is exposed to permanent deformations as a consequence to the pressure and flow stresses imposed by the cyclic cardiac activity. Singland et al. [2] studied the mobility of the custom-made endoprosthesis they developed in order to better understand their in-vivo solicitations when implanted in humans for the treatment of abdominal aortic aneurysm. They used dynamic tomodensitometry with electrocardiogram-gated modulation followed by numerical modelization of the stents skeleton in order to characterize the endoprosthesis degree of mobility and then to predict its risk of degradation related to the interaction between the stents and the polyester fabric. The numerical modelization studied the displacements of the sharp angles of the Gianturco stents, that were characterized as angular, radial, and longitudinal displacements. Their measurements showed a mean angular displacement of 4.5° ±1.5 (range: 2.8 to 7.1), a mean radial displacement of 0.6 mm

±0.4 (range: 0.2 to 1.5), and a mean longitudinal displacement of 0.4 mm ±0.2 (range: 0.2 to 0.9). The most important angular and radial displacements were observed at the level of proximal and distal necks. This can be explained by the fact that the necks are areas of transition between stressed stents in the aortic neck, and free-stents located in the aneurysmal sac for the angular displacement, and that at the level of the neck, the stent is stressed inside the arterial wall and its displacement follows those of the arterial wall because of its own compliance, since in the aneurysmal sac, the stents are not pre-stressed and do not move with the polyester fabric because they are not sutured together in this particular construction of endoprosthesis. The most important longitudinal displacements were observed on the body of the endoprosthesis, far from the necks. The authors did not find any relation between angular and radial displacements on one side and longitudinal displacements on the other side. However, they found that the behavior of the endoprostheses was heterogenous inside the group they studied. The limitations of this study consisted in the low number of cases and the different durations of implantation of the endoprostheses they studied, that unabled them to do correlations between the degree of angulation of the endoprostheses and the size of the aneurismal sac. Moreover, in this particular type of endoprosthesis, since the stents are inside the polyester fabric and not attached to it, it is impossible to consider that the fabric demonstrated the same displacement than the stents, excepted at the level of the necks. However, this study is the only one that tried to characterize in-vivo the deformations of an endoprosthesis during the cardiac cycle. Others characterized the aneurysm [3,4] but did not study the microdisplacements of the endoprosthesis itself.

These data about the microdeformations of the endoprosthesis and of the arterial wall in either the aneurismal sac or the necks, can explain the observations of endoprostheses migration. Umscheid et al. [5] studied displacements and shape modifications of the first generations of endoprostheses and proposed a relation between the microdisplacements related to the pulsatile arterial flow and the observation of shape and position modifications of the endoprosthesis. They emphasized the necessity to propose a global biomechanical approach for the understanding of the behavior of the aneurysm treated with an endoprosthesis in order to predict its long-term evolution. For the authors, the arterial systolic-diastolic flow creates an accordion motion on the endoprosthesis, that, because of the curved morphology of the aneurysmal aorto-iliac bifurcation, bends the endoprosthesis in the aneurysmal sac tugging its proximal and distal ends away from the necks. They also demonstrated that the size and an incomplete exclusion of the aneurysmal sac enhanced the mobility of the endoprosthesis and consequently its risk of migration. This hypothesis was not supported by a biomechanical study but showed the necessity to take into account the biomechanical characteristics of the endoprosthesis to insure long-term results.

Recent clinical studies reported the endoprostheses migration rate was about 20% [6-8]. The main clinical factors increasing the risk of migration are related, either to the characteristics of the artery itself, i.e. its properties at the time of the implantation or its modifications of properties during the implantation, or to the specific characteristics of the endoprosthesis. Some arterial wall characteristics can alter the quality of the endoprosthesis anchoring: a short and/or large proximal neck, a heavily calcified neck, or a neck with a thrombus layer. Other factors can increase the risk of migration by influencing the endoprosthesis biomechanics after its implantation: a highly angulated neck, a large aneurysmal sac with or without internal pressurization, and the morphology of the iliac arteries responsible for highly curvated endoprosthesis limbs. The most frequent secondary modification of the arterial wall is a neck dilatation that is found in about 50% of the cases when a migration is observed. It has been described that the proximal neck dilatation was more frequent with the use of endoprostheses constructed with a proximal self-expanding stent [9].

CLINICAL DATA ON BIOMATERIALS DEGRADATION PHENOMENONS AND STRUCTURE INTERACTIONS

The main advantage of a retrieval program of explanted prostheses in humans is to allow an early characterization of the degradation or ageing mechanisms of a particular type of device. However, such a program present an unavoidable selection bias since, because of its nature, it will mainly analyze devices explanted at the time of a reoperation for failure, and rarely unfailed devices retrieved at the time of an autopsy performed for a non device-related death. It is also very important to be able to differentiate observations related to a sporadic failure from those related to a degradation behavior of a specific model of device. Moreover, it is also important to differentiate observations related to a specific model of device from those related to the concept of endoprosthesis itself. The observations we done on explants of the first generations of tubular endoprostheses [10] showed dislocations of the stents skeleton related to ruptures of the ligatures linking the stents together that were found to be responsible for endoprosthesis migration and endoleaks. These observations showed the necessity to ensure a longitudinal stability to the endoprosthesis by creating a vertebral column to the stents skeleton. The polyester fabric of these endoprostheses showed openings of the woven structure responsible for endoleaks. A proposed hypothesis for these macroscopic observations was a mechanism of cyclic stress of both stents skeleton and polyester fabric by the aortic pulsatile flow. Then we proposed to characterize the phenomenon of microscopic degradation of the stents [11] and of the textile structures [12]. We found that stents showed corrosion phenomenon of nitinol with a decrease of the relative nickel concentration. Areas of corrosion consisted in small pits and more marked defects leading to stress fissures and total stent fractures. These corrosion phenomenons have also been described in other studies of explanted endoprostheses [13]. These observations demonstrated the necessity to construct endoprostheses with stents taking into account the cyclic in-vivo stress applied to them, and to realize appropriate surface treatments to keep them corrosion-proof. The analyses we performed on polyester fabrics taken from different models of endoprostheses demonstrated that the degradation phenomenons were influenced by the specific characteristics of the endoprostheses [12], one of the most important being the saturation index of the structure chosen for the polyester fabric. Low saturation index was responsible for openings of the woven structure and slipping of the warp yarns on the weft yarns (Fig. 1). These phenomenons increased with the increasing of the difference of saturation index between the warp and weft axes that led to highly anisotropic structure. These openings of the textile structure allowed the anchorage of the ligatures and of the stents struts, whose geometric shape was important, in the textile. The consequences of micro-movements and mechanical stresses related to the cardiac cycle were permanent interactions between the stents responsible for filaments wearing followed by yarns ruptures and macroscopic perforations of the fabric (Figs. 2-4). Zarins et al. [14] published the most important study of explanted endoprostheses where 120 explanted AneuRx endoprostheses were non-independently analyzed by the Medtronic company itself. The mean duration of implantation of the endoprostheses was 22±13 months (range: 1 to 61 months). They made similar observations to our study: stents fractures, ligatures ruptures, and le-

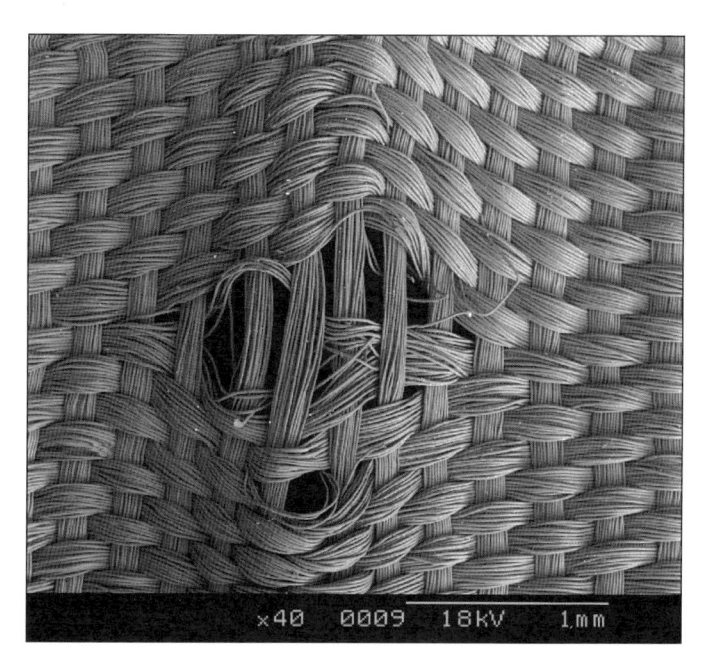

FIG. 1 Example of opening of the woven structure and slipping of the warp yarns on the weft yarns with a textile presenting a low saturation index.

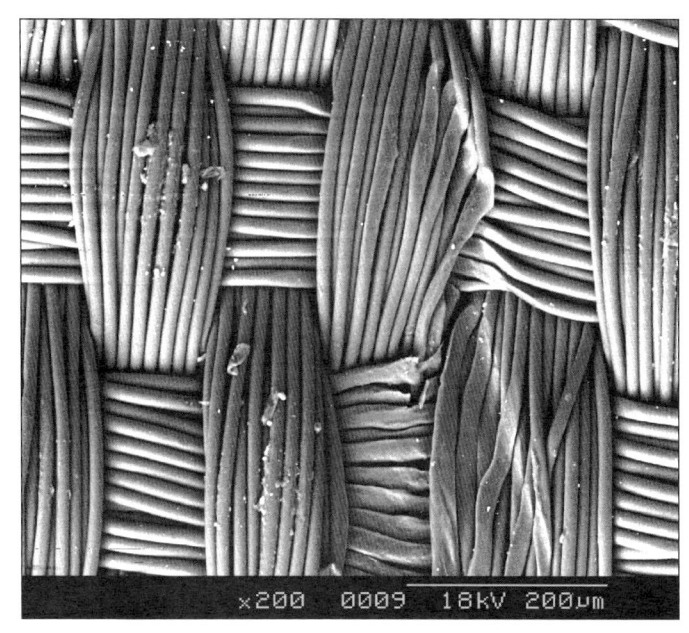

FIG. 2 Filaments crushed by a stent.

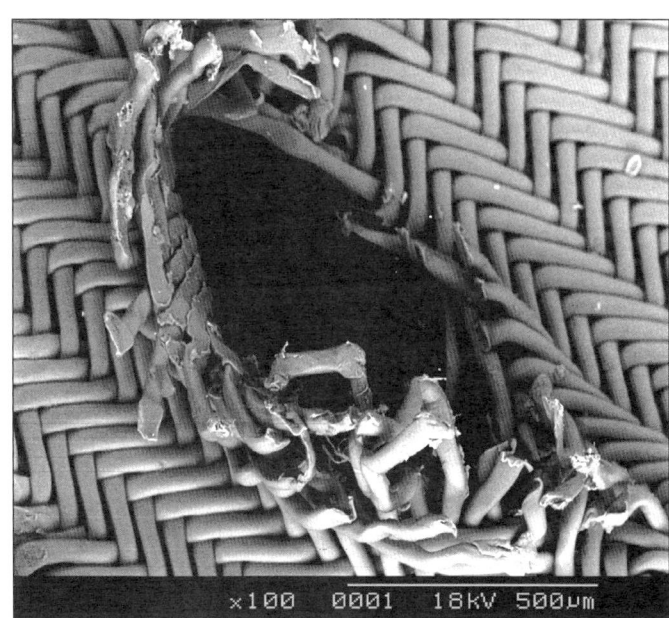

FIG. 3 Example of wearing phenomenons of a woven structure with fibrillation on ruptured yarns.

sions of the woven structure such as openings of the structure and phenomenons of yarns wearing with holes. These lesions were mainly observed after a 2-year duration of implantation, at the level of the bifurcation, and when the endoprosthesis had a high degree of angulation. There was no correlation between these lesions and the occurrence of an endoleak or a aneurysmal growth, but there was a correlation with the occurrence of a migration of the endoprosthesis.

How to predict endoprosthesis stability

Recent clinical data showed how the in-vivo behavior and the stability of the endoprostheses were difficult to predict. Basically, the different approaches available to predict the behavior of a new device and the impact of its characteristics on it, are: in-vitro and in-vivo experimental tests, numerical models of prediction, and fatigue bench-tests.

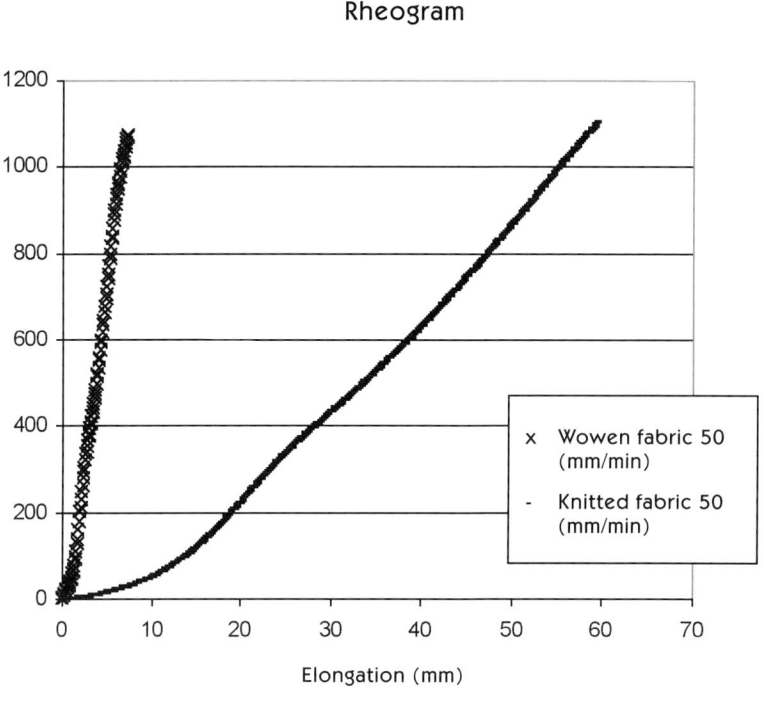

FIG. 4 Example of stress-strain curves taken from longitudinal traction tests and comparing a woven with a knitted structure. We easily observe that their behavior is totally different to reach the same level of stress.

EXPERIMENTAL STUDIES

The aim of these studies is to characterize the endoprosthesis behavior in experimental conditions as close as possible to the clinical conditions in order to be able to predict the occurrence of specific complications.

These studies tried to characterize the quality of the proximal fixation of the endoprosthesis and its risk of migration. Albertini et al. [15] developed a continuous and pulsatile flow model to evaluate the influence of the proximal neck angulation on the occurrence of periprosthetic endoleaks. They studied one size of a home-made endoprosthesis that was submitted to increasing angulations of the proximal neck from 0° to 70°. They demonstrated that endoleaks increased with the increasing of the angulation, but with a high inter-experimental variability of the results. However, characteristics of this experimental model were not representative of the in-vivo conditions and not transferable to other models of endoprostheses constructed with other types of stents and fabrics. In their study, the authors actually characterized the role of the angulation on the morphological reorganization of the proximal part of a specific endoprosthesis associating specific stents to a specific fabric. The high inter-experiment variability of the results on this specific model of endoprosthesis demonstrated that this reorganization is highly variable. Leigh et al. [16] demonstrated in-vitro that on straight necks, endoleaks decreased with the increase of the length of the neck, and that for short necks, endoleaks were more important with straight-edged fabric (fabric applied perpendicular to the stent and crossing the stents cells) than with zigzag-edged fabric (fabric applied in a zigzag configuration crossing the "Z" shape of the edge of the stents cells). Resch et al. [17] compared the stresses necessary to lead to the migration of different models of endoprostheses deployed in cadaver aortic necks. They found that the mean stress necessary to allow the endoprosthesis migration was related to the characteristics of its proximal stent. This mean stress was respectively 4.5 N for a nitinol self-expanding stent without hooks, 9.0 N for a nitinol self expanding stent with hooks, 12.5 N for a stainless-steel self expanding stent with hooks, 24.0 N for an other stainless-steel self expanding stent with hooks, and 25 N for a stainless-steel balloon-expanded stent. The stress necessary to pull out a textile prosthesis sutured to an aorta was 150 N. The arterial wall lesions created by the hooks were more important when they penetrated the entire aortic wall. Hinchliffe et al. [18] investigated the theoretical forces involved in and the nature of fixation between the modular components of a variety of aortic stent-grafts. The authors observed differences of behavior between the models with a maximum peak force of 36.0 N leading to the damage of the graft itself in one model, and average peak force of respectively 23.7 N, 7.3 N, 7.0 N, 5.4 N, and 2.4 N for the other models. The authors also analyzed the experimental stress-strain curves obtained during the tests and demonstrated differences of behavior related to the differences of the stents skeleton reorganization during the simplified traction tests they performed. Arko et al. [19] studied on an in-vivo animal model the importance of the length of iliac fixation on the forces necessary to generate the proximal neck migration of an endoprosthesis. Peak displacement forces to initiate migration were 30.2±5.5 N in animal with maximal iliac fixation compared with 18.1±3.7 N in those with minimum fixation. Liffman et al. [20] tried to determine, with an analytical mathematical modeling and an experimental benchtop, factors influencing the mobility and the risk of separation of modular stent-graft curved through 90°. Their benchtop allowed to control both pulsatile pressure characteristics inside the grafts and the pressure outside the graft mimicking the intra-aneurysmal sac pressure. The authors demonstrated that the curved stent-graft system oscillated transversally when there was zero mean pressure difference between the stent-graft and the aneurysm, mimicking a pressurized aneurysmal sac by an endoleak. Conversely, when the mean pressure difference increased, this condition mimicking an excluded aneurysmal sac, the transverse graft movement was damped and then disappeared, but with a higher risk of grafts separation. Curved thoracic endografts because of the specific conditions of thoracic aortic aneurysm treatment, are subject to forces that may cause migration or separation, the latter being more likely if the seal between the graft and the sac is blood-tight, if the blood pressure is high, and if the diameter of the graft is small and the sac large. These conditions impose a maximum overlap of the modular components of the endoprosthesis. This team [21] experimentally measured the effect of pressure and flow rate on the forces acting on a model of bifurcated endoluminal stent graft. These forces increased with the proximal or inlet pressure and the inlet area. These experimental data were consistent with the results of a mathematical model.

Another characteristic of the endoprosthesis that can act upon the durability of the treatment is the biomaterial chosen for the fabric. The properties of the fabric can act not only on the mechanical behavior of the endoprosthesis itself, but also on the biomechanical behavior of the aneuvrysm-to-endoprosthesis combination through the differences of pressure transmitted to the aneurysmal sac [22].

Mathematical models

Li et al. [23] used numerical simulation to describe the behavior of a representative stented abdominal aortic aneurysm model. They demonstrated that after EVAR, the stress applied to the aneurysmal wall was reduced by 90%. There were two drag forces acting on the endoprosthesis: one main downward component affecting the proximal neck fixation and exposing the body to distal migration, and a secondary transverse component with medial direction influencing the iliac fixations and exposing the limbs to a proximal migration. These forces are mainly generated by the net blood pressure and incidentally by the blood friction on the endoprosthesis wall. The authors showed that there were several factors which influence the endoprosthesis drag force to various degree. Drag force increases with the body diameter of the endoprosthesis, this one increasing from 2 N to 7 N when the body diameter increases from 18 mm to 32 mm, with the endoprosthesis-body-to-iliac-limb diameter ratio, this one increasing of 5.3 N when the ratio increases from 1.5 to 3, with the iliac limb angle, this one increasing from 3.8 N to 5.8 N when the angle increases from 23° to 90°, with the aortic neck angle, its effect being negligible when it is less than 40°, since drag forces significantly increase when it is higher than 40°, and with systolic pressure slope. In a previous study, the authors showed that increased intra-aneurysmal sac pressure decreased drag forces responsible for distal migration of the endoprosthesis [24]. Morris et al. [25] also developed a mathematical model in order to predict axial drag forces affecting the risk of migration of bifurcated endoprostheses. They showed similar results to others with forces increasing with body diameter of the endoprosthesis, these one showing a 220% increase when this diameter increased from 18 to 32 mm, with the limb angulation, these one showing a 52% increase when the angle increased from 10° to 80°, and with the arterial wall compliance. Howell et al. [26] used computational fluid dynamics to study on models of bifurcated endoprostheses derived from computed tomography in 4 patients who had previously undergone EVAR, to determine the forces applied to them during the cardiac cycle. They analyzed these forces on the overall endoprosthesis and on 3 areas: the body, the bifurcation, and the limbs. The authors demonstrated that these forces were influenced by the arterial pressure, the body diameter, and the angulation of the endoprosthesis. Moreover, they found that the most important axial forces were localized at the bifurcation, and that they decreased when the intra-aneurysmal sac pressure increased. Consequently, they concluded for clinical practice that it was recommended to implant endoprostheses with body diameter as small as possible, a long body with limbs as short as possible, and paradoxically to maintain a high intra-aneurysmal sac pressure, in order to prevent migration.

Canic et al. [27] used a mathematical modelisation to study the behavior of two different stent structures implanted in an arterial aneurysm: a Wallstent® self-expanding stent and an AneuRx® endoprosthesis. The Wallstent® stent demonstrated a high compliance with large radial and longitudinal displacements during each cardiac cycle, responsible for stent migration and arterial neck damages. The decrease of the compliance of the stent by superimposing stents in its central section decreased the risk of migration and arterial wall damage. In contrast, the AneuRx® endosprothesis, constructed with an external compliant nitinol stent skeleton covered by a fabric significantly less compliant than the arterial wall and the stents, demonstrated a lower risk of migration. In contrast, the combination of compliant stents to non compliant fabric increased the risk of interaction between these two different biomaterials and the risk of the onset fatigue phenomenons and ruptures.

FATIGUE TESTS

The first interest of a fatigue test would be to allow a comprehensive analysis of an endoprosthesis on a bench test completely representative of the in-vivo conditions of implantation in order to predict exactly its mid- and long-term behavior and durability. The small number of publications in this field shows how difficult it is to set up such a test that could be really predictive. Quite obviously, one factor at least cannot be reproduced with this type of test: time. Indeed, it is necessary to be able to speed up the cardiac cycle frequency in order to get a ratio allowing to predict the evolution of a 10-year implanted endoprosthesis after only a few months of testing. The realization of fatigue tests falls into the general scope of the pre-clinical tests imposed by the main institutions for standards and certification [28,29]. These institutions proposed to realize these tests in the worst conditions for the endoprostheses. One of the main problems for the test interpretation comes from the accelerated frequency of the bench test. This very high frequency, often close to 50Hz, does not allow a reorganization of the structures after being stressed as it occurs in-vivo. Even if the endoprosthesis deformation is controlled during the cyclic stress [30], the experimental conditions cannot be representative of the in-vivo conditions. Indeed, the only way to get a similar endoprosthesis displacement at a higher frequency is to increase the stress applied to it. Once the stress resulted in a deformation of the endoprosthesis, the latter will quickly go back to its initial state so as only the elastic component of the material and not its viscous component is investigated. Under these conditions, the presence of a potential creep cannot be investigated, making this test inappropriate. This high frequency does not generate an endoprosthesis fatigue representative of the conditions of implantation making the test results worthless. Few results or critical analyzes are given in the literature. Studies performed by companies reported that endoprostheses exposed to 380 million stress cycles did not present any damages [31]. Bench tests have also been proposed by companies marketing fatigue machines for biomedical applications [32], or are developed by academic institutions [33].

Conclusions about endoprostheses characteristics and durability

The introduction of the endoprostheses in the current therapeutic methods of modern vascular surgery generated specific problems particularly focused on their durability. This problematics of durability already existed with standard vascular prostheses but have often been underestimated or neglected. Endoprostheses are hybrid structures. In addition, they are exposed to interactions between soft and stiff materials that have probably been underestimated with the first generations of endoprostheses. The first observations of failures have been quickly taken into account, particularly because of their very early onset after implantation, and because of the immediate doubts related to the results of a technique in which very large amounts of money were invested with the hope of quick financial spin-offs.

Clinical trials demonstrated that the failures of this technique in terms of durability were particularly related to the endoprosthesis migration at the necks responsible for type I endoleaks, and to the materials degradation responsible for textile fabric perforations, stents ruptures, and migrations of the modular endoprosthesis components in the areas of overlapping leading to type III endoleaks. These endoleaks led to aneurysmal sac reperfusion and pressurization with a risk of secondary rupture.

Very quickly, new generations of endoprostheses have been proposed on the market. They integrated the increased knowledge on biomaterials interactions within an hybrid structure and on interaction between the endoprosthesis and the aneurysmal sac.

Most of the time, studies that tried to predict the risk of migration of the endoprosthesis at the level of the proximal neck amounted to a measure of the traction resistance of an endoprosthesis inserted in an experimental or cadaver aortic neck. These investigators compared the value of the peak force necessary to disconnection to the values of the axial drag forces applied to the endoprosthesis calculated through a numerical model. However, regardless of the experimental conditions that could not be accepted as representative to the in-vivo conditions, these studies only reported the peak force at the time of the disconnection and not the strain-stress curves of the test that could provide more information about the interactions between the endoprosthesis and the aortic neck (Fig. 4). Indeed, the results of these tests can be widely modified by the stent structure. A flexible stent, as a self-expanding stent, will have a tendency to deformation during a traction test. Its lengthening will lead to a decrease of its diameter and consequently to a decrease of the stress it applied to the neck, and then a decrease of the stress necessary to get the disconnection. A stiff stent, as a balloon-expandable stent, will not show a diameter modification during longitudinal traction, thus ensuring a constant stress on the neck during the test, the force necessary to disconnect the endoprosthesis decreasing with the gradual decrease of the surface of contact between the stent and the neck. It is therefore necessary to take into account the coupling between longitudinal deformation and radial deformation of the proximal stents. In these tests, most of the time only longitudinal displacements are mentioned despite radial displacements secondary to the longitudinal stresses applied to the endoprosthesis can modify the point of pressure and induce which can be currently called a loose.

The structural characteristics of the different types of proximal stents are very important for the understanding of the migration phenomenons since they lead to different interactions with the aortic neck. A self-expanding stent has to be implanted in the aortic neck with a variable degree of oversizing. Its fixation in the neck is caused by the stress that the stent applies on the arterial wall whose strain is unknown. The leakproofness is related to the stent stress on the artery. The aortic neck behavior is visco-elastoplastic. Once implanted, the stent will keep on to apply a continuous stress to the neck. If the stress is important enough, the neck will present a plastic deformation and its diameter will progressively increase. It squares with clinical trials observations. When the neck diameter increases, the simultaneous increase of the stent diameter will decrease the pressure that it applies to the neck. Consequently, the stent can move and migrate, and an endoleak can appear as soon as the arterial pressure will be higher than the pressure the stent applies to the aortic neck. In case of a balloon-expandable stent implantation, a known deformation of the aorta is done because of the stent deployement. However, the degree of stress applied to the neck is not known. The leackproofness of the area of fixation is caused by the pressure that the aorta will apply on the stent as a response to the deformation it underwent. Nevertheless, the aorta can adapt to this deformation and keep on to develop an aneuvrysmal reorganization by itself. Once again, if the pressure the aorta applies to the stent becomes lower than the arterial pressure, an endoleak can occur. It is difficult to know exactly what is the role of fixation devices, such as hooks or barbs, to avoid migration. Hooks can differently damage the artery according to the depth of penetration of the arterial wall. It is irrelevant to undertake tests comparing the ability to migration of an endoprosthesis having fixation device with a standard prosthesis sewn to an aortic neck, since this fixation corresponds to completely different types of biomechanical structure coupling. For surgical suture, the connection between the two structures consists in setting in compression the arterial and prosthetic structures by the running suture. It is the biomechanical coupling that is studied during traction test. Results of this test would be totally different if the suture had been done with the same number of stitches but with keeping the artery far from the prosthesis. When a fixation device is tested, it is the tearing of the arterial wall by the device that is studied. It corresponds to what we study when performing suture retention strength test as required by standards for vascular prostheses.

New generations of endoprostheses must present characteristics allowing them to be protected from the major and early degradation phenomenons observed on the textile fabric of the first generation. Our first studies demonstrated that some characteristics of the textiles could explain these phenomenons, particularly because of their low saturation index and of the high differences of saturation index between the warp and weft axes leading to a highly anisotropic structure. It is currently said in publications that it is necessary to avoid the onset of wearing phenomenons and if possible, to predict them with pre-clinical tests. The research program we undertake in our laboratory lets us think it is preferable to speak of ageing process rather than wearing phenomenons. Ageing is influenced by mechanical factors, to the level of stress and the type of solicitation such as cyclic solicitation, and to the biologic environment of the material. Ageing is a phenomenon that is coupled to chemical aspect with molecular chains ruptures, modification of the degree of polymerization, molecular reorganization with recrystallization phenomenons, leading to a less linked molecular structure. These phenomenons will determine a physical aspect without mass transfer, a typical structure reorganization with time (recrystallization), or with mass, the material releasing oligoelements predisposing to the reorganization. There is also a mechanical aspect to ageing concerning the visco-elastic behavior responsible for an energy exchange also modifying the structure and generating recrystallization phenomenons. Recrystallization creates material reorganization predisposing to the onset of fissurations increasing in turn ageing phenomenon of the material. We also showed that manufacturing process was an important factor for the onset of ageing phenomenon. In a textile structure, the metal-to-polymer contact leads to wearing phenomenons and to fissurations. In order to prevent too early ageing, we believe it is necessary to eliminate focused stress concentrations in bent areas of the endoprosthesis, particularly by controlling the saturation index of the textile and the stent morphology, to decrease the fibers specific surface by using preferentially large fibers with a diameter close to 20μ to 30μ, and to optimize the manufacturing process that must be controlled particularly on the textile to be sure of the lack of fissurations. It is very difficult to set up and to interpret experimental tests evaluating the friction of a stiff metallic structure on a textile. Furthermore, these tests have not really been developed by textile companies.

The set up of fatigue tests able to predict the long term behavior of an endoprosthesis is not established yet. As we previously said, these tests have to be accelerated in order to evaluate a 10-year life endoprosthesis, that is to say 380 million cycles, in 88 days. It is necessary to take into account the rheological behavior of the different components of the endoprosthesis and to be sure that the structure has enough time to follow the deformations in order to provide valuable informations from this test. It is also important to know exactly how to analyze the endoprosthesis to show degradation.

Conclusion

The specific characteristics of the structures used to construct an endoprosthesis can play a major role on their long term behavior. They influence the type of interactions between the endoprosthesis and the aortic wall, particularly at the neck, and then the risk of migration. They also influence the type of interactions between the soft and stiff materials that are used for their construction, and then the risk of degradation and poor-durability. The choice of not only the materials but also of their association, requires a preliminary detailed process of research and development. The complexity of endoprostheses biomechanics, still at the present time, makes difficult the set up of realistic and predictive test of their in-vivo behavior.

REFERENCES

1. Riepe G, Heintz C, Kaiser E et al. What can we learn from explanted endovascular devices. *Eur J Vasc Endovasc Surg* 2002; 24: 117-122.

2. Singland JD. Personal Communication.

3. van Herwaarden JA, Bartels LW, Muhs BE et al. Dynamic magnetic resonance angiography of the aneurysm neck: conformational changes during the cardiac cycle with possible consequences for endograft sizing and future design. *J Vasc Surg* 2006; 44: 22-28.

4. van Herwaarden JA, Muhs BE, Vincken KL et al. Aortic compliance following EVAR and the influence of different endografts: determination using dynamic MRA. *J Endovasc Ther* 2006; 13: 406-414.

5. Umscheid T, Stelter WJ. Time-related alterations in shape, position, and structure of self-expanding, modular aortic stent-grafts: A 4-year single-center follow-up. *J Endovasc Surg* 1999; 6: 17-32.

6. Zarins CK, Bloch DA, Crabtree T et al. Stent graft migration after endovascular aneurysm repair: importance of proximal fixation. *J Vasc Surg* 2003; 38: 1264-1272.

7. Sternbergh WC, Money SR, Greenberg RK et al. Influence of endograft oversizing on device migration, endoleak, aneurysm shrinkage, and aortic dilatation: Results of the Zenith multicenter trial. *J Vasc Surg* 2004; 39: 20-26.

8. Mohan IV, Harris PL, van Marrewijk CJ et al. Factors and forces influencing stent-graft migration after endovascular aneurysm repair. *J Endovasc Ther* 2002; 9: 748-755.

9. Dalainas I, Nano G, Bianchi P et al. Aortic neck dilatation and endograft migration are correlated with self-expanding endografts. *J Endovasc Ther* 2007; 14: 318-323.

10. Riepe G, Heilberger P, Umscheid T et al. Frame dislocation of body middle rings in endovascular stent tube grafts. *Eur J Vasc Endovasc Surg* 1999; 17: 28-34.

11. Heintz C, Riepe G, Birken L et al. Corroded nitinol wires in explanted aortic endografts: An important mechanism of failure? *J Endovasc Ther* 2001; 8: 248-253.

12. Chakfé N, Diéval F, Riepe G et al. Influence of textile structure on degradation of explanted aortic endoprostheses. *Eur J Vasc Endovasc Surg* 2004; 27: 33-41.

13. Major A, Guidoin R, Soulez G et al. Implant degradation and poor healing after endovascular repair of abdominal aortic aneurysms: An analysis of explanted stent-grafts. *J Endovasc Ther* 2006; 13: 457-467.

14. Zarins CK, Arko FR, Crabtree T et al. Explant analysis of AneuRx stent grafts: Relationship between structural findings and clinical outcome. *J Vasc Surg* 2004; 40: 1-11.

15. Albertini JN, Kaliafas S, Travis S et al. Pathophysiology of proximal vergraaft endoleak following endovascular repair of abdominal aortic aneurysms: A study using a flow model. *Eur J Vasc Endovasc Surg* 2001; 22: 53-56.

16. Leigh L, Rabkin D, Berbaum K et al. Impact of graft material configuration on stent-graft endoleak in-vitro. *J Vasc Interv Radiol* 2001; 12: 1423-1427.

17. Resch T, Malina M, Lindblad B et al. The impact of stent design on proximal stent-graft fixation in the abdominal aorta: An experimental study. *Eur J Vasc Endovasc Surg* 2000; 20: 190-195.

18. Hinchliffe RJ, Natarajan S, Hopkinson BR. In vitro analysis of modular aortic stent-graft failure. *J Endovasc Ther* 2006; 13: 77-84.

19. Arko FR, Heikkinen M, Lee ES et al. Iliac fixation length and resistente to in-vivo stent-graft displacement. *J Vasc Surg* 2005; 41: 664-671.

20. Liffman K, Sutalo ID, Lawrence-Brown MM et al. Movement and dislocation of modular stent-grafts due to pulsatile flow and the pressure difference between the stent-graft and the aneurysm sac. *J Endovasc Ther* 2006; 13: 51-61.

21. Sutalo ID, Liffman K, Lawrence-Brown MM et al. Experimental force measurements on a bifurcated endoluminal stent graft model: comparison with theory. *Vascular* 2005; 13: 98-106.

22. Trocciola SM, Dayal R, Chaer RA et al. The development of endotension is associated with increased transmission of pressure and serous components in porous expanded polytetrafluoroethylene stent-grafts: characterization using a canine model. *J Vasc Surg* 2006; 43: 109-116.

23. Li Z, Kleinstreuer C. Analysis of biomechanical factors affecting stent-graft migration in an abdominal aortic aneurysm model. *J Biomech* 2006; 39: 2264-2273.

24. Li Z, Kleinstreuer C, Farber M. Computational analysis of biomechanical contributors to possible endovascular graft failure. *Biomech Model Mechanobiol* 2005; 4: 221-224.

25. Morris L, Delassus P, Walsh M et al. A mathematical model to predict the in-vivo drag forces acting on bifurcated stent grafts used in endovascular treatment of abdominal aortic aneurysms (AAA). *J Biomech* 2004; 37: 1087-1095.

26. Howell BA, Kim T, Cheer A et al. Computational fluid dynamics within bifurcated abdominal aortic stent-grafts. *J Endovasc Ther* 2007; 14: 138-143.

27. Canic S, Ravi-Chandar K, Krajcer Z et al. Mathematical model analysis of Wallstent® and AneuRx®. Dynamic responses of bare-metal endoprosthesis compared with those of stent-graft. *Tex Heart Inst J* 2005; 32: 502-506.

28. ANSI/AAMI/ISO 25539-1:2003/A1:2005 www.aami.org/publication/CD/cdchart.html

29. Abel DB, Dehdashtian MM, Rodger ST et al. Evolution and future of preclinical testing for endovascular grafts. *J Endovasc Ther* 2006; 13: 649-659.

30. Kattekola B, Conti JC, Strope ER. High speed photographic verification of intravascular stent strains during accelerated durability testing. *Biomed Sci Instrum* 2004; 40: 219-224.

31. Schröder B, Kaufmann R. 50 Hz fatigue testing of large diameter stent grafts. *Medical Device Technol* 2007; 18: 58-60.

32. Anderson S. Bench testing to predict fatigue fracture of stents in the superficial femoral artery. In: Chakfé N, Durand B, Kretz JG, eds. *New technologies in vascular biomaterials: Fundamental about stents II*. Strasbourg: Editions Europrot, 2007: pp 107-116.

33. Singland JD. Evaluation mécanique et clinique des endoprothèses aortiques faites sur mesure. Thèse de Docteur de l'Ecole Nationale Supérieure d'Arts et Métiers, Paris, 2007, ENAM012. http://pastel.paristech.org/2999/.

4

DIFFERENT TYPES OF INFRARENAL (MODULAR, UNIBODY, AORTO-UNI-ILIAC) AND THORACIC ENDOGRAFTS: ADVANTAGES AND DRAWBACKS

GIANBATTISTA PARLANI, PAOLA DE RANGO, FABIO VERZINI
GIUSEPPE PANUCCIO, GUSTAVO IACONO, PIERGIORGIO CAO

Over the last decade, a succession of industry-manufactured endografts has been introduced into the market for the treatment of a broad spectrum of patients with abdominal aortic aneurysms (AAA) and thoracic aortic aneurysms (TAA). While the pioneers of endovascular aortic aneurysm repair (EVAR) used "home-made" endografts, a number of commercial devices, designed to gain approval from regulatory authorities either in Europe or in the USA, are being evaluated in clinical trials these days. Although the basic principles of EVAR are the same as those initially introduced in the nineties, today several devices are available to treat abdominal and thoracic aneurysm, differing with respect to design, modularity, metallic composition and structure of the stent, thickness, porosity, methods of attaching the fabric to the stent and the presence or absence of an active method of fixing the device to the aortic wall. The positive message from this decade of endograft evolution is that the overall performance among the current generations of aortic devices is quite similar and data appear to confirm low complication rate. However, long-term follow-up and a number of reinterventions are required.

The different device models available today should not be considered competitive but complementary. Indeed, since anatomic suitability is the main predictor of early and late EVAR success, the availability of a variety of models allows to enlarge the applicability of EVAR worldwide and guarantees durability. An ideal stent-graft incorporating all the advantages and no drawbacks is unreliable.

Summary of drawbacks and advantages according to general stent-graft characteristics

The primary objective of all aortic devices is to exclude the aneurysm sac from systemic arterial pressure. The ideal endograft should provide lifelong protection from rupture of the aneurysm without any risk of migration or displacement from the attachment sites. Components should be sufficiently robust and, at the same time, small enough to fit into a delivery system that can be negotiated easily through the access vessels. Different configuration, materials, and fixation systems in current endovascular devices allow for different potential drawbacks and advantages.

CONFIGURATION

Existing configurations of aortic stent-grafts include bifurcated endografts, aorto-aortic straight tubes and aorto-uni-iliac devices. Bifurcated endografts allowing sealing and attachment in both iliac arteries are the most frequently used today for AAA repair. Aorto-aortic straight tubes are mainly reserved for TAAs or aortic ulcer, while aorto-uni-iliac devices are for specific indications such as ruptured aneurysm, large iliac aneurysms, or iliac occlusive disease. Different designs include modular or unipiece systems. In modular design, the secondary segments are connected with the main aortic component of the endograft in-situ. Modular stent-grafts tend to be relatively user-friendly, adaptable to different anatomic configurations and aneurysm extension and highly conformable, although the junctions between the components carry an intrinsic risk of late disconnection, migration, and related endoleak. The introduction of bifurcated unipiece devices followed the potential to reduce those risks. However, deployment is complex: unipiece endografts have a cross-femoral wire to bring the "second limb" to the contralateral iliac artery.

The latest developments in stent-graft technology address previous limitations of the technique for the treatment of juxtarenal, suprarenal, and other complex aneurysms. Two approaches are being investigated, "fenestrated devices" and "branched endografts", both allowing the covered portion of the stent-graft to be extended above the visceral arteries, below the common iliac bifurcation or, in the case of TAA, proximal to the supra-aortic branches.

MATERIALS AND ADAPTATION OF STENT-GRAFTS

Differences are due to specific fabric and stent material, entirely stent-supported or largely unsupported structures, the endo or exo position of metallic frame, and the availability of a bare stent at the extremities of the prosthesis. The fabric consists of polyester or expanded polytetrafluoroethylene (ePTFE). Excessive thickness of the fabric reduces conformability while the excessive porosity leads to endotension and aneurysm growth. Most commercial endografts are fully supported by stents covering their entire length. The stents are usually constructed from two types of metal alloy, nitinol and stainless steel. Nitinol is a thermal memory alloy of nickel and titanium that increases in strength at body temperature. Elgiloy, used in some systems, is a modified version of stainless steel. The stent configuration may consist of continuous or separate rings, the latter allowing greater flexibility. Motion between fabric and stent materials has resulted in a high incidence of erosion of the fabric in some device brands. Thus, a firm connection between the two components made of different materials is essential.

For optimal long-term performance, the ability to adapt to morphologic changes - increased tortuosity or shortening of the aneurysm because of shrinking of the sac - is advantageous. Stiff grafts may be prone to late dislocation of modular segments or migration from the arterial attachment sites. Discontinuous stent rings or a helical stent may allow better adaptation to arterial angulations and to anatomical changes occurring after stent-graft implantation.

FIXATION

For proximal fixation several mechanisms are used including oversizing ("compression-fit"), radial force exerted by self-expanding stents, hooks, and barbs. Concerns about instability of the infrarenal necks, leading to migration, endoleak, and AAA growth, resulted in the development of suprarenal fixation by a bare stent ring connected to the proximal covered portion of the endograft for the treatment of AAA. This feature has become a key component of many of the current stent-graft systems, however, concerns about potential renal flow impairments have been raised, while they have not been substantiated by the available data. Finally, stent-graft systems are available in a range of lengths and diameters for proximal and distal fixation allowing for an optimal oversizing of the device (usually in the order of 20% for aneurismal disease, 10%-20% for dissections) in relation to the arterial diameter. Excessive oversizing should be avoided because it may result in pleating of the fabric with failure to seal.

Specific types of stent-grafts

AAA REPAIR

There are at least seven different companies offering bifurcated endografts of different design that have been approved by the regulatory authorities in Europe and the USA. Six stent grafts have modular configuration including AneuRx (Medtronic Inc., Santa Rosa, CA), Anaconda (Vascutek, Terumo, UK), Aorfix (Lombard Medical, Oxford, UK), Excluder (Gore & Associates, Flagstaff, AZ), Talent (Medtronic, Santa Rosa, CA) and Zenith (Cook Medical, Bloomington, IN). Only one, the Powerlink (Endologix, Irvine, CA) is a unibody bifurcated design. The main types of currently used AAA endografts and potential advantages and their downsides are summarized in Tables I and II. For almost all, substantial updates and changes in the original structure and device have been applied to overcome drawbacks of the original models that are not applicable in today's models.

BIFURCATED STENT-GRAFTS

Bifurcated modular endografts with infrarenal fixation

AneuRx. The Medtronic AneuRx stent graft (Medtronic Inc., Santa Rosa, CA) was one of the first modular devices and has the most clinical data in the USA. Its self-expanding, thin woven polyester graft material is externally supported by diamond-shaped nitinol structural elements (attached to the graft by individual polyester sutures) that supply radial force for sealing without barbs or hooks. A review in graft design in 1998 led to the original nitinol single-unit "stiff" body aortic module being replaced (under Food and Drug Administration [FDA] approval) by the currently available "flexible" aortic body composed of individual, discontinuous, 1 cm segmented nitinol rings joined end-to-end. Currently, FDA recommends computed tomography (CT) at 1 month, 6 months and then yearly after AneuRx implantation. Other important guidelines for this infrarenal fixed AAA endograft device include a proximal aortic neck of at least 15 mm, aortic neck angulation <45%, iliac seal zone >25 mm and 10% to 20% oversizing of the AneuRx graft.

Excluder. The Excluder is a self-expanding, bifurcated, two-component modular device composed of ePTFE with an outer self-expanding nitinol support structure. The ePTFE graft material is attached to the exoskeleton with an ePTFE fluorinated ethylene propylene composite film so that no sutures or holes are present in the graft. Strut design of the nitinol exoskeleton offers radial support and significant flexibility with the allowance of both longitudinal shortening and accommodating a large degree of vessel tortuosity. Seven pairs of downward-angled wire anchoring barbs are located at the cranial end (proximal margin) of the main stent body ("trunk ipsilateral component") to improve device fixation to infrarenal aortic neck. Delivery catheters require delivery through 18Fr (trunk ipsilateral) and 12Fr (contralateral limb) sheaths.

The Excluder device manufactured by WL Gore and Associates in Flagstaff, Arizona, was introduced in September 1997 and in November 2002 it became the third commercially available endograft approved by the US FDA. The original device has been substantially modified over the last 2 years after the alerts raised from the higher complication rates (sac hygroma, low flow endoleak, high graft porosity with sac growth) with the first generation device. Today a larger trunk and limb sizes as well as low porosity materials are provided. It could be estimated that by October 2005 over 3 000 Excluder endografts had been placed worldwide.

Anaconda. The endograft consists of a woven Dacron prosthesis supported by self-expanding nitinol ring stents. The proximal part of the aortic body has two nitinol rings at a variable distance from each other according to the diameter, with a saddle shape which is not intended for suprarenal positioning. The main body is not supported by other stents or longitudinal bars, while the iliac legs are fully supported. There is also a proximal active fixation system consisting of four pairs of hooks, two on the lateral margins and two on the front and rear margins. The proximal stent is connected to the release system by a series of wires that allow the device to collapse and be repositioned. The aortic device is also fitted with a guidewire

Table I TYPES OF CURRENTLY USED AAA ENDOGRAFTS

Device name	AneuRx	Excluder	Powerlink	Talent	Zenith	Aorfix	Anaconda	Endofit
Company	Medtronic	WL Gore	Endologix	Medtronic	Cook	Lombard Medical,	Vascutek Terumo	LeMaitre Vascular
Location	Santa Rosa, CA,USA	Flagstaff,AZ USA	Irvine,CA USA	Santa Rosa, CA,USA	Bloomington, IN, USA	Oxford,UK	UK	Burlington, MA,USA
CE	Yes	Yes	Yes	Yes	Yes	Yes	Yes	Yes
FDA	Yes	Yes	Yes	No	Yes	No	No	No
Device characteristics								
Configuration	Modular bifurcated	Modular bifurcated	Unipiece Bifurcated	Modular bifurcated; aorto-uni-iliac tapered	Modular bifurcated (Tri-Fab); Aorto-uni-iliac (Bi-Fab)	Modular bifurcated; Aorto-uni-iliac	Modular bifurcated	Aorto-uni-iliac
Graft material	Internal polyester	Internal PTFE	External PTFE	External polyester	Internal polyester	Internal polyester	External polyester	2 layers of PTFE encapsulating nitinol stents
Stent material	Nitinol	Nitinol	Elgiloy	Nitinol	Stainless steel	Nitinol	Nitinol	Nitinol
Aortic delivery system Fr	21.5	18	21-22	22-24	24	22	21	22
Fixation method	Compression-fit	Compression-fit and anchors	Compression-fit	Compression-fit	Compression-fit and barbs	Compression-fit and hooks	Compression-fit and hooks	Compression-fit long landing
Suprarenal stent	No	No	Optional	Yes	Yes	No	No	Yes
Maximum available size of aortic device	28	31	34	36	36	31	34	36
Maximum recommended infrarenal diameter that can be treated (mm)	29	28	32	32	32	29	31.5	32
Recommended aortic oversizing (%)	15-20	Maximum 20	15	15-20	15-20	10-20	10	10-20
Iliac limb diameter	12-20	12-20	16-20	12-24	10-24	10-20	9-18	16-18

Table II POTENTIAL ADVANTAGES AND DOWNSIDES OF CURRENTLY USED AAA ENDOGRAFTS

Device Name	AneuRx	Excluder	Powerlink	Talent	Zenith	Aorfix	Anaconda	Endofit
Potential Advantages	Largely studied; Modularity; Easy deployment	Modularity; Small sizes devices (fit for small vessels); Easy deployment	Disconnection and migration resistance; Optional suprarenal stent	Modularity; Suprarenal fixation; Large size for large necks	Modularity; Availability of stock products: versatility regards to size and lengths; Suprarenal fixation; Size for large neck	Conformability to short, angulated neck;	Possibility of repositioning after deployment; Easy cannulation system;	Smooth inner surface (decreased thrombogenicity); Hydrophilic sheath trackability in tortuous or calcified iliac arteries. Long stent for Suprarenal fixation;
Potential Limitations	Migration in hostile necks	AAAgrowth Porosity (old design)	Conformability in different anatomies; Fracture? (old device)	Renal coverage; Migration? (no hooks or barbs)	Renal coverage; Limb occlusion in tortuous iliac arteries	No much data available	Neck dilation (high radial force); No much data available	No much data available

with a magnet inside the controlateral gate, allowing easy cannulation by coupling with another magnet inserted from the opposite side. The standard configuration comprises a tri-piece modular device, with the aortic body with 2 equally short iliac limbs and two iliac legs.

Aorfix. The Aorfix stent-graft consists of a polyester fabric to which a continuous nitinol wire is embroidered in a circular fashion. Four double hooks are present at the proximal end in order to enhance fixation. Bifurcated or aorto-uni-iliac configurations are available. The delivery system consists of an outer sheath inside which the graft is constrained as well as two inner push-rods to which the proximal part of the graft is attached. The push-rods are released and the stent graft completely deployed.

Bifurcated modular endografts with suprarenal fixation

Zenith. The Cook Zenith endograft (Cook Inc, Bloomington, Indianapolis, USA) has multiple self-expandable stainless steel Z stents sutured to a dense woven polyester graft. It achieves suprarenal fixation with a bare stent with 10 caudally oriented barbs that hook proximal to the renal arteries to limit migration. Since its original introduction in 1993, the device has evolved into a modular "Tri-Fab" bifurcated endograft, including a bifurcated aortic main body and 2 iliac leg extensions. The system is constructed from a self-expanding stainless steal Z-stent skeletal framework; apart from the proximal and distal landing zones the metal scaffold resides on the external surface of the graft fabric, attached by multiple interrupted sutures providing a smooth interior surface for laminar blood flow.

The main body component is available in different lengths to position its bifurcation as close to the native aortic bifurcation as possible in order to minimize distal graft migration. The ipsilateral iliac stump is 30 mm longer than the contralateral that should be deployed about 15 mm above the aortic bifurcation.

Talent. The Talent aortic stent graft system (Medtronic Inc., Santa Rosa, CA) was first introduced in 1995 and has been deployed to date in over 25 000 patients worldwide. The device is a self-expanding modular system composed of serpentine shaped nitinol stents internally sutured to a woven polyester fabric in the aortic module and externally in the iliac limbs. The stents are spaced along a full-length uninterrupted nitinol spine. Since its original introduction, the graft has been repeatedly modified with the use of a thinner, low profile graft fabric, resulting in the Talent LPS and more recently, from 2002, in Talent Unidoc. To allow better conformability and to reduce the rate of graft kinking and limb thrombosis and connecting bar fracture, the lateral spine along the ipsilateral bifurcation limb was moved to the medial position. The use of transrenal FreeFlo Stent configuration with mini-support spring and the increased radial force by superelastic nitinol stent improved fixation and decreased infolding risk (Fig. 1).

Bifurcated unibody endografts

Powerlink. The PowerLink system (Endologix Inc., Irvine, California, USA) is so far the only authorized unibody bifurcated stent-graft. Its stents are formed from stainless steel cobalt chromium alloy and covered with ePTFE fabric. The stented endoskeleton is constructed as a shaped single-wire body woven into a double spine in the absence of sutures or welds. This infrastructure is covered by a thin-walled ePTFE fabric that is only sutured to the metal frame at the ends of the device. Proximal fixation may be infra- or suprarenal, the latter attained by means of a 2 cm uncovered bare metal stent segment option. It has to be introduced into the aorta, with one limb (the "contralateral limb") being manipulated into position by guide wires and pull-out wires directed across the aortic bifurcation by conventional interventional techniques.

Proximal cuff usage is frequent as the common strategy for deployment in Europe and in the USA. Indeed, the Powerlink has a long body (80 to 100 mm) prompting implantation of the device on the aortic bifurcation, rather than at the level of the renal arteries. This provides an anatomic barrier for potential graft migration, but necessarily includes placement of a proximal aortic cuff to achieve the infrarenal seal. The cuffs themselves are long providing an adequate overlap and protection from type III endoleak.

Aorto-uni-iliac endografts

The alternative strategy for aneurysm exclusion is to use an aorto-uni-iliac graft configuration (AUI). This requires blockage of the patent contralateral common iliac artery by means of a dedicated "plug" and a femorofemoral crossover

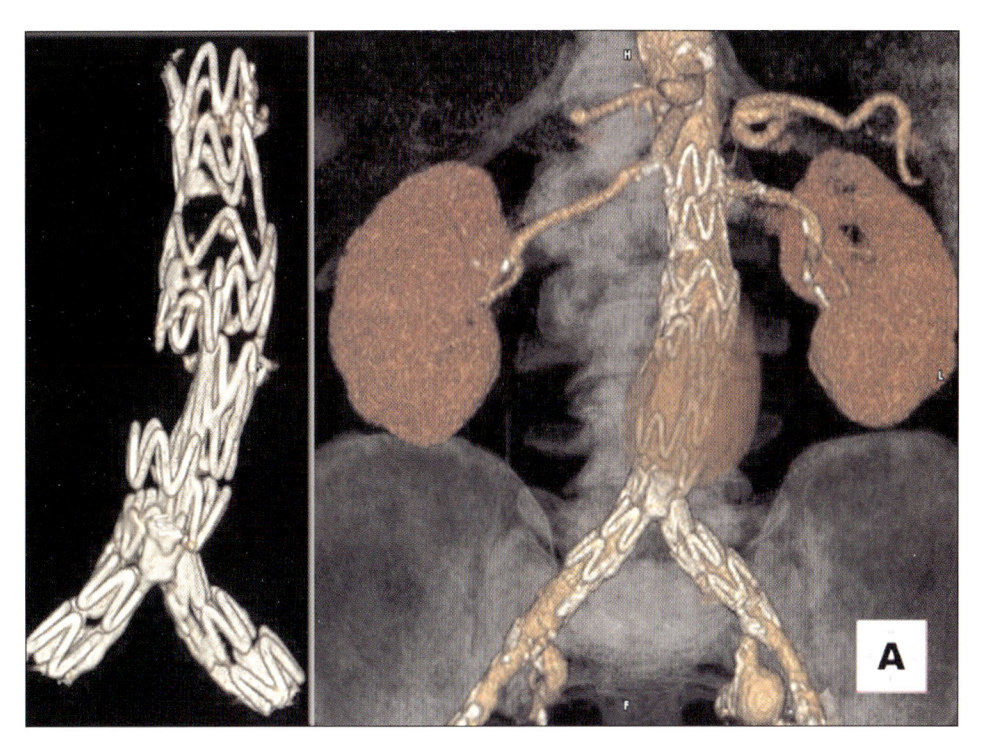

FIG. 1 One-month follow-up CT scan after EVAR (Talent, Medtronic). Complete exclusion of abdominal sac and graft patency with structural integrity of stent.

bypass in order to perfuse the contralateral leg. The perceived advantages of this approach are the technical simplicity, speed of deployment, and the fact that a greater proportion of cases are treatable. Indeed the use of AUI has been proposed to encompass some anatomical restrictions for bifurcated endografts including the presence of a narrow terminal aorta or a complex iliac anatomy (aneurismal, tortuosity or excessive calcification) precluding effective deployment or sealing of a contralateral iliac graft. Another advantage is the rapid aneurysm exclusion in cases of ruptured AAA. It has been argued that the additional extra-anatomic prosthetic bypass graft potentially increases the number of complications and limits the durability of aneurysm repair. However, many recent reports showed good patency rates, up to 99% at 4 years and 83% at 5 years [1,2] with low morbidity rates. Today many commercial AUI endografts have been approved for use in Europe and the USA and feature the same structural constructions of the bifurcated devices of the corresponding brands. The Talent Medtronic AUI graft has been studied within the Endograft treatment in Ruptured Aneurysm (ERA) multicenter trial for feasibility in AAA rupture (Fig. 2). Preliminary results of the new ERA trial show feasibility in half of ruptured AAA with mortality rates of 35% [3].

The EndoFit self-expanding device is the single type of endograft coming only in an AUI design, with conical nitinol frame and PTFE covering. The stent-graft fabric consists of 2 layers of PTFE that encapsulate the nitinol stents, making the inner surface smooth. This feature decreases the possible thrombogenicity of the luminal surface and contributes to easier introduction and advancement of wires and catheters via the graft.

Other supposed advantages of this specific graft are the 28-mm-long proximal bare stent attached to the main frame with only 2 steel bars, which avoids possible renal artery obstruction while enhancing proximal fixation in angulated or conical necks. Due to the quite long suprarenal stent and the increased radial force of the attachment zone, the manufacturer indicates a minimum 5 mm proximal neck length. The endograft is preloaded in a hydrophilic sheath for maximal trackability through tortuous or calcified iliac arteries.

Preliminary experiences in non-ruptured settings in high-risk patients are promising with a very low incidence of type I proximal endoleak even when dealing with short necks [4].

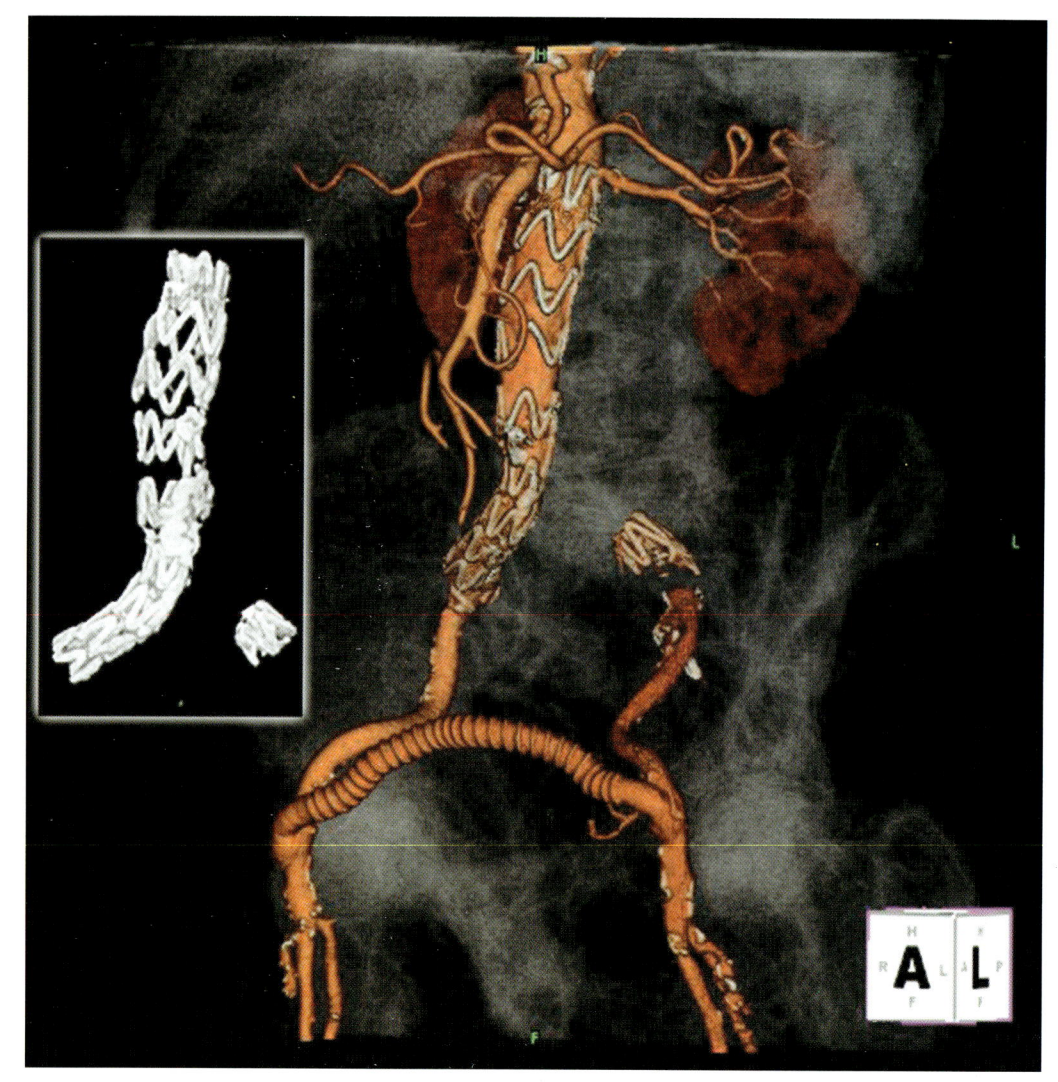

FIG. 2 Thirty-six month follow-up CT scan after EVAR. AAA treated with right aorto-uni-iliac endografting (Talent, Medtronic), left common iliac plug and fem-fem bypass.

Comparisons of different types of AAA endograft devices: advantages and drawbacks

A number of comparative data are becoming available today for contemporary EVAR devices from registries or large volume center series [5-10] suggestive of device-specific outcomes. It should be emphasized that these results should be evaluated with caution. The registries are affected by voluntary participation and incomplete reporting that could make comparative results less reliable. The large volume series are often retrospective and difficult to adjust for relevant confounder. Most of the device-specific drawbacks are related to old designs that today are substantially changed. It is clear that randomized trials comparing devices would not be simply challenging but also unreliable if not impossible given the different anatomical requirements specific for each device.

The main drawback of some devices with infrarenal fixation might be the poor compliance with challenging aortic necks. Tonnessen et al. [7] reported that the risk of migration is a time-dependent, device-dependent phenomenon. By comparing 77 AneuRx to 53 Zenith, freedom from migration rates at 1 and 4 years were 96% and 72% for the first and 100% and 97.6% for the last, respectively. In addition, the risk of secondary procedure was significantly higher in the AneuRx group. However, the AneuRx group involved an earlier practice of the authors with early device, experience and a longer follow-up period with respect to the Zenith group. The very low risk of migration in the Zenith devices has been reported in a number of other studies. Greenberg et al. [11] in a multicenter Zenith trial showed migration rates as low as 2.3% at 12 months which were mainly associated with inappropriate oversizing >30%. Endograft migration was 7% at 2 years and 19% at 3 years according to the large AneuRx multicenter trial and was mainly related to the presence of unfavorable neck anatomy [12-14]. Although migration rates as high as >27% at 3 years have been reported also with the AneuRx [12], most studies have relatively few patients with long follow-up, and variability in assess and definitions make these alerts unreliable. More recently, Fulton et al. [13] showed that unfavorable neck was a significant predictor of AneuRx migration (6% versus 42% at 4 years for favorable versus unfavorable neck), but more important, no death, rupture, or conversion were reported in secondary procedures required after migration, supporting the safety of the device even with challenging neck settings.

An inconclusive attempt to compare results between different EVAR devices within the patients enrolled in 2 randomized controlled trials (RCTs) on EVAR has been recently published [5]. Two bifurcated devices, Talent and Zenith, implanted within the EVAR 1 and 2 trials were compared. Obviously these results were affected by all the same confounders present in other series: only patients enrolled in one arm of the trials were examined (EVAR), therefore there was no balance in confounders among different devices and sample size was small. Indeed, a marked "center effect" (individual endovascular specialist preference for a single marketed endograft) drove the choice of one versus another device. Therefore, authors failed to find any convincing device-specific differences. Outcomes (at an average of 3.8 years) of 318 Zenith versus 187 Talent patients in low risk patients and 109 Zenith versus 34 Talent in high-risk patients were compared. Although authors reported reintervention rates (7% versus 9.4%), all cause mortality rates (8.5% versus 10.3%) and aneurysm-related mortality (1.2% versus 1.4%) higher in the Talent group, none of the differences attained statistical significance. More than one reason may explain these differences in outcomes: between others the Talent patients were less fit than the Zenith patients, Zenith was preferentially used in case of short infrarenal necks while Talent may have been generally selected in cases with wider necks and with significant angulation.

Several recent reports have also shown that the change in aneurysm size after EVAR may be device specific [6,8]. Aneurysm shrinkage has been reported to be more pronounced with thicker endografts than those constructed with more permeable materials. In trials, the Excluder and AneuRx devices had a sharply lower incidence of shrinkage when compared to other devices such as the Talent and the Zenith endografts. The clinical significance of these changes, however, is not entirely clear.

A four-center retrospective analysis by Bertges et al. [8] reported a relevant regression in size rate at 2 years in three quarter of the 78 Talent patients while regression was significantly lower in the 118 AneuRx (46%) and the 54 Excluder (44%) patients. For the AneuRx, most of these unfavorable outcomes are penalized by the fact that this was the earliest endograft to be used in only selected centers and reached longer follow-up.

The Excluder results were attributable to the high graft porosity today overcome with the new model device. Therefore, the alerts raised in a number of studies comparing Excluder with other competitors are no longer reliable [8,15]. Preliminary data with the new Excluder device are encouraging showing a significant increase in sac shrinkage during the first 12 months when compared to the old version 63.9% versus 25%; p<0.0001 [16]. Clearly long-term follow-up is needed to confirm the benefits of the new low porosity device over time.

The Zenith is constructed by using thick, impermeable Dacron and has been associated with aneurysm sac size regression at an early stage after its use. Greenberg et al. [11] reported a significant sac shrinkage (defined as a change in the size of the major axis 5 mm) rate of 68% at 1-year follow-up. Time to aneurysm shrinkage was also reported to be longer with the AneuRx (1.96 years) and the Talent (1.67 years) devices compared to the Zenith (1.01 years) in a single center experience with 167 EVAR using 5 different commercial devices [17]. However, substantial differences in follow-up lengths, anatomical characteristics, and population numbers among different devices were evident.

The Cleveland Clinic published a device specific outcome from their 6-year series including 703 EVAR treated with 5 devices: Ancure, AneuRx, Excluder, Talent, and Zenith. Again, the 12-month shrinkage was most common in the Zenith (about 55%) and Talent (52%) devices and was least in the Excluder group (15%). However, there were no differences in risk for aneurysm-related death, conversion, secondary intervention, migration, freedom from rupture, and type I or III endoleaks. Ouriel et al. [6] found a trend toward a higher microleak rate (4.0%; p=0.054) with the AneuRx, more type II endoleaks with the Excluder device (58%; p=0.001), and more modular separation with the Zenith (3.2%; p=0.03). Furthermore, the need for secondary intervention was significantly predicted by aneurysm size and date of the procedure and was independent from the brand of device.

The European Registry Eurostar compared the outcomes of 4 third generation models (AneuRx, Excluder, Talent and Zenith) versus EVT/Ancure, Stentor (MinTec, La Ciotat, France) and Vanguard (Boston Scientific, Natick, Ma, USA) in 6 787 patients. All new devices carried a low risk of migration, kinking, occlusion and secondary intervention, conversion. The AneuRx and Zenith also had a decreased risk for rupture [9]. Furthermore, the presence of severe neck angulation increased the risk for short-term proximal type I endoleak and migration for the Excluder and Zenith models, while the Talent device presented an increased long-term risk to proximal type I endoleak and secondary intervention.

A direct comparison between bifurcated versus AUI stent-graft may be very unreliable because it is recognized that AUI can be used to treat a large proportion of aneurysms, and are often used in older, unfit patients with larger aneurysms or in symptomatic or rupture settings. The RETA Registry reported alarmist unfavorable outcomes for the early outcomes in 263 AUI versus 733 bifurcated/tubular endografts implanted in UK centers. All in-hospital complications, reinterventions, conversions, and technical failure were significantly more frequent in the AUI group [10].

A recent single center comparison between the new generation devices showed that early and mid-term outcomes were similar in 86 patients treated with Talent bifurcated and 21 Endofit AUI; success rate was 96% versus 100%, respectively. However, endoleak rates were not significantly lower in the Talent group (4.65% versus 14.2%) [18].

Personal experience with AAA stent-graft

Between April 1997 and December 2007 a total of 956 consecutive patients with AAA were electively treated with EVAR at our Department.

A wide variety of endograft models were used. The AneuRx stent graft (Medtronic Inc., Santa Rosa, CA) was implanted in 237 procedures, the Zenith graft (William Cook Europe, Biaeverskow, Denmark) in 434, the Talent graft (World Medical-Medtronic, Sunrise, FL) in 136, the Excluder (WL Gore and Associates, Flagstaff, AZ) in 97, the Fortron (Cordis, Warren, NJ) in 35, the Anaconda in 13 (Vascutek, Terumo, UK), Powerlink (Endologix, Irvine, CA, USA) in 3, Endofit (Endomed, Phoenix, AZ, USA) in 1. Endograft configuration included 4 tubes, 931 bifurcated grafts, and 21 aorto-uni-iliac grafts combined with contralateral iliac occlusion and femoral-femoral bypass.

The peri-operative mortality rate was 1% (10/956), peri-operative conversion rate was 1.2% (12/956) and 30-day endoleak rate was 6% (57/956). At mean follow-up of 37 months (range 1-120) 8 ruptures (0.8%) were observed, three were fatal, for an overall aneurysm-related death of 1.4% (13/956). A total of 82 (9.5%) migrations of more than 10 mm were observed, late reinterventions were necessary in 139 patients (14.5%) including 38 (3.9%) late conversions to open repair. Actuarial rate of migration and late reintervention for the most employed device type are reported in Figs. 3,4. With regards to graft specific results, we were not able to find any statistically significant difference in terms of late device failure measured at 36 months interval, while a clear trend towards better results was evident for the newer generation endografts compared to the older ones.

Thoracic aorta repair

Endovascular technology is expected to result in more pronounced benefits in the treatment of diseases of the chest than in the abdomen because of the higher morbidity of thoracic aortic procedures. However, thoracic aorta presents a variety of pathologies that can be difficult to treat and therefore, despite introduction more than 10 years ago and different devices available today, thoracic endovascular aortic repair (TEVAR) treatment is

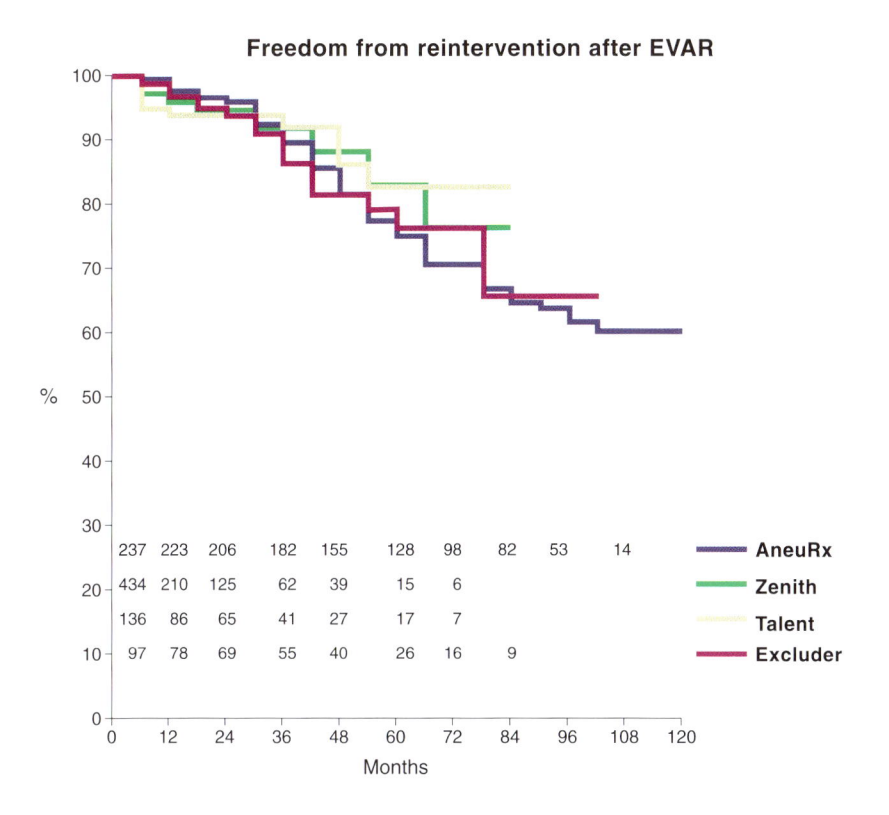

FIG. 3 Perugia Experience, freedom from reintervention after EVAR for different types of device.

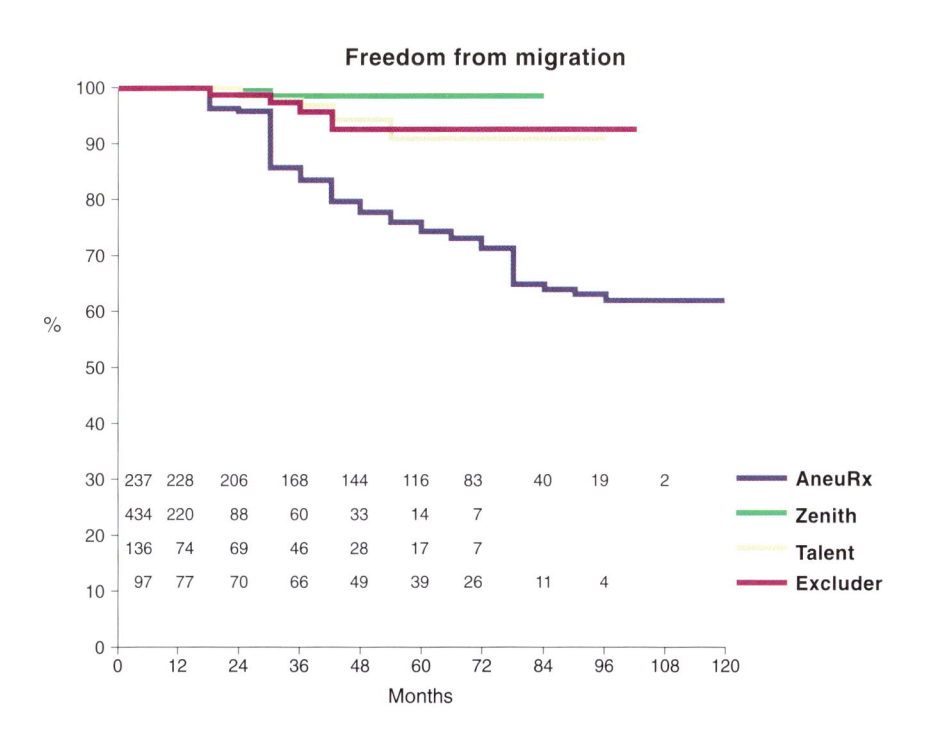

FIG. 4 Perugia Experience, freedom from migration after EVAR for different types of device.

still challenging and many controversial points are open.

Major challenges associated with TEVAR range from the relative rigidity and size of the delivery system, the ability to track from long distance through tortuous calcified vessels, the failure of the endografts to conform securely to the anatomy of the aortic arch. Other concerns regard the ability to provide accurate deployment counteracting high cardiac pressure, secure fixation and long-term durability. Finally, the same graft devices are used for both aneurysm and dissection despite the grossly different pathologies and required outcomes. Moreover, differently from AAA repair, TEVAR has not been compared to open surgery in randomized controlled trials. Today most data of the new generation TEVAR devices are from US FDA trials. Some new generation devices have been recently introduced, however, due to their close introduction, data are not available. No device-specific results are available yet and robust enough to assess the "ideal" device. Literature on TEVAR is very heterogeneous with case series or registry data, and information on different pathologies and different presentation (acute versus chronic) and no long follow-up. Although the results with the available TEVAR devices are encouraging, when compared to open repair, there is the need to further improve tractability, deployment, profile, and conformability.

TAG DEVICE

The TAG device (WL Gore and Associates) is a symmetrical expanded PTFE tube with an external nitinol self-expanding stent along the entire graft surface. A circumferential PTFE sealing cuff is located on the external surface of the endograft at the base of each flared, scalloped end. The major advantages of this stent are its flexibility, easiness and speed with which it can be deployed by pulling a ripcord that opens a sheath holding the device in place. Uniquely, deployment starts from the middle of the graft and rapidly extends toward both ends of the graft. This tends to prevent the device migrating distally caused by blood pressure forces. The device is pliable and can be successfully positioned in difficult, tortuous anatomy. The downside of this device is the low radial strength and the impossibility to adjust positioning during deployment. After the discovery of longitudinal wire fractures the device was modified (20 wire fractures in the original longitudinal spine in the Pivotal TAG trial) with its removal and a stronger PTFE was obtained with the addition of a low permeability film layer to prevent endotension. The modified device was then evaluated in the TAG Confirmatory trial, consisting of 51 patients with thoracic descending aneurysms compared with open surgical controls. At 2 years, TEVAR with TAG devices provided a survival advantage from aneurysm-related death in 97% of the TAG patients compared to 90% of the open controls. Also, freedom from major adverse events was better for the TAG endograft devices compared to open surgical controls, resulting as high as 48% in the TEVAR group and 20% in the open surgery group (Fig. 5) [19].

TALENT THORACIC AND VALIANT DEVICES

The Medtronic Talent thoracic endograft device is a polyester graft with fabric sewn to a self-expanding nitinol wire frame. The device is modular and accommodates the use of additional main sections as well as proximal and distal extensions. Today graft diameters can be manufactured up to 46 mm. The graft has been tested within the Valsartan/HCTZ Combination Therapy in Patients with Moderate to Severe Systolic Hypertension (VALOR) trial. Results on the 150 patients in the high-risk group have been presented. The thoracic aortic pathology treated included descending thoracic aneurysms (72%), dissecting aneurysms (9%), pseudo-aneurysm (9%), traumatic injury (6%), and complicated type B dissection (4%). Initial technical success rate was achieved in 98% of the patients. The mortality rate at 30 days was 8.4%. The stroke rate was 8%. The rate of paraplegia/paraparesis was 5.5% and two-thirds of the patients recovered in 6 months. The reported endoleak rate was 12% at 1 month and 10% at 6 months, with no ruptures, conversions, device migrations, or graft thromboses. Secondary interventions were performed in 2.8% of patients at 6 months. The Talent Thoracic Retrospective Registry represents the largest and longest experience with this device for disparate aortic pathologies including 457 patients followed-up to 5 years. In-hospital mortality was 4% in elective and 7.9% in acute. Estimates freedom from aneurysm-related deaths at 3 and 5 years were 94% and 90%, respectively; freedom from secondary procedures was 81% and 70% at the same intervals. In particular, 44 type I or III endoleaks and 7 migrations occurred [20].

Medtronic also has a third generation device, the Valiant thoracic stent graft. This device is simi-

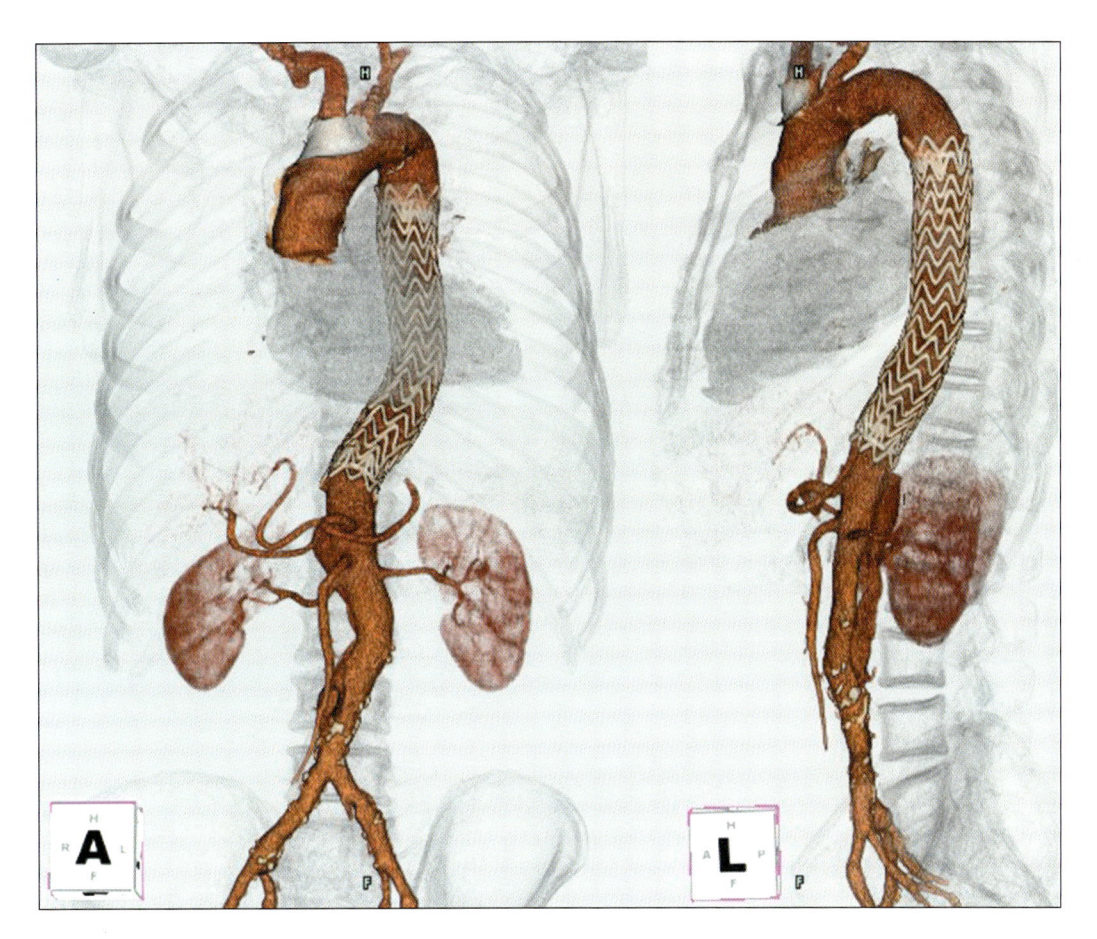

FIG. 5 Twenty-four month follow-up CT scan. TEVAR (TAG, Gore) for type B aortic dissection with complete thrombosis of false lumen in the thoracic aorta and residual flow in the abdominal segment without growth.

lar to the Talent thoracic stent graft in design and materials, however, the Valiant endograft has some design changes. First, the longitudinal connecting bar has been removed. Second, the proximal and distal attachment springs have been redesigned to be smaller and to distribute the attachment point force more equally. Third, the nitinol springs are attached to the outer surface of the graft to allow for better surface attachment and tissue incorporation. Fourth, the device has two proximal configurations, with or without a proximal bare stent. This device will be tested in the VALOR II trial, which started enrolling patients in December 2006. In addition, the VIRTUE registry for the evaluation of treatment in descending thoracic aortic dissections has started.

TX1 AND TX2 DEVICES

The Cook thoracic endograft is constructed from Dacron fabric sewn with braided polyester and monofilament polypropylene sutures to self-expanding stainless steel Z-stents. The device comes in two variants. The TX1 is a one-piece standalone graft (Fig. 6). The TX2 is a two-piece modular device. The proximal portion (TX2P) is covered and includes 5 mm-long, caudally oriented barbs to prevent distal migration. The distal portion (TX2D) has a two-stent overlap zone in which the stents are internalized and an uncovered Gianturco Z-stent with barbs distally to help prevent proximal migration. The proximal components can be either tapered or non-tapered. A 30 mm landing zone are required as opposed to 20 mm for the other devices.

The Zenith TX2 device is being tested clinically in the STARZ-TX2 trial which enrolled 160 patients treated with the TX2 device and 70 patients as open surgical controls. Preliminary results of the TX2 pivotal trial showed peroperative mortality was 1.9% in the TEVAR group, compared to

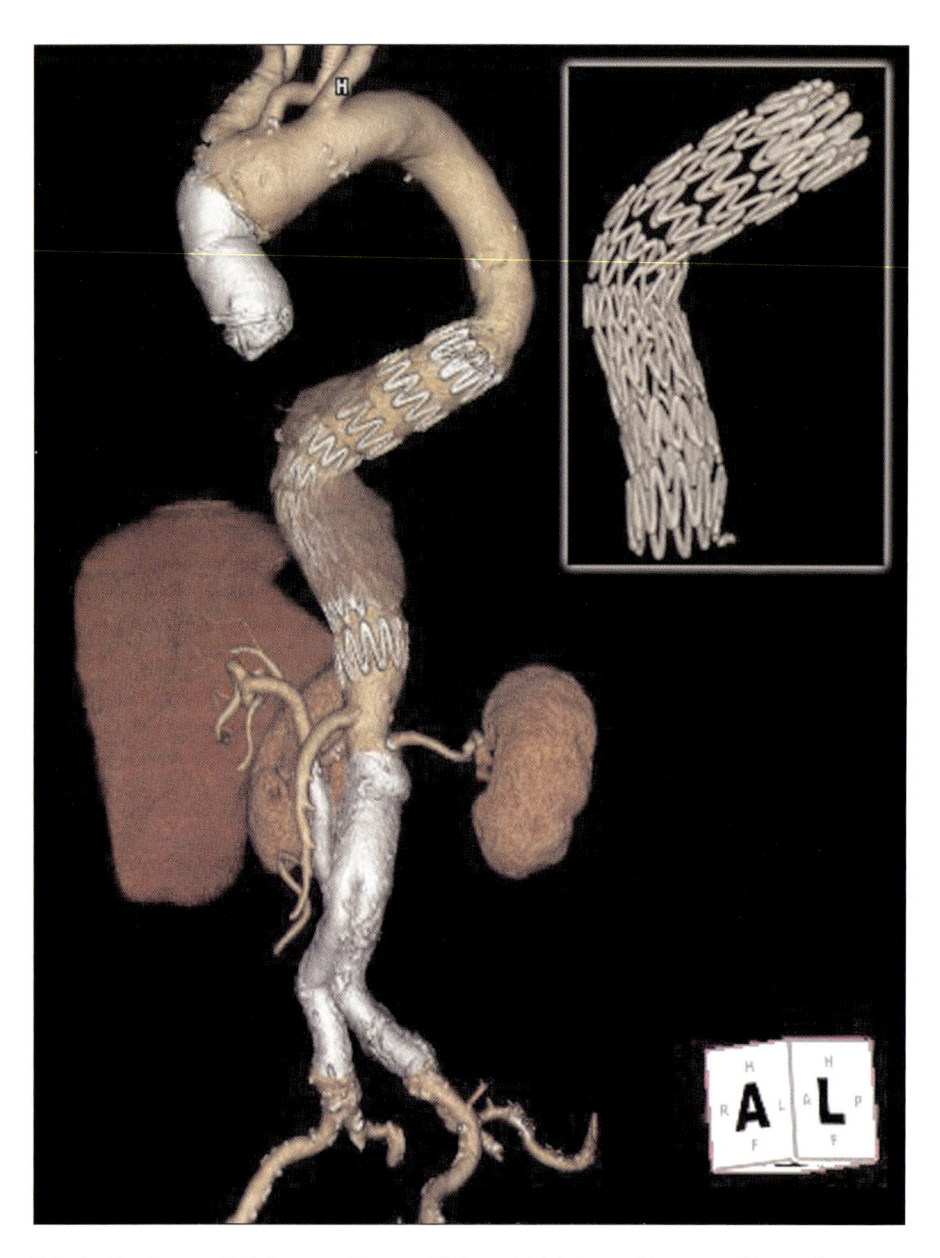

FIG. 6 Twelve month follow-up CT scan. TAA and AAA treated by aorto-iliac replacement, aorto-hepatic by-pass and TEVAR (TX1, Cook) with coverage of celiac trunk in patient with previous aortic valve and ascending aorta replacement. In the box structural analysis that shows integrity of the stent graft.

5.7% in the open control. The stroke rate in the TEVAR group was 2.5% versus 7.1%, and paraplegia in 1.3% of the TEVAR patients and 5.7% of the open surgical patients. Finally, renal failure requiring dialysis was noted in 1.3% versus 4.3% in the control group.

The new Zenith Dissection endovascular system, which combines a covered proximal endograft (TX2) with an uncovered open mesh distal component (TZD), has been recently introduced for the treatment of acute dissection. This system has been proposed to facilitate remodelling of the aorta with effective closure of the entry site without coverage of a long length aorta.

Relay device

The Relay device created by Bolton Medical consists of self-expanding nitinol stents sutured to a polyester fabric graft. The nickel titanium stents are sinusoidal in shape and are serially placed along the length of the polyester graft fabric. An additional curved nitinol wire is sutured to the outer curve of the endograft to provide longitudinal support. This device has currently completed phase 1 of the safety trials and has commenced a pivotal trial. The phase 1 study for the Relay device, as of November 2005, had enrolled 20 patients, 18 with thoracic aortic aneurysms and 2 with penetrating ulcers. Technical success was achieved in all but 3 cases. In the remaining 17 successful deployments, the aneurysms were excluded angiographically 100% of the time.

ENDOFIT DEVICE

One of the latest devices for the thoracic aorta, the Endofit manufactured by Endomed, is made from a nitinol stent covered with PTFE and provides a bare stent proximally. It has been noted that the device suffers a lack of column strength therefore distal migration can occur particularly in the presence of tortuous anatomy when the device needs to be deployed in the distal part of the aortic arch. This migration does not appear to be a problem when the device is deployed in the descending thoracic aorta, the only indication accepted today. The devices have been recently modified and produced without the bare spring.

Conclusion

Aortic endograft technology has rapidly improved after the early use of first generation devices, and the available models today show very promising early and mid term success rates. Comparative results with historic surgical series in the treatment of thoracic aortic pathologies and randomized trials for AAA are suggesting that endovascular treatment can soon become the first line therapy for most cases with suitable anatomy. Device durability should however be confirmed in longer term studies and indefinite clinical and imaging follow-up are still mandatory.

Up to date there is no evidence of any superiority of a single device model over the others and probably this will never be reached. Each device has in fact peculiarities that make it more useful in specific settings, and operator experience with a specific model of endograft is often responsible for much of the favorable results in single graft series.

An experienced endovascular specialist should be able to take advantages of the specific features of different models in order to choose the best graft for the anatomic characteristics of any single patient. Therefore deep knowledge of different graft designs and results for specific anatomical subsets is imperative to afford the best long-term success in patients with different aortic pathologies.

REFERENCES

1. Hinchliffe RJ, Alric PA, Wenham PW et al. Durability of femoro-femoral bypass grafting after aortouniiliac endovascular aneurysm repair. *J Vasc Surg* 2003; 38: 498-503.
2. Lipsitz EC, Ohki T, Veith FJ et al. Patency rates of femorofemoral bypasses associated with endovascular aneurysm repair surpass those performed for occlusive disease. *J Endovasc Ther* 2003; 10: 1061-1065.
3. Peppelenbosch N, Geelkerken RH, Soong C et al. Endograft treatment of ruptured abdominal aortic aneurysm using the Talent aortouniiliac system: an international multicenter study. *J Vasc Surg* 2006; 43: 1111-1123.
4. Saratzis N, Melas N, Lazaridis J et al. Endovascular AAA repair with the aortomonoiliac EndoFit stent-graft: two years' experience. *J Endovasc Ther* 2005; 12: 280-287.
5. Brown LC, Greenhalgh RM, Kwong GP et al. Secondary interventions and mortality following Endovascular Aortic Aneurysm Repair: device specific results from the UK EVAR Trials. *Eur J Vasc Endovasc Surg* 2007; 34: 281-290.
6. Ouriel K, Clair DG, Greenberg RK et al. Endovascular repair of abdominal aortic aneurysm: device specific outcome. *J Vasc Surg* 2003; 37: 991-998.
7. Tonnessen BH, Sternbergh WC, Money SR. Mid and long-term device migration after endovascular abdominal aortic aneurysm repair: a comparison of AneuRx and Zenith endografts. *J Vasc Surg* 2005; 42: 392-401.
8. Bertges DJ, Chow K, Wyers MC et al. Abdominal aortic aneurysm size regression after endovascular repair is endograft dependent. *J Vasc Surg* 2003; 37: 716-723.
9. Van Marrewijk CJ, Leurs LJ, Vallabhaneni SR et al. Risk-adjusted outcome analysis of endovascular abdominal aortic aneurysm repair in a large population: how do stent-graft compare? *J Endovasc Ther* 2005; 12: 417-429.
10. Thomas SM, Beard JD, Ireland M et al. Results from the prospective registry of endovascular treatment of abdominal aortic aneurysm (RETA): mid term results to five years. *Eur J Vasc Endovasc Surg* 2005; 29: 563-570.
11. Greenberg RK, Chuter TA, Sternbergh WC et al. Zenith AAA endovascular graft: intermediate-term results of the US multicenter trial. *J Vasc Surg* 2004; 39: 1209-1218.
12. Zarins CK; AneuRx Clinical Investigators. The Us AneuRx clinical trial: 6-year clinical update 2002. *J Vasc Surg* 2003; 37: 904-908.

13. Fulton JJ, Farber MA, Sanchez LA et al. Effect of challenging neck anatomy on mid-term migration rates in AneuRx endografts. *J Vasc Surg* 2006; 44: 932-937.
14. Cao P, Verzini F, Zannetti S et al. Device migration after endoluminal abdominal aortic repair: analysis of 113 cases with a minimum follow-up period of 2 years. *J Vasc Surg* 2002; 35: 229-235.
15. Hobo R, Buth J; EUROSTAR collaborators. Secondary interventions following endovascular abdominal aortic aneurysm repair using current endografts. A EUROSTAR report. *J Vasc Surg* 2006; 43: 896-902.
16. Tanski W 3rd, Fillinger M. Outcome of original and low permeability Gore Excluder endoprosthesis for endovascular abdominal aortic aneurysm repair. *J Vasc Surg* 2007; 45: 243-249.
17. Biebl M, Hakaim AG, Oldenburg WA et al. Midterm results of a single-center experience with commercially available devices for endovascular aneurysm repair. *Mt Sinai J Med* 2005: 72: 127-135.
18. Dalainas I, Moros I, Gerasimidis T et al. Mid-term comparison of bifurcated modular endograft versus aorto-uni-iliac endograft in patients with abdominal aortic aneurysm. *Ann Vasc Surg* 2007; 21: 339-345.
19. Makaroun MS, Dillavou ED, Kee ST et al. Endovascular treatment of thoracic aortic aneurysm: results of the phase II multicenter trial of the GORE TAG thoracic endoprosthesis. *J Vasc Surg* 2005; 41: 1-9.
20. Fattori R, Nienaber CA, Rousseau H et al. Results of endovascular repair of the thoracic aorta with the Talent thoracic stent graft: the Talent Thoracic Retrospective Registry. *J Thorac Cardiovasc Surg* 2006; 132: 332-339.

PREOPERATIVE ASSESSMENT FOR DESCENDING THORACIC AORTIC ENDOGRAFTING

PIERRE ALRIC, LUDOVIC CANAUD, FREDERIC JOYEUX
PASCAL BRANCHEREAU, CHARLES MARTY-ANE, JEAN-PHILIPPE BERTHET

In 1994 Dake et al. [1] demonstrated the feasibility of endovascular treatment of descending thoracic aortic aneurysms by reporting implantation of self-expandable covered endografts in 13 patients. In that era only limited number of patients (only 8% of thoracic aneurysms in Dake's experience) were eligible for endovascular treatment, whereas almost 15 years later this technique has evolved from experimental treatment of selected cases to an established modality for a wide range of acute and chronic thoracic aortic pathologies: aneurysms, false aneurysms, dissections, traumatic ruptures, ulcerations, intramural hematomas and aortitis. Initially these endovascular techniques were only considered in patients at high surgical risks but they have rapidly become the treatment of choice in most patients. The evident and immediate advantages of covered endografts directly relate to the avoidance of surgical access, selective intubation with single lung ventilation, extra corporeal circulation and proximal aortic cross clamping in patients with a high incidence of serious comorbidities or associated traumatic lesions. The majority of studies demonstrate a reduction of morbidity after endovascular treatment as compared to open surgery. However, endovascular therapy comprises specific complications including different types of endoleaks, migration, dislocation, kinking, collapse and stent fractures. Non-specific complications are related to contrast agents and arterial lesions caused by introducing the devices.

Endovascular treatment of descending thoracic aortic pathologies requires a preoperatively determined interventional strategy. Strict selection of patients is indispensable for successful endovascular treatment. The preoperative plan is based on specific assessment, addressing endovascular accessibility, the morphology and all necessary measurements determining graft selection and dimensions. The choice of an endovascular technique should also anticipate potential complications like accidental coverage of aortic side branches. Finally, the choice of endograft depends on the type of pathology, demanding knowledge of the entire spectrum of available endovascular material.

Preoperative imaging

Vascular access problems should meticulously be explored by a complete morphologic assessment of the entire aorta, iliac and femoral arteries. If necessary, surgical access of the common iliac artery, infrarenal aorta, descending thoracic aorta, ascending thoracic aorta or common carotid artery has to be anticipated in order to introduce and advance the endograft to the target lesion.

Preoperative imaging should include the aortic arch prior to implantation to evaluate the risk of accidental migration of atherosclerotic debris with subsequent peri-operative cerebral or peripheral embolization. In case aortic arch embolic sources are identified it should be considered to modify the surgical strategy and avoid passage of guide wires and angiography catheters by brachial or supra-aortic vessel access: peri-operative angiography can then be performed via the contralateral femoral access.

The main imaging techniques currently available include computed tomography angiography (CTA), CTA with 3D-reconstruction, arteriography and magnetic resonance angiography (MRA). MRA with gadolinium allows complete morphologic assessment, avoiding nephrotoxicity in patients with renal insufficiency [2] but is not applicable in emergency setting. Quality heterogeneity and variable accessibility make MRA a second choice imaging technique at this moment.

At present, CTA is the technique of choice for preoperative measurement [3]. A 64 multi-slice scanner can perform an entire thoraco-abdominal-pelvic acquisition within 15 to 20 seconds with only 100 mL of contrast injection. It is well known that arterial diameter measurements can be overestimated if the studied image is not perpendicular to the vessel axis. Measurements of length can be difficult due to angulations and tortuosity of arteries. Angiography allows excellent information on length and vascular tortuosity, however, reliable diameter assessment or visualization of aortic calcifications and mural thrombus are not possible [4].

CTA with 3D-reconstructions with images perpendicular to the central lumen line are currently common use, especially in the difficult areas like the aortic arch. In the majority of centers, 3D CTA is the only imaging technique necessary to perform all required measurements. Several studies comparing this technique with CTA without reconstruction demonstrate the additional value of vascular reconstructions in patients with marked angulations and tortuous vessels (greater than 60°). It appears that 3D CTA overestimates measurements of vessel length and that the technique is reliable in patients with limited tortuous arteries [4-6].

The value of dynamic CTA and MRA remains to be demonstrated. With aortic compliance, aortic diameters vary during cardiac cycles. Aortic diameter variations between systole and diastole can reach 17.8% in specific segments [7]. These differences can have the consequence that 10%-15% overseizing of the endograft is not enough to achieve adequate apposition.

We believe that thoraco-abdominal-pelvic CTA is the technique of choice to perform all aortic measurements and assess aorta-iliac access. It is extremely important that preoperative measurements are performed by the surgeon himself.

Deliberate covering of the left subclavian artery and the celiac artery

SUBCLAVIAN ARTERY

Extension of all descending thoracic aortic pathology towards major aortic side branches represents a limiting factor of endovascular treatment. Fenestrated endografts and side branch technology for the treatment of aortic arch and thoraco-abdominal aortic aneurysms are currently explored in experimental clinical research. Extra-anatomic bypasses allow extension of endovascular indications at the proximal and distal level of the thoracic aorta. In several cases the proximal or distal neck is not long enough (equal or superior to 20 mm) and deliberate coverage of the left subclavian artery (LSA) or celiac artery (CA) necessary. In emergency patients, this decision is not discussed if coverage is indispensable for adequate anchoring. In elective cases, eventual coverage of the LSA or CA should be discussed and decided prior to treatment.

Several studies report on the relatively harmlessness of deliberate LSA coverage by an aortic endograft. However, recent literature demonstrates a change of attitude in several groups who have reviewed their results and realized that revascularization of the LSA was more frequently necessary as assumed.

A meta-analysis of Peterson et al. [8] showed 23% complication rate in patients with LSA coverage as compared to only 3% in patients in whom the LSA was revascularized prior to endovascular treatment. In the experience of Reece et al. [9], more than 40% of patients with deliberate LSA coverage required pre- or postoperative revascularization. Several arguments to revascularize the LSA prior to endovascular aortic repair include:

1. Dominant left vertebral artery and/or associated lesions of other supra-aortic arteries; in these cases, LSA revascularization is justified to reduce the rate of postoperative cerebral vascular accidents [10].
2. Hypoplastic, absent or terminal left vertebral artery and a distinct cerebellar branch of the basilar trunk; the risk of left arm ischemia is significant and especially in young and left-handed patients, LSA revascularization should be considered.
3. Endoleak following endografting: the left vertebro-subclavian steal flow assumed to vascularize the left arm might cause a type II periprosthetic endoleak or persistent perfusion of a false dissection lumen. This problem can be solved by occluding the LSA during endografting.
4. Spinal cord ischemia: there is a major risk of spinal cord ischemia in case of LSA coverage [8,11]. The cervical segments C1-C4 are perfused by the anterior spinal artery which is the first side branch of the intracranial portion of the vertebral artery. The last four cervical segments and the two first thoracic segments are vascularized by two to four radico-medullar arteries originating from ascending and deep vertebral and cervical arteries. Vascularization of that region can be responsible for the dorsal superior territory of T3-T8. In case of extensive descending aortic coverage and exclusion of the LSA there is a major interest for LSA revascularization in order to reduce the risk of paraplegia.
5. Left internal mammary coronary artery bypass: patients who will have or already underwent left internal mammary coronary artery bypass should receive LSA revascularization. In these patients a left carotid-LSA bypass is preferred in order to avoid dangerous internal mammary clampage of flow. In all other cases a LSA-carotid artery transposition should be preferred since efficacy and long-term patency are better as compared to the outcome of bypasses [12]. In all elective or semi-urgent patients, if circumstances allow, we prefer to perform LSA transposition just prior to aortic endograft deployment. In case of urgency (ruptured aneurysm, hemodynamic instable traumatic rupture) the endograft is implanted first and LSA revascularization performed in a second stage and only if clinically necessary.

CELIAC ARTERY

If the distal neck for endograft implantation is too short, the liberate coverage of the CA with preservation of the superior mesenteric artery (SMA) has been described. Few studies report on this kind of treatment. Vaddineni et al. [13] reported on 46 patients treated with endovascular repair for descending thoracic aortic aneurysms of whom 7 had deliberate coverage of the CA. Except for one distal type 1 periprosthetic endoleak, no other complication or death were encountered. The authors recommend preoperative arteriography to confirm adequate collateral circulation via the gastroduodenal artery and between the SMA and the CA before considering coverage of the latter. In fact it is dangerous to assume that CA coverage only carries limited risks of complications. In case preoperative arteriography via the SMA does not visualize rapid re-injection of the hepatic artery and CA, revascularization of the CA prior to endografting should be realized. If arteriography demonstrates adequate collateral flow, the endograft can be positioned over the CA, however, if postoperative clinically related problems occur, rapid surgical revascularization should be performed.

Spinal cord ischemic risk assessment

Paraplegia rate following descending thoracic aortic endografting, including all pathologies, varies between 2% and 6.5% [14]. In the absence of controlled randomized studies it is difficult to proof lower paraplegia rates as compared to open repair but the data from literature demonstrate higher neurological complications following surgery.

Theoretical explications for this relatively low paraplegia rate after endovascular repair include absence of clamping, minimal perioperative hemodynamic changes, possibility to tolerate higher arterial pressures in these patients without thoracotomy or thoracolaparotomy with aorta-prosthetic sutures, less and lighter anesthesia allowing more rapid neurological assessment and progressive and non-immediate periprosthetic thrombosis.

Prior to conventional surgery, spinal cord perfusion can be depicted by selective angiography, visualizing the responsible intercostal arteries, which can subsequently be re-implanted in the aortic tube graft. Another option is systematic revascularization of all back bleeding intercostal arteries without preoperative spinal arteriography. Endovascular treatment does not allow intercostal artery revascularization. Therefore, the value of spinal cord angiography is of limited value. In an attempt to predict neurological complications, some groups have used motor evoked potentials during and after aortic occlusion by means of inflating an intra-aortic balloon during 15 minutes or after deployment of the endograft during 20 minutes. The complexity and associated risks of embolization do not really support the use of this modality [15,16].

Pathophysiology

Several mechanisms of spinal cord ischemia after endovascular thoracic aortic repair can be identified, allowing introduction of strategies to prevent paraplegia:
1. The risk of paraplegia increases with the number of covered intercostal arteries, especially in thoracic pathologies between T8 and T12. Sacrificing more than 10 intercostal arteries or covering an aortic segment larger than 20 cm are major risk factors for the development of spinal cord ischemia [16]. Therefore it is recommended to limit the length of endografts as much as possible. The use of covered endografts with proximal and distal non-covered stents reduces the extension of covered aorta.
2. It has been observed that the risk of paraplegia is higher in patients who already underwent abdominal aortic aneurysm repair due to overserving of lumbar arteries being part of the collateral network to the spinal cord [15-18]. The same accounts for the left subclavian artery which therefore should be preserved as much as possible.
3. Like in open thoracic-abdominal aortic surgery, cerebrospinal fluid (CSF) drainage reduces intrathecal hypertension during and after the procedure. The majority of teams recommend CSF drainage during 24 to 72 hours with a pressure less than 10 mmHg, especially in patients with previous abdominal aortic surgery, patients requiring extensive thoracic coverage (longer than 20 cm) and endograft placement between T8 and T12. In case of delayed paraplegia, CSF drainage should be performed, despite unproven efficacy of this measure.
4. Perioperative arterial hypotension is a risk factor for spinal cord hypoperfusion and subsequent cord infarction. It is recommended to strive for a mean arterial pressure of at least 70 mmHg during the first postoperative days [16,19].

Choice of aortic endoprosthesis

Measurements

The choice of diameter and length of the endograft are based on the preoperative aortic measurements. It is recommended to include at least 20 mm of length for the proximal and distal fixation. Some endografts do have a length of more than 20 cm but most often several endografts are used as a "trombone" technique with an overlap of approximately 5 cm.

The majority of endovascular teams oversize the endoprosthesis with a diameter being 10%-20% larger than the proximal aortic neck. In case of substantial diameter difference between the proximal and distal neck it is possible to apply a tapered endograft or use two grafts with different diameters. In the latter case the smaller endograft should be implanted first.

In emergency settings the ideal diameter graft might not be available. In these circumstances it is recommended to implant a little larger endograft rather than a little smaller diameter endograft.

In centers with thoracic aortic endovascular experience the availability of endografts with different lengths and diameters has increased and become common practice. In addition, deliverance of specific endografts can currently be arranged within 24 hours in the majority of cases.

TYPE OF AORTIC ENDOPROSTHESIS

At present, five thoracic endoprostheses are commercially available in France: TAG (W.L. Gore & Associates, Flagstaff, Arizona, USA); Valiant (Medtronic Vascular, Santa Rosa, CA, USA); Zenith TX (Cook Inc., Bloomington, IN, USA); Endofit (LeMaitre Vascular, Burlington, MA, USA); Relay (Bolton Medical, Sunrise, FL, USA). They all have differences in material, deliverance, release, anchoring and concepts. The first three devices already had important precedence and underwent several modifications of the first generation version.

The TAG endograft consists of straight internal polytetrafluoroethylene (PTFE) graft and a supporting external structure of nitinol. The proximal and distal segments are covered stents.

The Valiant graft is constructed of a nitinol frame covered with a woven polyester, either straight or cone-shaped. The different stents are sutured to the prosthesis. The proximal end can have a non-covered stent to improve the quality of proximal fixation.

The Zenith TX consists of a Dacron graft, straight or cone-shaped, externally supported by stainless steel stents. The proximal extremity is covered and has hooks which anchor the endograft directly in the aortic wall.

The Endofit device is composed of a straight or conical tube with interrupted nitinol stents sealed between two PTFE layers, with or without non-covered proximal stent.

The Relay endoprosthesis has nitinol stents sutured to a straight or conical polyester prosthesis. The frame consists of sinusoidal series of stents along the entire length of the prosthesis. A nitinol wire at the external curvature of the endograft provides longitudinal support. The proximal end of the device has a non-covered stent.

DECISION-MAKING

The choice of an aortic endoprosthesis is not determined by consensus. At present, only the experience with the different devices can be used to define some proposals for use. In aortic dissections it seems that the most recommended endograft is the TAG-device, probably because of its flexibility and limited traumatic impact on the aortic wall.

The Zenith endograft is perhaps less appropriate for acute dissections because of the proximal and distal hooks which might perforate the aortic intimal flap. In angulated areas of the aorta, especially at the isthmus, the Valiant seems to have the best radial force characteristics and is less subject to endograft collapse, as described with the TAG-device [20].

This impression had been confirmed by an experimental work which we recently performed in human cadavers, studying the behavior of different aortic endografts with respect to aortic arch angulations. In distal descending thoracic aneurysms, in case of a short distal neck just above the celiac artery, the highest precision is obtained with the Zenith device due to the accurate distal release.

Conclusion

Endovascular treatment of descending thoracic aortic pathologies requires accurate preoperative planning. CTA allows the choice of access, assessment of aortic arch atherosclerotic plaques and thrombus not to be crossed and measurements necessary for the choice of graft. Depending on the level of pathology, deliberate coverage of aortic side branches should be decided prior to the procedure or carefully be avoided in order to reduce major morbidity, especially cerebral embolization and spinal cord ischemia. The choice of aortic endograft depends on the aortic pathology, anatomic features, level of disease and knowledge of available devices.

REFERENCES

1. Dake MD, Miller DC, Semba CP et al. Transluminal placement of endovascular stent-grafts for the treatment of descending thoracic aortic aneurysms. *N Engl J Med* 1994; 331: 1729-1734.
2. Neschis DG, Velazquez OC, Baum RA et al. The role of magnetic resonance angiography for endoprosthetic design. *J Vasc Surg* 2001; 33: 488-494.
3. van Herwaarden JA, Bartels LW, Muhs BE et al. Dynamic magnetic resonance angiography of the aneurysm neck: confor-

mational changes during the cardiac cycle with possible consequences for endograft sizing and future design. *J Vasc Surg* 2006; 44: 22-28.

4 Parker MV, O'Donnell SD, Chang AS et al. What imaging studies are necessary for abdominal aortic endograft sizing? A prospective blinded study using conventional computed tomography, aortography, and three-dimensional computed tomography. *J Vasc Surg* 2005; 41: 199-205.

5 Sprouse LR 2nd, Meier GH 3rd, Parent FN et al. Is three-dimensional computed tomography reconstruction justified before endovascular aortic aneurysm repair? *J Vasc Surg* 2004; 40: 443-447.

6 de Gracia MM, Rodríguez-Vigil B, Garzón-Möll G et al. Correlation between the measurement of transverse diameter in the proximal neck on computed tomography and on aortography before endovascular treatment of infrarenal aortic aneurysm. *Ann Vasc Surg* 2006; 20: 488-495.

7 Muhs BE, Vincken KL, van Prehn J et al. Dynamic cine-CT angiography for the evaluation of the thoracic aorta; insight in dynamic changes with implications for thoracic endograft treatment. *Eur J Vasc Endovasc Surg* 2006; 32: 532-536.

8 Peterson BG, Eskandari MK, Gleason TG et al. Utility of left subclavian artery revascularization in association with endoluminal repair of acute and chronic thoracic aortic pathology. *J Vasc Surg* 2006; 43: 433-439.

9 Reece TB, Gazoni LM, Cherry KJ et al. Reevaluating the need for left subclavian artery revascularization with thoracic endovascular aortic repair. *Ann Thorac Surg* 2007; 84: 1201-1205.

10 Feezor RJ, Martin TD, Hess PJ et al. Risk factors for perioperative stroke during thoracic endovascular aortic repairs (TEVAR). *J Endovasc Ther* 2007; 14: 568-573.

11 Ferreira M, Monteiro M, Lanziotti L et al. Deliberate subclavian artery occlusion during aortic endovascular repair: is it really that safe? *Eur J Vasc Endovasc Surg* 2007; 33: 664-667.

12 Cinà CS, Safar HA, Lagana A et al. Subclavian carotid transposition and bypass grafting: consecutive cohort study and systematic review. *J Vasc Surg* 2002; 35: 422-429.

13 Vaddineni SK, Taylor SM, Patterson MA et al. Outcome after celiac artery coverage during endovascular thoracic aortic aneurysm repair: preliminary results. *J Vasc Surg* 2007; 45: 467-471.

14 Bavaria JE, Appoo JJ, Makaroun MS et al. Endovascular stent grafting versus open surgical repair of descending thoracic aortic aneurysms in low-risk patients: a multicenter comparative trial. *J Thorac Cardiovasc Surg* 2007; 133: 285-288.

15 Gravereaux EC, Faries PL, Burks JA et al. Risk of spinal cord ischemia after endograft repair of thoracic aortic aneurysms. *J Vasc Surg* 2001; 34: 997-1003.

16 Chiesa R, Melissano G, Marrocco-Trischitta MM et al. Spinal cord ischemia after elective stent-graft repair of the thoracic aorta. *J Vasc Surg* 2005; 42: 11-17.

17 Carroccio A, Marin ML, Ellozy S et al. Pathophysiology of paraplegia following endovascular thoracic aortic aneurysm repair. *J Card Surg* 2003; 18: 359-366.

18 Kawaharada N, Morishita K, Kurimoto Y et al. Spinal cord ischemia after elective endovascular stent-graft repair of the thoracic aorta. *Eur J Cardiothorac Surg* 2007; 31: 998-1003.

19 Etz CD, Homann TM, Plestis KA et al. Spinal cord perfusion after extensive segmental artery sacrifice: can paraplegia be prevented? *Eur J Cardiothorac Surg* 2007; 31: 643-648.

20 Muhs BE, Balm R, White GH et al. Anatomic factors associated with acute endograft collapse after Gore TAG treatment of thoracic aortic dissection or traumatic rupture. *J Vasc Surg* 2007; 45: 655-661.

6

THE ARTERIAL APPROACHES FOR ENDOVASCULAR AORTIC GRAFTING

AYSEL CAN, GIOVANNI TORSELLO, THOMAS UMSCHEID

Endovascular repair of abdominal aortic aneurysms (EVAR) has become a widely accepted treatment modality. Today, abdominal aortic aneurysms (AAA) can be treated without major surgical procedures. Many studies have demonstrated feasibility and effectiveness of endografting in the treatment of AAA reducing the risks associated with laparotomy, aortic clamping and blood transfusion [1].

One main reason for failure of the endovascular procedure is inability to gain access into the aorta with a large introducer sheath. Thus, access may be limited by severe calcified or tortuous iliac vessels. For this reason some patients are excluded from the endovascular therapy. In addition, arterial exposure and passing the access system through the iliac arteries are independent risk factors for technical failure and increased morbidity and mortality after EVAR.

Since the first introduction of EVAR, there have been many improvements in stentgraft diameter and trackability. Quality of introducer sheaths has received an increasing attention by the manufactory companies to allow performing EVAR also in patients with severe iliac disease.

Surgical approach techniques are also crucial to reduce morbidity and increase quality of life after EVAR. With the objective of further decreasing the invasiveness of the procedure, the preclosing technique has been developed using Prostar XL for complete percutaneous endovascular aneurysm repair [2-5]. In our experience complete percutaneous endovascular aortic grafting is feasible in most patients [5]. In this chapter we present various surgical arterial approaches for endovascular aortic grafting as well as the complete percutaneous technique for EVAR. We describe the criteria for patient selection as well as early and late complications of each approach.

Standard surgical access

Arterial access for endovascular aortic aneurysm repair is usually gained through cutdown of the common femoral artery (CFA). One or both common femoral arteries are surgically exposed through a longitudinal or oblique groin skin incision. Proximal and distal control of the vessel is obtained with vessel loops and/or vascular clamps. A guidewire and angiography catheter are first introduced through a 5-8F sheath via a CFA anterior wall puncture. Advancement of wires, catheters and sheaths must be done carefully to avoid dissection of the vessel wall and thrombo-embolism. The reason for resistance during advancement of guidewires or catheters must be investigated by fluoroscopy. Directly or after arteriotomy of the CFA the introducer containing the stentgraft is advanced into the aorta using a stiff wire. After the introducer has been removed, the artery is repaired with fine monofilament sutures. Vacuum drains are usually placed in the wound, which is closed in layers.

Alternative surgical access and additional maneuvers

Additional maneuvers are necessary in patients with severe occlusive disease (Fig. 1) or aneurysm of the common femoral artery. Endarterectomy with or without patch or replacement of the common femoral artery using alloplastic graft (Fig. 2) must be performed in such cases before or after EVAR.

In case of severe aorto-iliac calcification of the iliac arteries and/or aortic bifurcation it is recom-

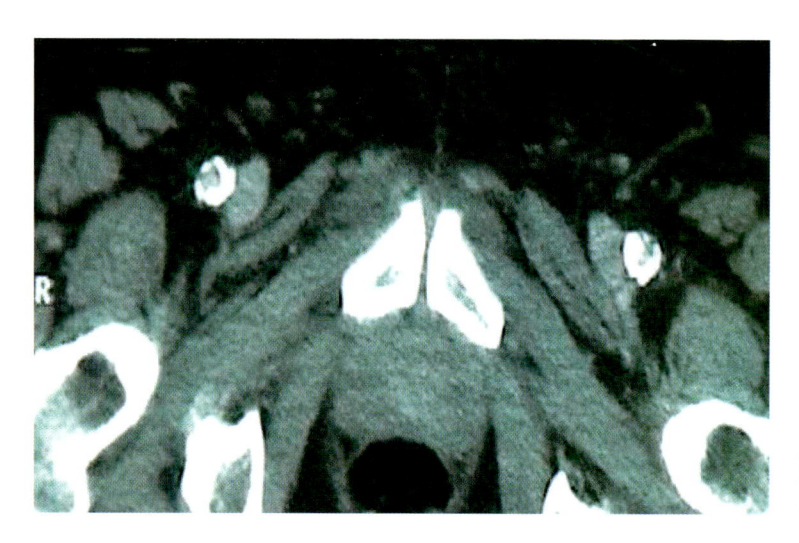

FIG. 1 CT scan of a patient with AAA and severe calcification of both common femoral arteries.

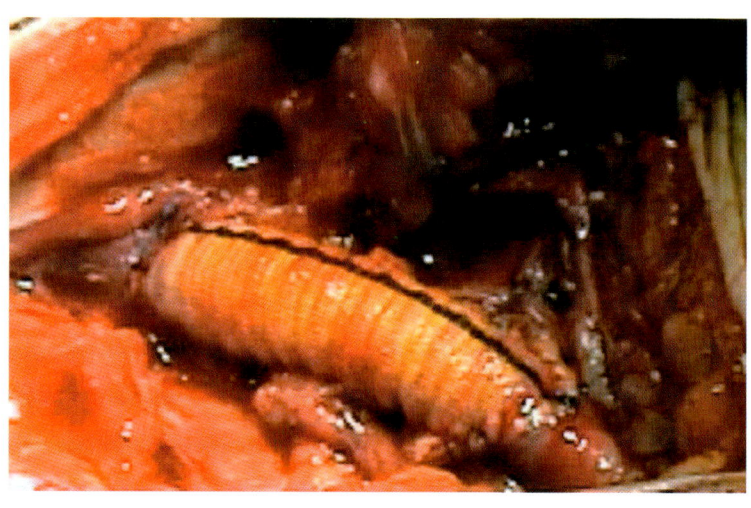

FIG. 2 Replacement of the common femoral artery using alloplastic graft soaked with rifampicin. The patient was treated for a mycotic aneurysm of the common femoral artery and aneurysm of the descending aorta.

mended to proof the trackability of the introducer system of the stentgraft using vascular dilators up to 24 F. With this method we dilate the vessel and avoid to damage or waste the expensive stentgraft if its passage through is not possible. To facilitate the maneuver it is also possible to stretch the iliac segment manually while advancing carefully the stentgraft.

Percutaneous transluminal angioplasty (PTA) or surgical reconstruction of the external iliac artery or common iliac artery must be performed in some patients with severe iliac occlusive disease. In our experience, stents should not be implanted before passing the stentgraft through the iliac artery to avoid their dislodgement into the aorta and higher friction for the introducer system.

In case of surgical exposure of the aorto-iliac vessels, a prosthesis is used either as a temporary conduit, or it is subsequently left in place as an iliac/aorto-femoral or cross over bypass graft [6-9]. If prosthetic grafts are used as conduits, the diameter should be 8 mm or more to allow the introduction of sheaths of large diameter. To overcome an unfavorable angulation between the common iliac artery and the delivery sheath the technique of the transabdominal wall tunnel can be used [9]. After retroperitoneal exposure of the common iliac artery, a puncture site is chosen inferolateral to the surgical incision. A cannula is then advanced in alignment with the common iliac artery through the anterior abdominal wall into the retroperitoneal space. Serial dilatation is performed over a guide wire placed through the cannula to create the subcutaneous tract. The common iliac artery is punctured under direct vision and a guidewire is then advanced into the proximal aorta. A common iliac artery arteriotomy is performed and the delivery system introduced over the guidewire through the tunnel into the iliac artery.

In case of extensive tortuosity of the external iliac artery (Fig. 3), surgical shortening via a retroperitoneal approach can be performed. The authors prefer the "through and through approach" using a brachiofemoral stiff wire for straightening the iliac arteries enhancing the trackability of the stentgraft (Fig. 4). In case of both tortuosity and severe calcification this technique is not recommended because of possible vessel wall rupture.

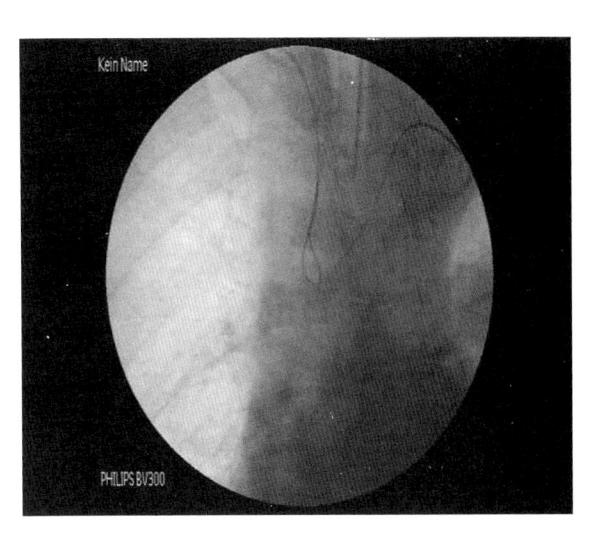

FIG. 4 For the "Through and through approach" it is necessary to catch the stiff wire at the level of the aortic arch using a transbrachial goose neck catheter for straightening the iliac arteries.

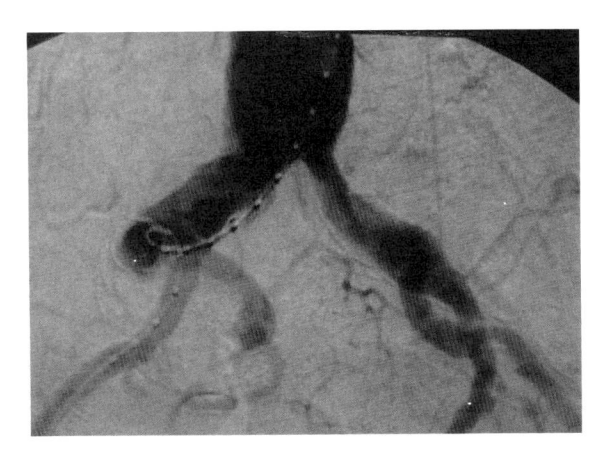

FIG. 3 Angiography of a patient with AAA and kinking of the right iliac artery.

Percutaneous procedure

As technology trends toward less invasive methods and sheath sizes become smaller, the use of a total percutaneous approach for the endovascular aortic grafting is becoming more common. Since 1999 an increasing number of reports have described the preclose technique using Prostar XL for complete percutaneous endovascular aneurysm repair [3,5,10-14]. Prostar XL is a suture based closure device and has been used for more than 9 years at our institution in more than 800 patients after a wide variety of percutaneous interventions. Until today, many studies have been published analyzing the advantages and disadvantages of this device as well as the procedure related complications.

Device description and preclose technique

The Perclose device is made up of two components. The first one is a sheath containing four nitinol needles which are connected at their tips to two suture loops. The second component includes a deployment ring and a barrel. This is positioned above the artery to guide the needle through the subcutaneous tissue once the sutures have been pulled through the arterial wall from inside out.

Arterial access is achieved with an 18 gauge needle by introducing an 8F sheath into the common femoral artery. The puncture should be performed at level of the inguinal ligament to avoid placement of the introducers in the superficial femoral artery or profunda artery. Then, the sheath is exchanged over a guide wire for a 10F Prostar XL, ensuring that the needles penetrate the arterial wall before the arteriotomy is enlarged by the use of sheaths up to 24F [5,10,11,15]. The use of this device requires enlargement of the skin incision and subcutaneous dilation at the puncture site. The sutures are fastened at the end of the procedure after removing the introducer sheath of the stentgraft. Hemostasis is achieved by sliding a self-locking knot to the artery with adjustment of the knot position using a knot pusher. The skin incision is approximated by a single stitch knot or sterile strips.

Patient selection

The feasibility, safety and efficacy of the complete percutaneous approach depend on the appropriate selection of patients and correct puncture and suture technique. Major risk factors that can affect the success of this method and present a limitation for its use are obesity, calcification of the femoral artery, presence of an inguinal arterial prosthesis or aneurysm of the femoral artery. However, Starnes et al. [16] showed that percutaneous vessel closures were successfully achieved also in arteries with anterior calcification.

Access site complications

Complications after surgical exposure

Bleeding, paresthesia, lymphoceles and healing disorders including graft infections are typical complications of wounds in the groin. These complications can necessitate surgical revision leading to prolonged hospital stay. Additionally, the scars make redo treatments for endoleaks or graft limb occlusion more difficult.

Percutaneous approach: complications and trouble shooting

Based on the stage of the procedure we distinguish several sources of complications.

Device introduction

If the femoral puncture has been made too low, the introduction of large introducers through the superficial femoral or profunda artery would tear the vessel wall. Therefore, it is important to identify the common femoral artery by taking into account the pre-operative imaging (Duplex scan, CT or angiography) or by performing an angiography during the procedure. We recommend a puncture at level of the inguinal ligament.

In the presence of tortuosity of the iliac arteries or of the aneurysm neck, the forced advancement of Prostar XL can be dangerous, leading to peripheral embolism or rupture of the arterial wall. If kinking of the aorto-iliac segment is severe we do not exceptionally remove the guidewire before the tip of the Prostar XL has passed the tortuosity.

Needle deployment

In case of a scarred groin or calcification of the anterior vessel wall, the flexible nitinol needles can deflect while retracting the handle. To remove the device the handle should be pushed back into the hub. After the guidewire has been re-inserted, the Prostar XL device can be removed. If this maneuver is not possible, the needle should be identified by fluoroscopy and removed using a clamp or needle holder after enlargement of the skin incision. A digital exploration should be avoided.

Getting flow through the marker lumen

If no pulsatile flow through the marker lumen is achievable, the needles will not grasp the arterial wall. In this case, it is not advisable to retract the handle. Especially, in obese patients it is mandatory to create a sufficient subcutaneous tunnel between the skin and the vessel wall. In case of unsufficient back flow we recommend to flush the port and to slightly rotate the device to exclude mechanical obstruction of the marker lumen.

Knot slipping

Disruption of the vessel wall during slipping of the fisherman knot can be avoided by preventing twisting of the sutures and testing the free run before performing the knot. Additionally, we recommend to irrigate the multifilament sutures and remove accurately fibrin and debris from the suture surface.

It is also helpful to pull gently the long end of the suture in the right direction while slipping the knot and using the knot pusher for advancing the knot to the vessel wall.

When feeling resistance while advancing the knot, the reason should be carefully evaluated.

Final bleeding control

The guidewire should be removed first after successful bleeding control has been achieved. If this is not sufficient, the knot should be hold against the vessel wall with the knot pusher for a while compressing manually the artery above the puncture site. High blood pressure should be normalized. If the above mentioned measures are not effective, a felt pledget can be sewn using the sutures of Prostar XL. This technique, well known from open cardiovascular surgery, is useful to avoid surgical exploration of the femoral vessel.

Conclusion

The technical feasibility of endovascular repair depends on adequate arterial approach. Since large bore introducer sheaths are required, access to the femoral artery through open inguinal incision is the most commonly used approach for aortic endografting. In case of severe diseased iliofemoral vessels, alternative approaches increase the technical success rate of EVAR.

The percutaneous endovascular aneurysm repair provides a less invasive access to the aorta in contrast to the surgical cutdown of the femoral arteries. The percutaneous closure technique enables the physician to perform the complete endovascular procedure in local or regional anesthesia. Especially, the treatment of ruptured aortic aneurysms benefits from this alternative. However, satisfactory hemostasis after use of large introducer sheaths depends on a careful patient selection, an appropriate suture technique and trouble shooting.

Success rates of percutaneous endograft implantation without conversion to an open groin incision described in earlier clinical studies ranges between 46.2% to 93% [2,3,5,10-13].

Recently performed prospective study at our institution showed that the success rate mainly depends on the learning curve of the physician.

Pseudoaneurysm, arteriovenous fistula as well as arterial occlusion or stenosis are possible complications of this technique. In a recent prospective study Watelet et al. [14] described one pseudoaneurysm and three bleedings in four out of 29 cases which healed spontaneously. No late complication was detected after a mean follow-up of 17.5 months. The incidence of infection after placement of percutaneous suture-mediated devices is low. As consequences of this complication may be disastrous, prevention is best provided by peri-procedural antibiotics, together with a sterile technique and environment. We further recommend a Duplex scan of the groin before to select the patients eligible for percutaneous technique and after the procedure to maintain adequate follow-up.

A prospective randomized study comparing both procedures showed no difference in terms of complications and costs. The surgical cutdown approach necessitates a longer mean operation time and longer postoperative hospital stay associated with higher hospital costs [5]. The additional cost for the Prostar device appears to justify its use for endovascular grafting. in the treatment of most patients with aortic aneurysm.

REFERENCES

1. Torsello G, Osada N, Florek HJ et al. Long-term outcome after Talent endograft implantation for aneurysms of the abdominal aorta: A multicenter retrospective study. *J Vasc Surg* 2006; 43: 277-284.

2. Börner G, Ivancev K, Sonesson B et al. Percutaneous AAA repair: Is it safe? *J Endovasc Ther* 2004; 11: 621-626.

3. Howell M, Villareal R, Krajcer Z. Percutaneous access and closure of femoral artery access site associated with endoluminal repair of abdominal aortic aneurysm. *J Endovasc Ther* 2001; 8: 68-74.

4. Lee WA, Brown MP, Nelson PR et al. Total percutaneous access for endovascular aortic aneurysm repair ("Preclose technique"). *J Vasc Surg* 2007; 45: 1095-1101.

5. Torsello G, Kasprzak B, Klenk E et al. Endovascular suture versus cutdown for endovascular aneurysm repair: A prospective randomized pilot study. *J Vasc Surg* 2003; 38: 78-82.

6. Abu-Ghaida AM, Clair DG, Greenberg RK et al. Broadening the applicability of endovascular aneurysm repair: the use of iliac conduits. *J Vasc Surg* 2002; 36: 111-117.

7. Criado FJ. Iliac arterial conduits for endovascular access: technical considerations. *J Endovasc Ther* 2007; 14: 347-351.

8. Lee WA, Berceli SA, Huber TS et al. Morbidity with retroperitoneal procedures during endovascular abdominal aortic aneurysm repair. *J Vasc Surg* 2003; 38: 459-463.

9. Macdonald S, Byrne D, Rogers P et al. Common iliac artery access during endovascular thoracic aortic repair facilitated by a transabdominal wall tunnel. *J Endovasc Ther* 2001; 8: 135-8.

10. Howell M, Doughtery K, Strickmann N et al. Percutaneous repair of abdominal aortic aneurysms using the AneuRx stent graft and the percutaneous vascular surgery device. *Cathet Cardiovasc Intervent* 2002; 55: 281-287.

11. Rachel ES, Bergamini TM, Kinney EV et al. Percutaneous endovascular abdominal aortic aneurysm repair. *Ann Vasc Surg* 2002; 16: 43-49.

12. Teh LG, Sieunarine K, van Schie G et al. Use of the percutaneous vascular surgery device for closure of femoral access sites during endovascular aneurysm repair: lessons from our experience. *Eur J Vasc Endovasc Surg* 2001; 22: 418-423.

13. Traul DK, Clair DG, Gray B et al. Percutaneous endovascular repair of infrarenal abdominal aortic aneurysms: a feasibility study. *J Vasc Surg* 2000; 32: 770-776.

14. Watelet J, Gallot JC, Thomas P et al. Percutaneous Repair of Aortic Aneurysms: A Prospective Study of Suture-Mediated Closure Devices. *Eur J Vasc Endovasc Surg* 2006; 32: 261-265.

15. Haas PC, Krajcer Z, Diethrich EB. Closure of large percutaneous access sites using Prostar XL percutaneous vascular surgery device. *J Endovasc Surg* 1999; 6: 168-170.

16. Starnes BW, O'Donnell SD, Gillespie DL et al. Percutaneous arterial closure in peripheral vascular disease: A prospective randomized evaluation of the Perclose device. *J Vasc Surg* 2003: 38; 263-271.

7

MANAGEMENT OF INTRA-PROCEDURAL PROBLEMS

MARTIN MALINA, TIM RESCH, BJÖRN SONESSON

Most intra-operative complications of aortic stentgrafting are avoidable by adequate preoperative imaging and planning. This chapter outlines problems that we encountered in our experience of more than a thousand aortic stent graft (SG) implantations which we feel may happen again. We have focused on problems associated with access, sizing and deployment of standard, commercially available SGs.

Access

Access problems comprise some of the most frequent reasons for failed aortic stent grafting [1,2] in spite of modern pre-operative imaging such as computer tomography (CT) and magnetic resonance (MR) and improved profile of the available devices. It is mainly the inability to cross the iliac vessels with large sheaths and subsequent life threatening hemorrhage from iliac rupture which might occur. Endovascular procedures are still often refused or abandoned unnecessarily due to access problems.

We regard the abortion of an endovascular procedure due to limited iliac access a serious complication. It puts the patient at risk of remaining untreated or undergoing the greater trauma of open repair. Iliac access problems are avoidable in the vast majority of cases and ought not to be a limiting factor for endovascular aortic repair.

HEMORRHAGE FROM IATROGENIC ILIAC RUPTURE

Iliac rupture from violent attempts to insert large bore sheaths occurs more frequently in female patients due to the smaller diameter of female iliac arteries. It is more common in patients with circumferential calcifications or exophytic plaques that are likely to catch the sheath. Iliac rupture may also occur during dilation of the distal end of an aorto-iliac SG when the oversized balloon is mistakenly allowed to protrude into the native vessel beyond the SG.

Iliac rupture should rarely affect the rapid recovery of the patient and does not necessitate open surgery or general anesthesia – provided it is correctly handled! Although iliac rupture remains a cause of death in endovascular aortic interventions, it does not need to be extremely dangerous. Rupture must, however, be recognized in time and the surgeon must be adequately trained and equipped to deal with it. Iatrogenic iliac rupture often remains overlooked for too long. Sudden hypotension or tachycardia during manipulation with large bore iliac sheaths should always evoke suspicion of hemorrhage and prompt for immediate iliac arteriography to rule out extravasation. The rupture is typically unmasked towards the end of a lengthy procedure upon withdrawal of the large introducer sheath (Fig. 1). Until then, the sheath obliterates the narrow iliac vessel and prevents bleeding. The surgeon tends to be less alert at this moment because he may already consider the operation successfully completed. Complications should, however, be anticipated when the insertion of the sheath had been difficult.

Panicy withdrawal of the guide wire upon iliac rupture is a bad mistake. An iliac occlusion balloon, inflated proximal to the rupture site, will stabilize the patient instantly. The large sheath itself usually obliterates the stenotic distal external iliac artery sufficiently to prevent excessive backbleeding.

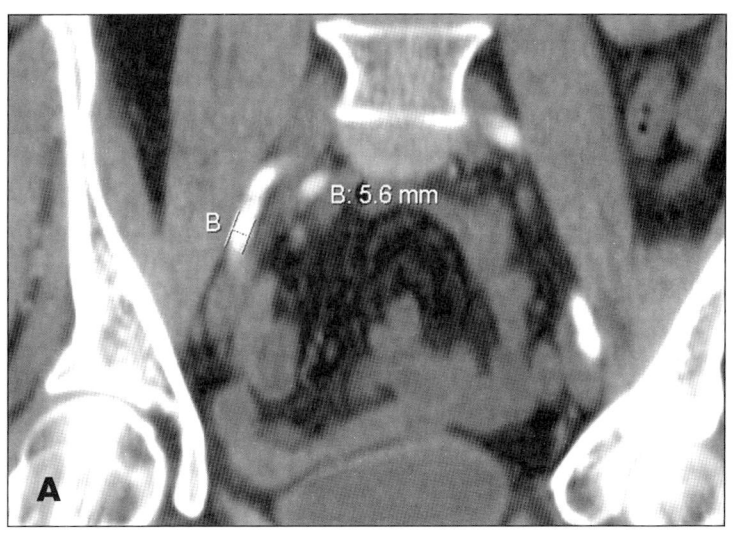

FIG. 1 5.6 mm wide external iliac arteries (A) in a female patient who required a large thoracic SG. The patient became hemodynamically unstable after the large bore introducer sheath was retracted into the external iliac artery (arrow) (B). Instant contrast injection reveals massive extravasation. An occlusion balloon is inflated in the distal aorta from the contralateral side. The iliac rupture was successfully excluded with covered stents (C).

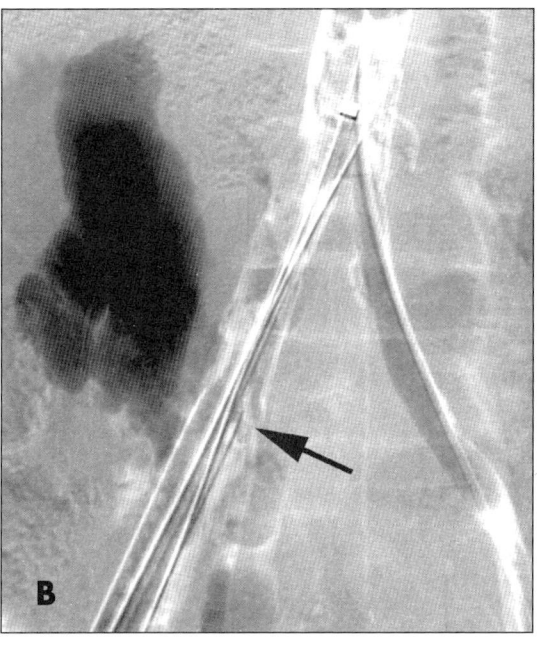

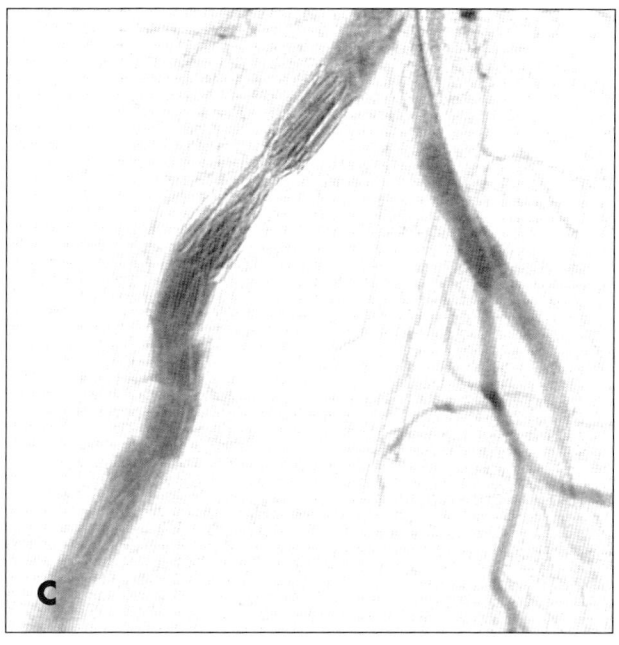

Arterial rupture at the level of the iliac bifurcation is occasionally associated with hypogastric backbleeding that may require more proximal cross clamping with an aortic occlusion balloon. The aortic balloon is preferably passed from the contralateral side. Thereby, the ipsilateral sheath may still be used to treat the rupture site. An aortic balloon is also recommended whenever it is deemed that excessive bleeding will occur during the short period of time it takes to exchange an ipsilateral iliac occlusion balloon for a covered stent.

Once hemorrhage has been arrested and the lesion is accurately defined by contrast injection via the sheath, an appropriate covered stent is selected and prepared. The stent is hurriedly deployed after rapid deflation and exchange of the iliac occlusion balloon. The use of a distal aortic occlusion balloon from the contralateral side offers more time for the deployment.

The originally planned SG procedure can be continued in spite of an iliac rupture unless the condition of the patient deteriorated due to the blood loss before the lesion was adequately treated.

Iliac stenosis

Virtually no iliac stenosis is impossible to cross with a large introducer sheath. Several sequential steps can be applied until the lesion is crossed. The potential risks of each step should be carefully considered and weighed against the risk of alternate treatment options.

We dilate the iliac arteries gently with hydrophilic dilators whenever the device cannot pass easily. Accessibility from the contra lateral side is explored at an early stage. Resistant lesions are dilated more aggressively with percutaneous transluminal angioplasty (PTA) balloons until the required sheath does cross or until iliac rupture seems imminent.

Before intentionally rupturing the iliac artery, the vessel should be lined ("paved") with covered stents [3]. Once the vessel has been paved, it can be violently dilated ("cracked") to any desired diameter with a high pressure PTA balloon. We prefer balloon expanded covered stents with a high radial strength that withstands recoil. A final vessel diameter of 10 mm will normally suffice to accept sheaths of any size.

The rather thin fabric of most covered stents may rift during violent "cracking" of narrow and calcified vessels. It is therefore prudent to keep spare covered stents at hand.

An alternate approach is to bypass the stenotic iliac segment by inserting the large introducer sheath directly into the common iliac artery or distal aorta via a retroperitoneal incision. The retroperitoneal SG insertion has been mainly abandoned after the advent of the aforementioned "paving and cracking" technique because it requires a rather large incision. Furthermore, the retroperitoneal insertion of a large and rigid introducer sheath is awkward due to the unfavorable perpendicular angle between the introducer sheath and the common iliac artery. This can be avoided by supplementing the retroperitoneal incision with a small groin incision and passing the sheath from the groin parallel to the external iliac artery. The common iliac artery is thereby reached at a more favorable angle that facilitates insertion of the sheath. A graft conduit, proximally anastomosed to the common iliac artery, also facilitates the retroperitoneal insertion of a SG. After completion of the aortic SG deployment, the conduit is distally anastomosed to the femoral artery in order to bypass the stenotic external iliac vessel.

Iliac and aortic tortuosity

Attempts to push a large stiff sheath through excessively tortuous vessels tend to buckle the arteries which aggravates the tortuosity, making it even harder for the sheath to cross (Figs. 2-3).

The first step that needs to be explored in such cases is the use of a stiffer guide wire. External manual compression of the iliac fossa may also support the iliac kink and help guide the introducer sheath into the aorta.

A so called body floss wire (through-and-through wire) is advocated as the next step [4]. Typically, a brachial wire is passed into the descending thoracic aorta, captured from below with a large snare and exteriorized in the groin. The mildest tension at any such body floss wire will facilitate the crossing of tortuous vessels remarkably. The aortic arch needs to be protected from the guide wire with a brachial sheath to prevent potential cheese cutting injury.

Another adjunct for extremely tortuous access with high friction, such as in relining a kinked SG, deserves to be mentioned. Instead of pushing from below, the sheath may be towed from above. "A snake should be pulled, not pushed, through a keyhole". Traction at the sheath is readily achieved by clamping the body floss wire as it emerges from the distal end of the sheath and then pulling at the wire from the arm (Fig. 3).

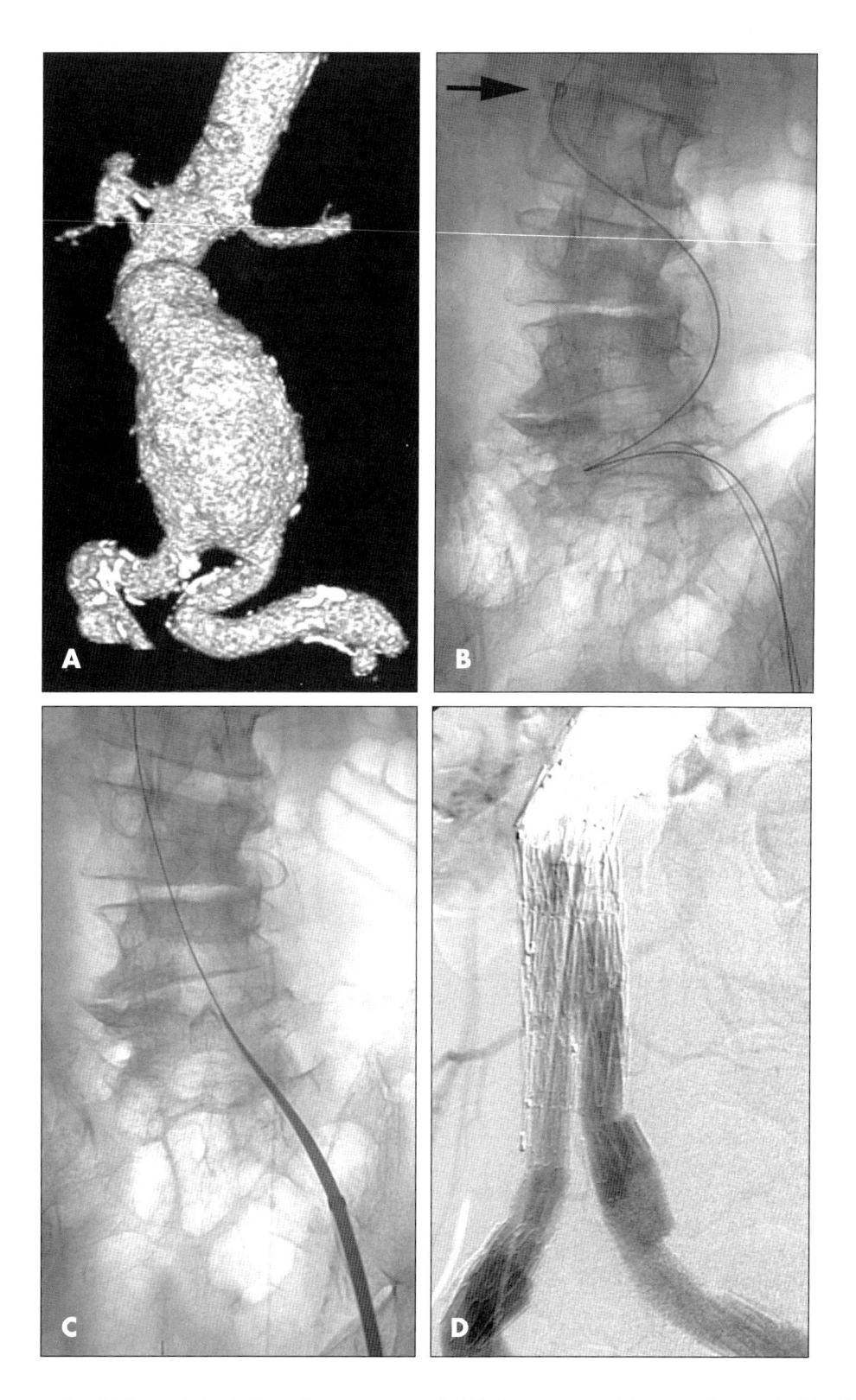

FIG. 2 Preoperative CT demonstrates tortuous iliac access vessels (A). Attempt to straighten out the vessels (B) with a 7 F introducer sheath (arrow) on a Lunderqvist wire fails. The iliac segment is straightened out by gentle traction on a brachial-femoral body floss wire (C) and allows safe insertion of a large introducer sheath. The limb of an aorto-iliac SG maintains the straightened iliac course after withdrawal of the Lunderqvist wire (D).

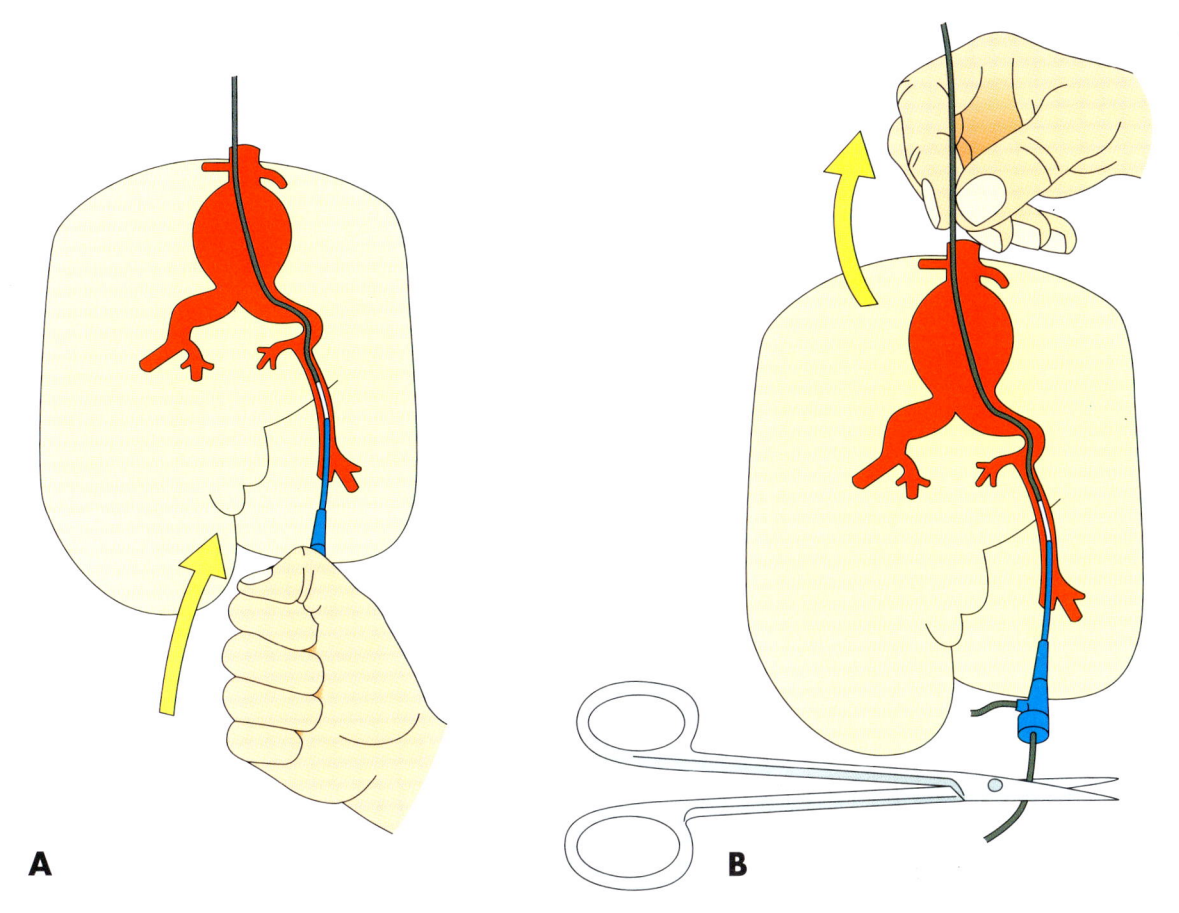

FIG. 3 A - Pushing the sheath from below tends to buckle a tortuous or stenotic iliac vessel. B - Pulling the sheath from above by clamping the guide wire at the distal end of the sheath straightens out the vessel.

Suboptimal stent graft sizing

There are multiple reasons for erroneous sizing of a SG. Solutions to some of the more common mistakes are suggested in the following.

UNDERSIZED PROXIMAL SG DIAMETER

Generous SG oversizing is recommended in the aorta. Potential leakage from excessive folding of the fabric can be "ironed" with an additional balloon expanded stent as described below.

An undersized SG diameter, however, is a serious problem that may cause a type I endoleak. A larger diameter proximal extension piece should be inserted on such occasions if there is room enough within the neck. Even moderate undersizing may eventually develop a late endoleak if the neck dilates over time.

Unfortunately, the undersized SG usually occupies the whole length of the aneurysmal neck, leaving no room for a larger extension piece. One may attempt to dislocate the SG distally in order to make room for the larger extension piece. A femoro-femoral body floss wire may serve to pull down an aorto-bi-iliac device. Attempts to dislocate an aortic SG can also be made with large balloon catheters. Any such manipulation should be performed with great caution so as not to rupture the fixation site of destroy the SG.

The presence of proximal barbs and a bare top stent will often prevent safe distal repositioning of the SG. A proximal extension with a fenestrated SG is then necessary. It is, however, most challenging to implant a fenestrated SG within an existing device. The excess of radiopaque markers renders orientation confusing and repositioning during deployment may be impaired if the devices hook into each other.

Undersized distal SG diameter

An undersized iliac limb with a subsequent distal type I endoleak is treated with a larger distal extension piece. It is, however, more difficult to seal off the leak if the undersized limb reaches all the way to the iliac bifurcation. This typically occurs when an aorto-bi-iliac SG is implanted without leaving room for the intended extension piece in a short common iliac artery (Fig. 4). Simple extension of the limb into the external iliac artery will not resolve persistent backflow from the hypogastric artery. It is worth to attempt pushing the distal end of the limb cranially to buckle the aortic SG and make room for a larger extension piece that will seal off the common iliac artery. If buckling fails, the hypogastric artery may need to be coil embolized prior to extending the undersized limb into the external iliac artery.

Oversized SG diameter

Restrained SG oversizing should be applied in small blood vessels because the bulky folds of the fabric may obstruct the lumen. While 5-8 mm oversizing is appropriate for an aortic SG it may jam a narrow external iliac artery. Additional stenting will be necessary to restore the lumen and may involve "cracking" of the artery to accommodate the oversized device.

Collapse of the thoracic SG

An infamous exception to the rule of generous oversizing of the aortic SG is the acutely angulated ("gothic") arch [5,6], particularly in patients with a small aortic diameter. Young victims of road traffic accidents with aortic transection comprise a special group of such patients. Excessive oversizing of the thoracic SG may provoke collapse of the device

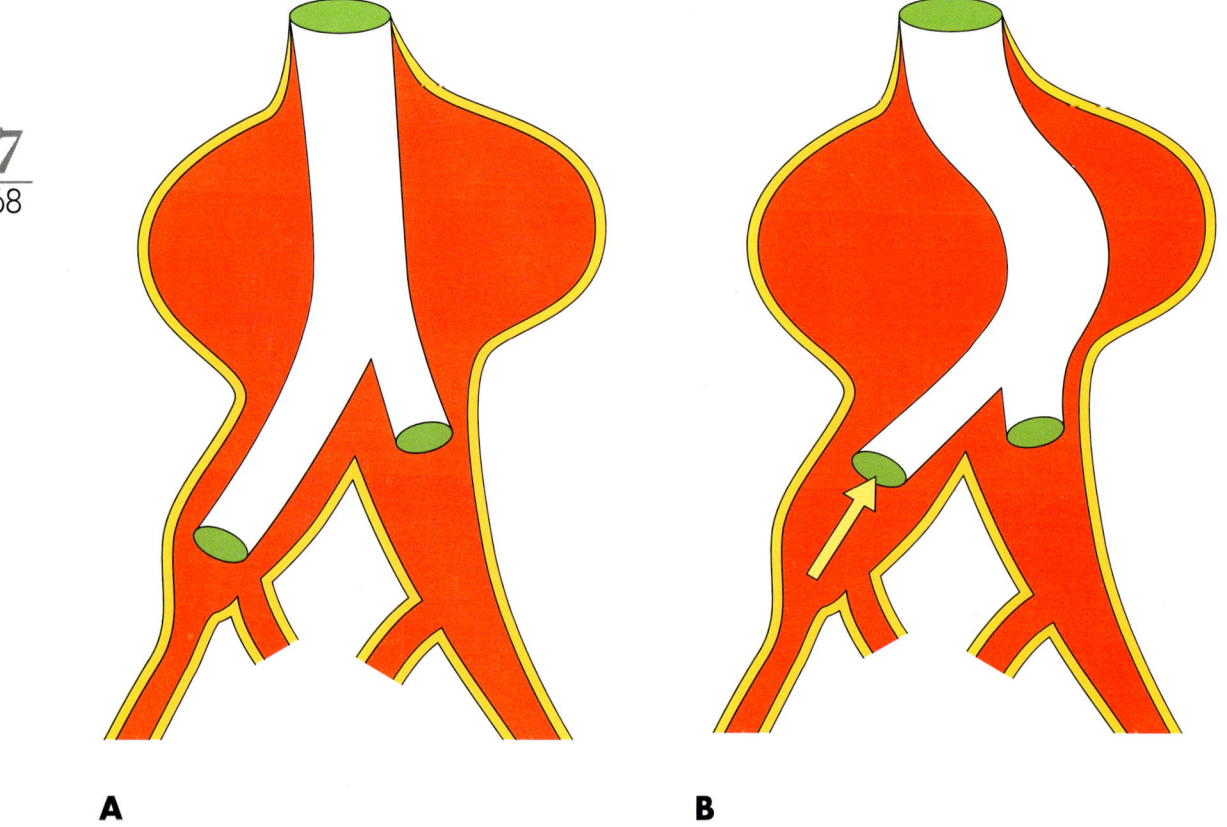

A **B**

FIG. 4 A - The ipsilateral limb of an aorto-bi-iliac device reaches all the way to the iliac bifurcation leaving no room for a larger extension piece that was initially intended to seal off the wide common iliac artery. B - Pushing the limb cranially buckles the entire SG and makes room for the extension piece in the common iliac artery.

with subsequent aortic occlusion. While collapse and folding can be re-stented safely in other settings, adjunctive manipulation in the aortic arch is dangerous with a risk of cerebral emboli and retrograde aortic dissection.

Misplaced stent graft

An extension piece should be inserted whenever the cranial end of a SG is deployed too distally or the caudal end too proximally. These mistakes are relatively simple to manage but underline the necessity of keeping spare SGs on the shelf. The following misplacements are more challenging.

Too proximal implantation of the cranial end

Accidental overstenting of the visceral arteries or the left common carotid artery are the most serious types of misplacement of an aortic SG. Attempts to reposition the aortic SG distally as described above may prove useful. Some SGs are equipped with a distal safety wire and until that wire has been released, significant traction can still be applied on the SG. If the accidentally overstented side branch cannot be uncovered it should be recatheterized and stented.

The renal arteries can usually be re-catheterized and stented instantly unless excessive overstenting has occurred. Partial coverage can be overcome via a femoral approach but the brachial access may prove helpful in more severe cases. Balloon expanded stents are preferred for greater radial force.

If the superior mesenteric artery (SMA) is overstented and antegrade attempts to re-catheterize it from within the aorta fail, it can still be salvaged instantly by a procedure that combines endovascular and open techniques as follows [7]: a peripheral branch of the SMA is isolated and punctured via a laparotomy. a long 0.014" or 0.018" guide wire is passed retrograde into the aortic lumen in spite of the fact that the origin of the SMA is covered by the aortic SG (Fig. 5). The wire is snared in the aorta from a brachial approach and the SMA can then

FIG. 5 The guide wire has been passed retrograde from the accidentally overstented SMA into the aorta and snared from the arm. An introducer sheath has then been passed into the SMA and now makes it possible to stent the SMA in order to provide a so-called chimney graft.

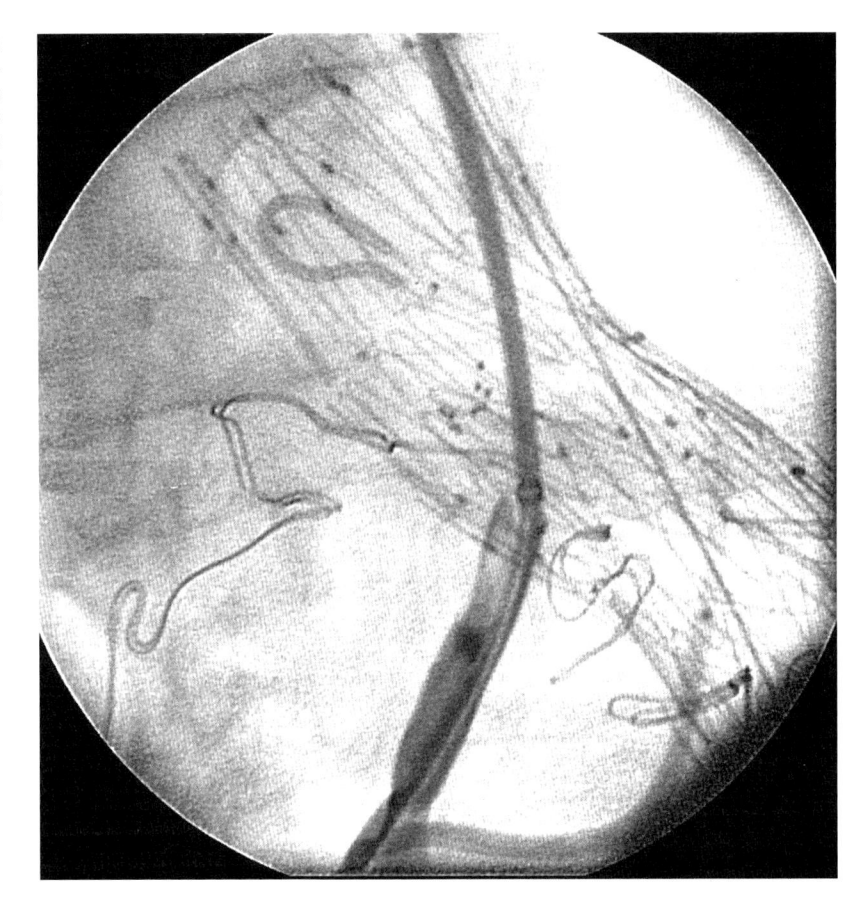

be stented from the arm over the brachial-SMA body floss wire. A so called chimney graft is thereby acquired [8]. Both arteriotomy or clamping of the SMA are avoided as the mesenteric puncture site is supplied with just one suture.

A similar technique can be used when the left common carotid artery is accidentally covered by a thoracic SG (Fig. 6): The common carotid artery is exposed and a retrograde wire is passed into the ascending aorta. The wire is snared from the groin to obtain a carotid-femoral body floss wire but the stent is preferably inserted from the carotid artery itself. The risk associated with brief cross clamping of the common carotid artery is low while there is collateral perfusion from the external carotid artery. Prior to stenting of the carotid artery, great care should be taken to confirm that the vessel is truly overstented. Misinterpretation of the angiography from parallax is common in the arch (Fig. 7).

Too distal implantation of the caudal end

The celiac trunk may get accidentally covered by the distal end of a thoracic SG and could, potentially, be salvaged in a similar way as described above for the SMA. It is unclear whether that is necessary. Most patients tolerate sacrifice of the celiac trunk although lethal complications from liver and gastric ischemia have occurred. We advocate that the overstented celiac trunk need not be treated if selective injection of contrast in the SMA confirms adequate collateral perfusion of the hepatic artery.

The accidentally overstented hypogastric artery during abdominal stentgrafting poses a different problem. The risk for end organ ischemia is limited but there is a risk for significant back bleeding from the hypogastric artery into the aortic aneurysm outside the SG. Continued pressurization and expansion of the aneurysm sac may ensue. The overstented hypogastric artery can be catheterized from the contralateral side if the mistake is identified prior to the insertion of the contralateral limb of the aorto-bi-iliac SG. If the mistake is identified at a later stage, it may be necessary to catheterize the hypogastric artery with a catheter passing outside the ipsilateral limb. This is not always feasible and retroperitoneal ligation of the hypogastric artery may prove necessary.

Inability to catheterize the contralateral limb of the biliac device

It sometimes proves difficult to catheterize the short contralateral limb of a modular aorto-bi-iliac SG from below. This may be due to excessive ves-

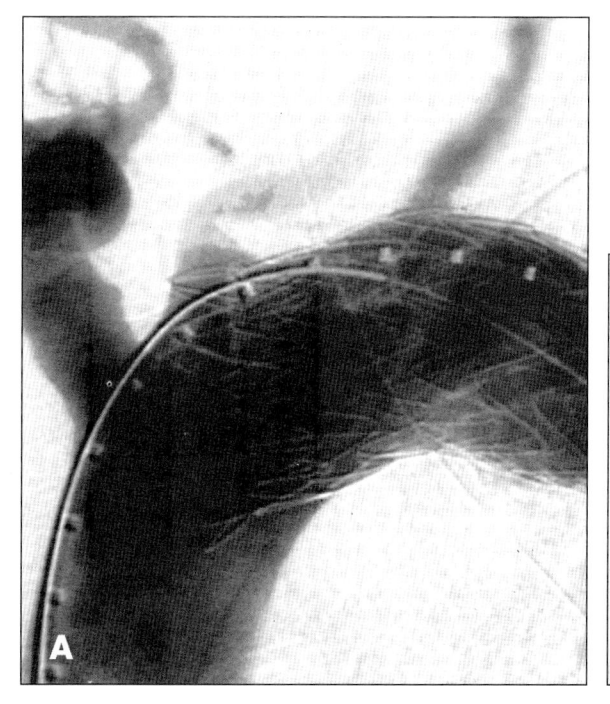

FIG. 6 Accidentally overstented left carotid artery (A). A carotid-femoral body floss wire has been obtained (arrow) (B) and the left common carotid artery has been reconstituted with a stent.

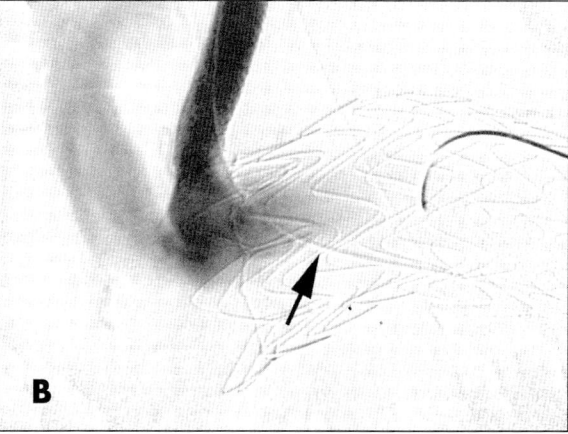

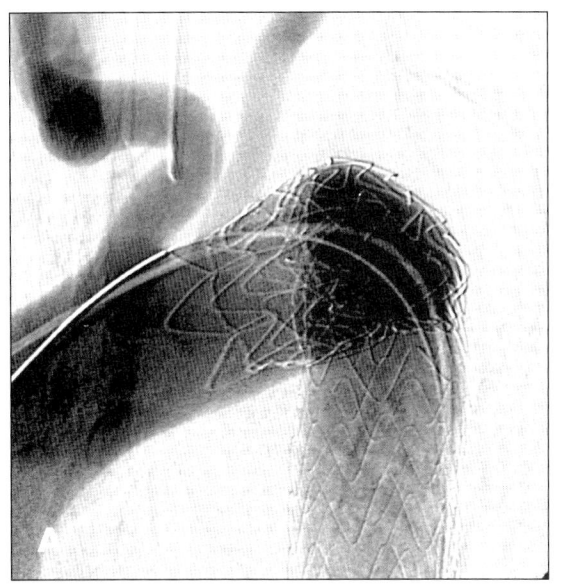

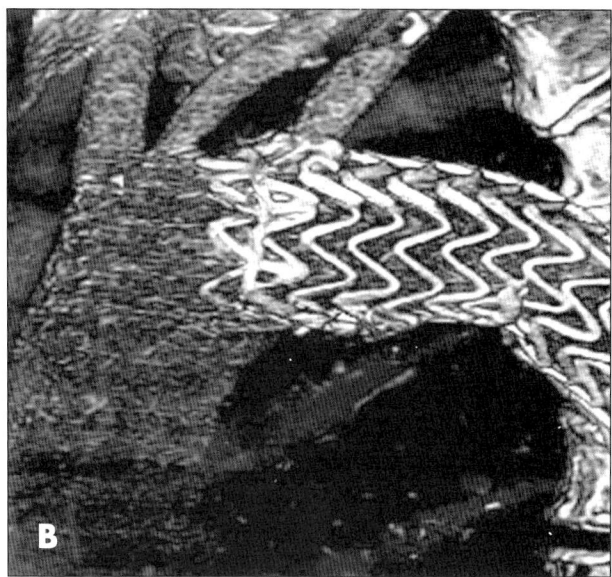

FIG. 7 Completion angiography after implantation of a thoracic SG (A) falsely suggests that the left common carotid artery is overstented. The postoperative CT reconstruction (B) proves that the carotid artery was not covered.

sel tortuosity or unfortunate positioning of the contralateral stump. A long hydrophilic wire can, however, be passed from the ipsilateral side over the flow divider. The tip of the wire is then snared within the aneurysmal sack with a large snare from the contralateral side and exteriorized in the groin.

Transforming the aorto-bi-iliac device into a uni-liac SG by relining it with a short aorto-uni-iliac SG is an option that is used on rare occasions when the insertion of a contralateral limb fails completely.

Poor stent graft apposition in the neck with type I endoleak

SGs are notoriously rigid and comply poorly with angulation or irregularities at the neck [9]. A proximal type I endoleak may persist in spite of repeat moulding of the SG with balloon catheters. Excessive folding of the graft fabric may also cause a proximal type I endoleak.

The placement of an adjunctive balloon expanded stent inside the neck has proven efficient to seal off these types of endoleak. The stent will either straighten out the neck or mould the SG to provide better apposition to the aortic wall. The long-term efficacy of a large Palmaz stent in the neck is not known.

The large stent is mounted on a balloon catheter manually. We have used the Palmaz 4014 stent mounted on a valvuloplasty balloon catheter or, lately, on a compliant balloon (Coda, Cook). The stent slips easily off the balloon and should be advanced through an introducer sheath to the implantation site. The balloon expanded stent will foreshorten significantly upon inflation and should be centered just below the proximal edge of the graft fabric. Manual expansion ought to be applied and carefully observed under fluoroscopy in order to prevent iatrogenic rupture of the neck. Rupture is extremely unusual with this technique. It is necessary to keep at hand a large volume of diluted contrast for inflation of the large balloon because incomplete or interrupted expansion may lead to slippage of the stent.

Thrombosis

Massive intra-arterial thrombosis is a serious complication during any endovascular procedure and needs to be prevented. In general, thrombosis poses a greater threat to endovascular interventions than hemorrhage and aggressive heparinization ought to be applied.

Intra-operative thrombosis of the abdominal aortic SG is particularly likely to occur in patients with an occluded hypogastric artery or whenever the iliac limb is extended into the external iliac artery. The reason for that is that there may be no flow through the limb while the external iliac artery remains obliterated by the large introducer sheath or during subsequent repair of the femoral artery.

This type of limb thrombosis can be avoided by restoring flow as quickly as possible, by repeat flushing of the sheath and by aggressive heparinization.

Whenever limb flow cannot be restored expediently it is prudent to create a temporary arteriovenous fistula. The fistula is easily obtained by inserting the side arm of the large femoral sheath into the valve of a small introducer sheath in the femoral vein.

Intra-operative SG thrombosis that occurs in spite of all precautions needs to be treated aggressively. Instant massive heparinization and distal cross clamping may prevent peripheral trash. Embolectomy should be attempted gently under fluoroscopic guidance with a double lumen catheter over a stiff wire in order to avoid dislocation of the newly implanted SG or spill over into the contra lateral limb. The result should be confirmed angiographically and persistent mural thrombi should be stented with long, selfexpanding stents. Since flow must be restored immediately after successful thrombectomy, any femoral lesion should be repaired first. It is for example unsuitable to leave an aortic SG obstructed for an hour while inserting a femoral patch.

The alternative option to embolectomy is femoro-femoral cross over bypass. It should be considered in unilateral thrombosis that seems technically difficult to resolve without jeopardizing the SG.

Patients undergoing endovascular repair of a ruptured aortic aneurysm are particularly at risk for SG trombosis. Coagulopathy is present in the emergency setting while heparinization is postponed for understandable reasons. We tend to heparinize even this group of patients gradually as increasing amounts of thrombogenic material are inserted and final exclusion of the ruptured aneurysm is anticipated.

Iliac obstruction

Iliac obstruction from kinking or dissection is not uncommon after aortic stent grafting. It needs to be identified intra operatively and instantly repaired in order to avoid subsequent SG thrombosis.

Iliac outflow should be confirmed by a completion angiography at two perpendicular projections after implantation of the aortic SG. Simultaneous aspiration through the large femoral introducer sheath during contrast injection is required if the sheath obstructs femoral outflow. The stiff guide wire ought to be replaced with a catheter prior to the completion angiography to unmask unexpected kinking after removal of the wire.

Kinks typically arise within the limb of the SG or at the transition between the rigid limb and a tortuous native iliac artery — especially if the SG is extended into the external iliac arteries. Significant iliac kinks or dissections require adjunctive stenting. When in doubt, insert more stents! The intra operative addition of an iliac stent is a minor issue compared to sudden late thrombosis of the entire SG.

Conclusion

Intra-operative complications and unexpected difficulties will always arise during aortic stent grafting in spite of careful pre-operative imaging and planning. The most frequent complications are associated with access problems, misplacement of the SG or suboptimal sizing of the device. The majority of these complications can be managed endovascularly. The adjunctive maneuvers necessitate more advanced endovascular skills and well equipped laboratories with excellent imaging and a wide range of spare parts such as various stents, SGs, catheters, guide wires etc. This also underlines the need for complete endovascular training of the vascular specialist.

REFERENCES

1 Gabrielli L, Baudo A, Molinari A et al. Early complications in endovascular treatment of abdominal aortic aneurysm. *Acta Chir Belg* 2004; 104: 519-526.

2 Cuypers PW, Laheij R, Buth J. Which factors increase the risk of conversion to open surgery following endovascular abdominal aortic aneurysm repair? *Eur J Vasc Endovasc Surg* 2000; 20: 183-189.

3 Hinchliffe RJ, Ivancev K, Sonesson B et al. Paving and Crack-

ing: An Endovascular technique to facilitate the introduction of aortic stent-grafts through stenosed iliac arteries. *J Endovasc Ther* 2007; 14: 630-633.

4. Malina M, Sonesson B, Lindblad B et al. Hybrid procedures and homemade devices for aortic repair. In: Branchereau A, Jacobs M, eds. *Hybrid vascular procedures*. Oxford: Blackwell Publishing, 2004: pp 143-155.

5. Mestres G, Maeso J, Fernandez V et al. Symptomatic collapse of a thoracic aorta endoprosthesis. *J Vasc Surg* 2006; 43: 1270-1273.

6. Steinbauer MG, Stehr A, Pfister K et al. Endovascular repair of proximal endograft collapse after treatment for thoracic aortic disease. *J Vasc Surg* 2006; 43: 609-612.

7. Sonesson B, Hinchliffe RJ, Dias NV et al. Hybrid recanalization of superior mesenteric artery occlusion in acute mesenteric ischemia. *J Endovasc Ther* 2008; 15: 129-132.

8. Malina M, Sonesson B, Dias N et al. How to fashion a homemade fenestrated stent graft: An option for urgent aneurysms with an inadequate neck. In: Becquemin JP, Alimi Y (eds). *Controversies and updates in vascular surgery*. Torino: Edizioni Minerva Medica, 2007: pp 143-148.

9. Dias NV, Resch T, Malina M et al. Intraoperative proximal endoleaks during AAA stent-graft repair: evaluation of risk factors and treatment with Palmaz stents. *J Endovasc Ther* 2001; 8: 268-273.

8

EVAR AND TEVAR: ENDOLEAKS AND ENDOTENSION

GEOFFREY GILLING-SMITH

The introduction of new technology follows a predictable pattern. Initial enthusiasm is soon tempered by reports of failure. Those who find change uncomfortable are quick to condemn the new technology and remind all who will listen of the benefits of the tried and tested "gold standard". Undeterred, the enthusiasts examine the modes of failure, refine and develop the technology until eventually a "plateau of realism" is reached. The limitations of the new technique are understood, its indications are defined and its role alongside existing technology assured.

So it was with endovascular repair of aortic aneurysm. The concept seemed simple: endovascular relining of the abdominal or thoracic aorta with a covered stent graft would isolate the aneurysm from the circulation and prevent rupture. However, it soon became apparent that grafts sometimes failed to isolate the aneurysm from the circulation. Follow-up imaging revealed persistent or recurrent perfusion of the aneurysm sac and in some cases continued expansion of the aneurysm. More worryingly, there were also reports of late rupture and death. The opponents of the endovascular revolution crowed, the enthusiasts went back to the drawing board.

Since those early days, stent graft technology has evolved and the limitations of the technique have been understood and accepted. Perhaps more importantly we now have a much better understanding of the modes of failure and their causes. We can often anticipate and prevent complications before the patient is at risk. Secondary intervention to prevent late rupture is not without risk, however, and debate continues about the significance of certain "complications" and the indications for secondary intervention.

This chapter reviews the meaning, clinical significance and management of two such "complications": endoleak and endotension.

Definitions

In 1997, Geoff White [1] proposed the term "endoleak" to describe *"persistent or recurrent flow of blood within the aneurysm sac but outside the stent graft"*. He differentiated between early or primary endoleak (present from the time of the intervention) and late or secondary endoleak (developing at some time during follow up). He also proposed a classification of endoleak, which has proved clinically useful and has largely stood the test of time.

Since endovascular repair was intended to isolate the aneurysm from the circulation, it was at first believed that the presence of any type of endoleak was evidence of failure whereas "freedom from endoleak" was evidence of success. It was noted, however, that some aneurysms continued to expand despite the absence of endoleak on routine follow-up imaging while others shrank even though an endoleak was present. This focused attention on the importance of pressure within the aneurysm sac and in 1999, the author proposed the term endotension [2] to describe *"continued or recurrent pressurization of the aneurysm sac"* The term was derived from *endo* meaning "within" and *tension*, which in English describes the state of the wall of an aneurysm that is pressurized (as in "under tension") while in French it means "blood pressure".

There have since been alternative definitions proposed for the term endotension. One such – *expansion of the aneurysm in the absence of endoleak* – is, in the author's opinion, unhelpful and possibly misleading since it again focuses attention on the presence or absence of endoleak and morphological change rather than the presence or absence of significant intra-sac pressure. Perhaps more worryingly, by describing expansion as a distinct clinical entity, such a definition tends to reinforce a commonly held (but incorrect) view that expansion is evidence of sufficient pressure to cause rupture (which it is not) and therefore an indication for secondary intervention. This may lead to unnecessary and potentially harmful endovascular or even open surgical intervention.

It should also be noted that differentiation between patients with and without endoleak is only clinically useful if one can be confident that an endoleak is or is not present and that unfortunately is not the case. Indeed at a recent international scientific meeting, one speaker proposed that the term endotension (used incorrectly) was irrelevant since with modern imaging techniques it was possible to demonstrate an endoleak in most cases of expansion. It was left to a very eminent member of the audience to point out to the speaker that he had missed the point completely. What matters is not whether or not the aneurysm is expanding or whether or not blood can be seen flowing (very slowly) within the aneurysm sac: what matters is whether or not the patient remains or is again at risk of death from aneurysm rupture and that depends primarily on whether or not the aneurysm is pressurized (i.e. whether or not endotension is present).

Basic principles

The aim of endovascular repair of abdominal or thoracic aortic aneurysms is quite simply to prevent death from rupture. Since it is pressure within the aneurysm that causes expansion and ultimately rupture of the aneurysm while it is the flow of blood within the aneurysm that results in hemorrhage and death if rupture occurs, it follows that prevention of fatal rupture relies on isolation of the aneurysm from both pressure and flow.

It should be noted, however, that flow of blood within the aneurysm (endoleak) is of no clinical significance unless there is sufficient pressure to cause rupture. On the other hand it may be argued that pressure within the aneurysm (endotension) is of no clinical significance unless there is blood flowing within the aneurysm since rupture is likely to be a benign event. Indeed, some have proposed "fenestration" of an enlarging aneurysm in which there is no evidence of endoleak in order to depressurize the sac and thus prevent further expansion.

At all events, the relationship between endoleak and endotension is more complex than it might at first seem and secondary intervention to treat the cause of either or both phenomena without careful consideration of their clinical significance of is in most cases inappropriate.

Endoleak

Although the classification of endoleak proposed by White was developed to categorize endoleak complicating endovascular repair of the abdominal aorta (EVAR), the classification can equally well be employed to describe endoleak after endovascular repair of the descending thoracic aorta (TEVAR).

ANASTOMOTIC ENDOLEAK (TYPE I)
Clinical significance

Blood may leak into the aneurysm sac at the proximal or distal sites of endograft attachment either because of a primary failure to establish an adequate seal between the stent graft and the aorta or iliac artery (primary endoleak) or because following successful isolation of the aneurysm, caudal migration of the endograft and/or disengagement of the endograft from the distal aortic neck or iliac arteries has resulted in late failure of seal (secondary endoleak).

Type I endoleaks are at systemic pressure and although it remains unproven, it is prudent to assume that they cause significant pressurization of the aneurysm sac which remains or is again at risk of rupture. Indeed it may be argued that the flow of blood at systemic pressure into an otherwise closed aneurysm sac is if anything more dangerous than the flow of blood through an untreated aneurysm so that the risk of rupture is actually greater than if the aneurysm had not been treated. Furthermore, if the endoleak develops some time during follow-up after previously successful isolation of the aneurysm and a period of depressurization and shrinkage, it is possible that the risk of rupture is increased since the period of depressurization may have allowed the aneurysm wall to atrophy and weaken.

At all events, the aneurysm is at risk of rupture and in most cases rupture will result in significant hemorrhage. For these reasons, early intervention to treat such endoleaks is advisable in most cases. A possible exception to this rule is the patient in whom there persists a very small proximal endoleak on completion angiography despite ballooning and/or stenting of the aortic neck. If an appropriate cuff is not immediately available in the author's opinion it is reasonable to observe such patients for up to two weeks while a cuff is ordered. If the leak is still present on CT scan after this time, the cuff should be deployed. If the leak has sealed, the patient may be observed but an increased frequency of clinical and radiographic review may be advisable since pressure can be transmitted through thrombus sealing an endoleak (see below).

Management of primary proximal type I endoleak

If the seal between the aortic neck and the endograft is inadequate, management options include balloon dilatation of the endograft within the neck of the aneurysm, deployment of a Palmaz stent within the neck of the aneurysm, deployment of a covered stent graft cuff or conversion to open repair.

The choice of treatment depends on the cause of the problem. It is always worth trying to balloon dilate the graft within the neck of the aneurysm in an attempt to mould the graft to the aorta. If this is successful, the deployment of a Palmaz stent to maintain the effect of balloon dilatation may be advisable but if the graft is too small or has been deployed too low these techniques will not help. Indeed, deployment of a Palmaz stent may preclude other options.

If the endograft has been sized correctly but inadvertently deployed too low or if with hindsight it seems that the neck of the aneurysm is too short, diseased or calcified, it will be necessary to extend the repair proximally.

EVAR: If there is an adequate length of neck below the renal artery origins, deployment of a short endograft cuff up to the renal arteries may be all that is required. If, however, the neck is short, consideration must be given either to deployment of a fenestrated cuff or to conversion to open repair. The decision will depend on the general fitness of the patient, the magnitude of the leak and the physicians' familiarity with fenestrated stent graft technology. If the patient is relatively fit and/or the leak is significant, the delay inherent in planning and ordering a fenestrated cuff may be considered unacceptable and the risks of conversion to open surgical repair may seem preferable. If not, a cuff should be planned or the patient should be referred to a specialist unit.

If the graft has been deployed correctly but is too small, deployment of a standard cuff within the neck of the endograft is unlikely to be successful since the cuff will be constrained by the endograft. The options then are deployment of a fenestrated cuff (extending the repair into the supra-renal aorta) or conversion to open surgical repair. The choice will depend on the general fitness of the patient, the magnitude of the leak and the physicians' familiarity with fenestrated stent graft technology as above.

TEVAR: It will usually be necessary to extend the repair by deploying a further endograft across the left subclavian and sometimes the left carotid artery origins. Although many believe that one can safely cover the left subclavian, there is undoubtedly a risk of upper limb and/or hind brain ischemia and one should not of course occlude the left subclavian if the left internal mammary artery has been employed to revascularize the coronary circulation. In the author's opinion therefore one should in general try to restore flow into the left subclavian artery either by in-situ fenestration of the graft via the brachial artery or by extra-anatomic carotid to subclavian bypass. This will in any case be necessary if the graft encroaches on the left carotid origin.

Management of secondary proximal type I endoleak

The development of a proximal endoleak during follow-up is usually evidence of caudal migration of the endograft. This in turn is evidence either of the inadequacy of fixation or of dilatation of the neck of the aneurysm. Balloon dilatation and/or deployment of a Palmaz stent is unlikely to be efficacious and the choice therefore is between deployment of a cuff, proximal extension of the repair across the renal (EVAR) or subclavian (TEVAR) artery origins or conversion to open repair. If an endovascular solution is preferred, it is in general advisable to consider extending the repair proximally since a standard cuff deployed to the same level as the original endograft is likely to suffer the same fate as the endograft.

Management of distal type I endoleak

EVAR: The management of either primary or secondary distal endoleak is in general relatively straightforward. In most cases it is sufficient simply to extend the endograft into the distal common or proximal external iliac artery by deploying an appropriately sized endograft limb. If extending into the external iliac artery, consideration should be given to embolization of the proximal internal iliac artery to prevent backbleeding into the aneurysm sac. If the contralateral internal iliac artery is occluded, it may be advisable to reimplant the ipsilateral internal iliac artery so as to secure flow of blood to the pelvic organs.

TEVAR: The management of distal endoleak after endovascular repair of the descending thoracic aorta may be complicated by the need to maintain flow into the celiac and/or superior mesenteric arteries. If there is an insufficient length of relatively normal aorta proximal to the celiac axis it may be necessary to employ a short fenestrated endograft.

SIDEBRANCH ENDOLEAK (TYPE II)

Backbleeding from lumbar, inferior mesenteric or accessory renal arteries is common after EVAR and is always primary. The observation of type II endoleak on imaging performed some time after endovascular repair in a patient in whom no such endoleak was observed on completion angiography or on imaging performed early after operation is not of course evidence that a previously occluded sidebranch has become patent. It is simply evidence either that previous imaging was inadequate or that there has been a change in the pattern of blood flow within the aneurysm sac.

Backbleeding from intercostal arteries has been documented after TEVAR but it seems to occur much less frequently than sidebranch reperfusion after EVAR and consequently has received much less attention. The following discussion will therefore focus on type II endoleak after EVAR but the principles can be applied to the management of type II endoleak after TEVAR.

Clinical significance of type II endoleak

This remains perhaps the most disputed issue in endografting. Many believe that type II endoleaks are nearly always benign and advocate a policy of observation. Others argue that such endoleaks can occasionally cause rupture and death and should therefore be treated.

Sidebranch reperfusion is observed on post-operative imaging in 15%-20% of patients [3-5], the reported incidence depending on the interval between operation and first scan. Between 50% and 80% of such leaks thrombose spontaneously within the first six months after operation [4,5] but a minority persist for at least six months and it is these which seem to cause most concern.

Although it is perhaps understandable that the absence of a previously noted sidebranch endoleak on follow-up imaging should be reassuring, it should be noted that failure to demonstrate a sidebranch endoleak may simply reflect inadequate imaging. More importantly, it is important to understand that persistence of a sidebranch endoleak is not evidence that it imparts significant pressure to the aneurysm sac or that the patient is at risk. It is simply evidence that there is more than one patent sidebranch (and that blood can flow between sidebranches across at least part of the aneurysm sac) or that a patent sidebranch is acting as outflow vessel for a graft related endoleak.

There is good evidence that sidebranch endoleaks are in general at less than systemic pressure [6,7] and that the pressure within the aneurysm thrombus (and therefore the pressure adjacent to the aneurysm wall) is less than the pressure within the endoleak track [7]. Unsurprisingly, continued expansion of the aneurysm is more common in patients with persistent type II endoleak than in those with no endoleak [4,5,8] but expansion is not evidence that the pressure within the aneurysm is sufficient to cause rupture. Indeed, Dias et al. [7] recorded an intra-sac pressure of between 58% and 87% of systemic pressure in patients with type II endoleak and expanding aneurysm. Although it may be argued that some of these patients were at risk of rupture, it is clear that many were not. This is perhaps the reason that rupture in association with type II endoleak remains a very rare occurrence [5,9].

Management of type II endoleak

Intervention is indicated if it is thought that there is a significant risk that the endoleak will lead to rupture and significant loss of blood.

Although there have been reports of rupture in association with type II endoleak within six months of operation, such an event is very rare indeed and most endovascular specialists believe that intervention to treat type II endoleak is not indicated unless the leak persists for more than six months. In addition, intervention is probably not indicated if the aneurysm is shrinking or relatively small and stable. The question therefore is whether or not to intervene if the aneurysm is expanding.

In the author's opinion (and practice) persistent type II endoleaks can in general be observed even if the aneurysm is expanding. It is vitally important, however, to be certain that there is no graft related endoleak and/or other cause of expansion and all previous follow-up imaging should be reviewed carefully to ensure that there is no evidence of migration, iliac limb disengagement or deformation of the endograft. Occasionally, if the patient is young and/or the aneurysm is very large it may be prudent to consider intervention but this may benefit the physician more than the patient. It is a sad fact of modern medical practice that a complication from an unnecessary intervention is far less likely to precipitate litigation than rupture of an aneurysm in a patient in whom the physician has decided not to intervene.

At all events, in such cases, one should first measure the pressure within the aneurysm sac either by direct translumbar puncture or by means of a catheter introduced via one or other femoral artery and passed alongside the iliac limbs. If the mean pressure is low (less than 70% of the systemic mean), the patient can be spared an unnecessary intervention. If it is high one can proceed to intervention with a degree of confidence that the decision to intervene is based on some evidence of risk.

A variety of methods have been proposed to abolish sidebranch reperfusion:
- transarterial embolization of the sidebranch(es);
- translumbar embolization of the endoleak track;
- laparoscopic clipping of the sidebranch(es);
- laparotomy and ligation of the feeding sidebranch(es);
- laparotomy and under-running of the sidebranch ostia from within the aneurysm sac leaving the endograft undisturbed;
- conversion to open surgical repair.

Embolization by transarterial or translumbar routes is the least invasive option and should perhaps be considered before any of the more invasive treatments. Interestingly the translumbar approach is reportedly much more likely to succeed than the transarterial approach [10,11]. Should embolization fail, the author advocates under-running of the sidebranch ostia from within the aneurysm sac. This affords an opportunity to inspect the endograft and assure the integrity of the repair. Conversion should not be undertaken unless there are other problems.

TYPE III ENDOLEAK

Type III endoleaks are perhaps the most dangerous of all leaks. They occur late following initially successful isolation of the aneurysm and are due either to perforation of the graft fabric by a fractured stent or disconnection of the components of a modular graft. In all cases, blood can flow directly from the aorta into the aneurysm sac. This is very likely to lead to early rupture and this in turn is likely to result in significant blood loss. Urgent intervention is therefore indicated in most cases.

Modular disconnection can usually be treated by endovascular deployment of a covered stent to bridge the gap between the two components that have separated. It should be noted, however, that disconnection often occurs as a result of migration and angulation of the endograft so that consideration may occasionally need to be given to conversion to open repair.

Perforation of the graft fabric can only be treated by relining the endograft (secondary endografting) or by conversion to open repair.

Type IV endoleak

Occasionally, the late phase of a contrast enhanced CT will reveal a blush of contrast around the endograft. This is believed to result from graft porosity (leakage of contrast through the interstices of the endograft fabric) or "microleaks" through the holes made in the graft fabric to suture the fabric to the stent skeleton.

The significance of type IV endoleaks is unknown. The author has never seen a type IV endoleak and is unaware of any reports of late rupture due to such leaks. Although such leaks could transmit significant pressure to the aneurysm sac, it is very unlikely that rupture would result in significant hemorrhage and in general such leaks can probably be safely observed. It is important, however, to review all imaging carefully to exclude any alternative cause for the blush of contrast.

Endotension

Clinical significance

The term endotension was intended to describe "sufficient pressure to cause rupture". By definition, therefore, endotension is clinically significant in all cases since the aneurysm remains or is at risk of rupture. The problem is that we do not know how much pressure is necessary to cause rupture, nor do we know if continuous pressure is less or as hazardous as pressure that varies throughout the cardiac cycle (i.e. a pulsatile waveform). Furthermore, we know that the pressure can vary throughout the aneurysm [12] and that there is significant variation in the tensile strength of the aneurysm wall both within and between patients [12]. Thus in any individual patient we really have no idea whether or not there is sufficient pressure to cause rupture and the management decision must be based on estimations of risk.

An additional consideration is the presence or absence of endoleak. In the presence of a low flow endoleak or even no endoleak at all, it is very unlikely that rupture will lead to hemorrhage and death. It should be noted, however, that continued expansion of the aneurysm may lead to shortening and dilatation of the aneurysm neck (effacement) so that the proximal anastomosis becomes insecure. This may lead to migration of the endograft and late proximal endoleak.

Causes of endotension

The aneurysm sac may be pressurized directly via an endoleak or indirectly via thrombus. Pressure may for example be transmitted via thrombus sealing an endoleak or through thrombus sealing the interstices of a porous graft. It is also likely that pulsation of the endograft within a closed space (the aneurysm sac) can result in pressurization of the sac although this has not been demonstrated in-vivo and the magnitude of such an effect remains unknown.

Diagnosis of endotension

Endotension may be assumed if there is a graft related endoleak (type I or type III). Endotension may not, however, be assumed in the presence of type II or type IV endoleak, nor may it be assumed simply because the aneurysm is expanding. Expansion of the aneurysm is evidence only that the pressure within the aneurysm is greater than the pressure within the surrounding tissues. If it is thought that the patient would be at risk if the aneurysm was at systemic pressure, it is necessary to measure the pressure within the aneurysm sac either by direct translumbar puncture of the aneurysm sac under fluoroscopic control or by passing a catheter into the aneurysm via one or other iliac artery passing between the stent graft and the artery wall. The problem is that neither technique is wholly reliable. At the very least one must try to measure the pressure in more than one location and preferably close to the aneurysm wall rather than close to the endograft or within an endoleak track.

Management of endotension

If the pressure within the aneurysm sac is the same as or close to systemic pressure, there is clearly a risk of rupture and consideration should be given to intervention (balancing the risk of intervention against the risk of hemorrhage and death should rupture occur). Conversely, if the pressure is very low (40 mmHg or less) one may safely assume that all is well. The problem comes between these two extremes. What does it mean if the pressure is around 50%-60% of the systemic mean? Is there a risk of rupture? Should one intervene?

It will be for the reader to decide whether or not the following guidelines are reasonable, as they are based on no evidence:
- the risk of aneurysm rupture is probably very low if the mean intra-sac pressure is less than 70% of mean systemic pressure;
- for any given mean intra-sac pressure, the risk of rupture is probably higher if there is significant variation in pressure throughout the cardiac cycle than if the pressure wave is relatively flat;
- for any given mean intra-sac pressure, the risk of rupture is probably higher if there is evidence to suggest that a previously depressurized aneurysm is again pressurized (i.e. the risk is probably higher in an aneurysm that is expanding following a period of shrinkage than it is in an aneurysm that has continued to expand since endovascular repair);

The options for treatment of graft related and sidebranch endoleak have been discussed above. If there is no endoleak but the aneurysm is continuing to expand and the pressure within the aneurysm sac is high, consideration may be given to further intervention. The options are, however, somewhat limited. One may either reline the endograft (secondary endografting) or convert to open surgical repair. Neither procedure is free from risk and it is in the author's opinion difficult to justify any intervention unless there is evidence of another problem (shortening and widening of the aneurysm neck or kinking of the endograft for example). If there is no evidence of any other problem it is very unlikely that the patient will come to harm. Even if rupture occurs this is likely to be a benign event (there are even those who advocate fenestration of such an aneurysm to permit depressurization [13] and to date the author has never offered secondary intervention to treat expansion in the absence of endoleak.

Implications for surveillance

Endovascular repair mandates life long surveillance to assure the continued efficacy of the repair and/or to detect complications that may threaten the patient (i.e. complications which may, if left untreated, result in rupture of the aneurysm and death of the patient). Surveillance does, however, impose a significant burden on the patient who must regularly attend the hospital as well as the medical staff who must review the images. It also has important cost implications. Endovascular repair offers many advantages over conventional open surgical repair and there is level I evidence of reduced morbidity and mortality. It is not cost effective and a large part of the reason for this is the cost of surveillance and secondary intervention. It is vitally important therefore that we refine our surveillance protocols to ensure that they are as reliable, safe and cost effective as possible. It is also important that we strive to rationalize the indications for secondary intervention. In the author's opinion there have been a huge number of unnecessary interventions performed over the last ten years to treat type II endoleaks and expansion in the absence of endoleak. These have caused significant morbidity and mortality. They have also lent weight to the argument that endovascular repair is not cost effective and in the current climate of limited health care resources that threatens the future of endovascular repair.

Any surveillance program must reliably detect graft related endoleak, change in aneurysm morphology, migration and reduction in renal and lower limb blood flow. The detection and management of migration are discussed elsewhere in this book but graft related endoleak and expansion can reliably be detected by Duplex ultrasound. There are those who argue that one should nonetheless subject the patient to serial CT scanning since this more reliably detects low flow type II endoleak [14]. There are even those who advocate contrast enhanced magnetic resonance imaging to identify microleaks.

The author finds it very difficult to understand the rationale behind these arguments. Does it matter if the chosen method of surveillance does not reliably detect complications which do not threaten the patient? In Liverpool, patients routinely undergo baseline CT scanning, Duplex ultrasound and plain radiography within one month of endovascular repair. Thereafter, surveillance relies on duplex ultrasound and plain radiography at one year intervals and CT scanning is only performed if Duplex ultrasound is technically unsatisfactory or reveals a problem. We take the view that we do not need to identify low flow type II or type IV endoleaks unless the aneurysm is expanding. Even then, we will in most cases manage the patient conservatively.

Summary

Graft related endoleaks (type I and type III) are a significant cause of endotension and there is a significant risk of hemorrhage if the aneurysm ruptures. In general therefore, such endoleaks should be treated by secondary intervention.

Sidebranch reperfusion (type II endoleak) is in most cases benign and can be observed. Expansion in the presence of persistent type II endoleak is an indication for further investigation to exclude alternative causes of expansion and to determine the pressure within the aneurysm sac. If the pressure is high, consideration should be given to intervention to treat the endoleak but only after careful consideration of the risk of the proposed intervention and the risk of fatal hemorrhage should rupture occur.

Expansion in the absence of endoleak is an indication for further investigation to identify possible sources of pressurization and to measure the pressure within the aneurysm sac. If this is high, consideration may be given to secondary intervention although the only rational imperative for intervention is the observation of shortening or widening of the aneurysm neck.

REFERENCES

1. White GH, Yu W, May J et al. Endoleaks as a complication of endoluminal grafting of abdominal aortic aneurysms: classification, incidence, diagnosis and management. *J Endovasc Surg* 1997; 4: 152-168.

2. Gilling-Smith GL, Brennan JA, Harris PL et al. Endotension after endovascular aneurysm repair: definition, classification and strategies for surveillance and intervention. *J Endovasc Surg* 1999; 6: 305-307.

3. Silverberg D, Baril DT, Ellzy SH et al. An 8 year experience with type II endoleaks: natural history suggests selective intervention is a safe approach. *J Vasc Surg* 2006; 44: 453-459.

4. Higashiura W, Greenberg RK, Katz E et al. Predictive factors, morphologic effects and proposed treatment paradigm for type II endoleak after repair of infrarenal abdominal aortic aneurysms. *J Vasc Interv Radiol* 2007; 18: 975-981.

5. Jones JE, Atkins MD, Brewster DC et al. Persistent Type II endoleak after endovascular repair of abdominal aortic aneurysm is associated with adverse late outcomes. *J Vasc Surg* 2007; 46: 1-8.

6. Vallabhaneni SR, Gilling-Smith GL, How TV et al. Aortic side branch perfusion alone does not account for high intra-sac pressure after endovascular repair in the absence of graft related endoleak. *Eur J Vasc Endovasc Surg* 2003; 25: 354-359.

7. Dias NV, Ivancev K, Resch TA et al. Endoleaks after endovascular aneurysm repair lead to nonuniform intra-aneurysm sac pressure. *J Vasc Surg* 2007; 46: 197-203.

8. Van Marrewijk CJ, Fransen G, Laheij RJ et al. Is a Type II endoleak after EVAR a harbinger of risk? Causes and outcome of open conversion and aneurysm rupture during follow up. *Eur J Vasc Endovasc Surg* 2004; 27: 128-137.

9. Harris PL, Vallabhaneni SR, Desgranges P et al. Incidence and risk factors of late rupture, conversion and death after endovascular repair of infrarenal aortic aneurysms: the Eurostar experience. *J Vasc Surg* 2000; 32: 739-749.

10. Baum RA, Carpenter JP, Golden MA et al. Treatment of Type II endoleaks after endovascular repair of abdominal aortic aneurysms: comparison of transarterial and translumbar techniques. *J Vasc Surg* 2002; 35: 23-29.

11. Timaran CH, Ohki T, Rhee SJ et al. Predicting aneurysm enlargement in patients with persistent type II endoleaks. *J Vasc Surg* 2004; 39: 1157-1162.

12. Vallabhaneni SR, Gilling-Smith GL, Brennan JA et al. Can intrasac pressure monitoring reliably predict failure of endovascular aneurysm repair? *J Endovasc Ther* 2003; 10: 524-530.

13. Van Nes JG, Hendriks JM, Tseng LN et al. Endoscopic aneurysm sac fenestration as a treatment option for growing aneurysms due to type II endoleak or endotension. *J Endovasc Ther* 2005; 12: 430-434.

14. AbuRahma AF. Fate of endoleaks detected by CT angiography and missed by color duplex ultrasound in endovascular grafts for abdominal aortic aneurysms. *J Endovasc Ther* 2006; 13: 490-495.

9

MIGRATION AND DISLOCATION OF AORTIC DEVICES DURING FOLLOW-UP

ANDREW ENGLAND, RICHARD MCWILLIAMS

The pulsatile blood flow within the aorta exerts relentless displacement forces on any implanted stent-graft. The device must be sufficiently well-designed to resist these displacement forces and oppose movement. Device migration and the dislocation of stent-graft components are potentially two of the more serious complications following endovascular aneurysm repair (EVAR). Both can lead to reperfusion of the aneurysm sac and aneurysm rupture. There are a number of fixation methods available on commercial stent-grafts which attempt to resist these displacement forces, including radial force, hooks and barbs, and longitudinal columnar support [1]. Despite this, migration has been reported with all commercially available stent-grafts. This chapter aims to highlight the problem of stent-graft movement within the aorta and discusses the issues surrounding the diagnosis and management of stent-graft migration and limb dislocation.

Definition

Device migration can simply be defined as the movement of an endograft from one position to another over time [1]. The most common scenarios involve caudal movement at the proximal attachment site or cranial movement of the distal attachment. With increasing interest in migration there are many proposed definitions, currently the most widely used definition is from the reporting standards of the Society of Vascular Surgery (SVS) which defines migration as ≥10 mm of stent-graft movement relative to anatomical landmarks or any migration leading to symptoms or requiring reintervention [2]. The definition of migration is in itself complex; factors such as the imaging modality, assessment methodology and experience of the observer can limit the ability to identify small changes in stent-graft position. Greenberg et al. [3] argue that a stricter definition of migration is needed and define migration as movement of more than two

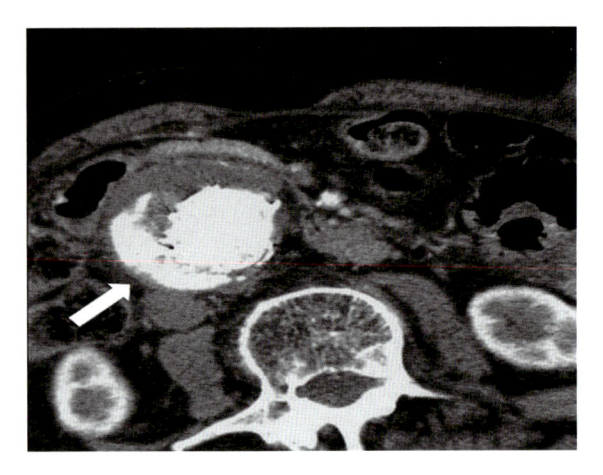

FIG. 1 A follow-up CT scan of a patient at 24-months demonstrating a large proximal type I endoleak (arrow) resulting from caudal device migration.

Diagnosis

The early years of EVAR saw a major emphasis on the detection and management of endoleak and on the assessment of changes in aortic sac morphology. Device migration has not occupied center-stage and, in the authors' experience, surveillance examinations are not routinely scrutinized for evidence of migration in many centers. The aims of surveillance should include the detection of evidence of impending failure due to progressive device migration. Once detected this allows for pre-emptive secondary intervention to avoid the possibility of late attachment site endoleak and rupture.

Stent-graft migration may be detected on several imaging modalities. The commonest surveillance imaging test after EVAR is a multi-slice CT scan. Migration is best assessed by review of the 3D-dataset at a dedicated workstation where reconstructed 3D images allow the distances between the cranial (Fig. 2) and caudal (Fig. 3) attachment sites to be calculated in relation to fixed aortic and iliac reference points such as the renal arteries, superior mesenteric arteries (SMA) and hypogastric arteries.

Litwinski et al. [4] report that elongation of the infra-renal aortic neck may result in artefactual stent-graft migration. In such cases, although the distance between the renal arteries and the stent-graft increases, this is due to elongation of the aor-

times the reconstructed resolution of the imaging study, for example if using a 5 mm reconstructed slice thickness the definition of migration would be movement of ≥10 mm. It is our experience that more subtle endograft positional changes can be identified when analyzing computed tomography (CT) datasets using 3-D workstations. The diagnosis of stent-graft migration also requires that the remaining aortic neck should be taken into consideration together with the presence or absence of an endoleak (Fig. 1) which in turn reflects the risk of aneurysm sac pressurization and can guide management.

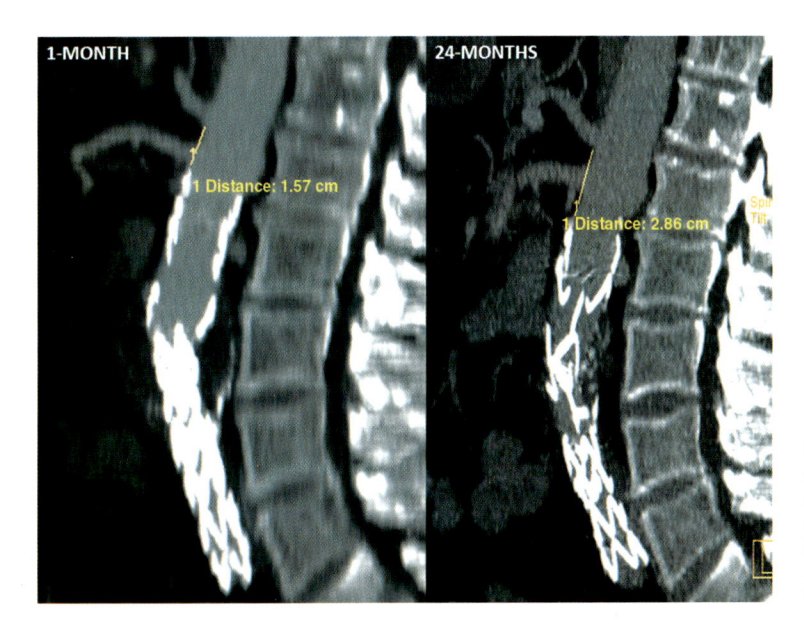

FIG. 2 Follow-up sagittal CT reformatted images showing the distance between the celiac axis and the proximal portion of the stent-graft on the 1-month and 24-month follow-up scans. There has been 12.9 mm of caudal stent-graft migration during the follow-up period.

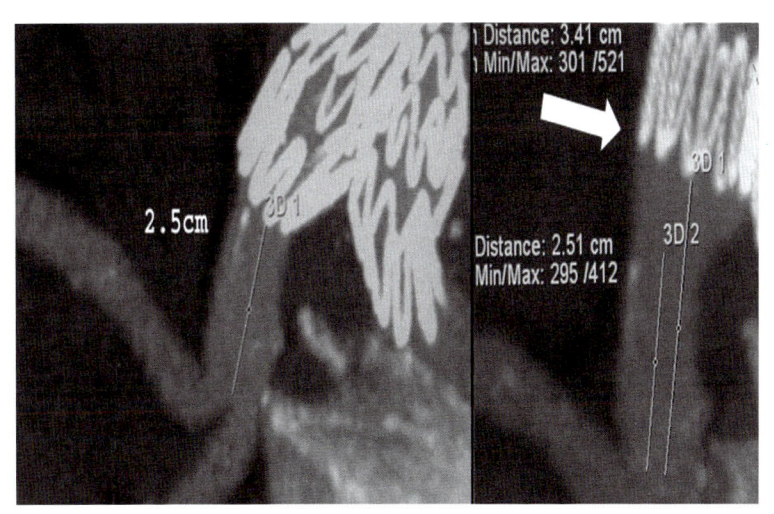

FIG. 3 Oblique reformatted CT images showing dilatation of the right common iliac artery with subsequent cranial migration of the iliac limb (arrow).

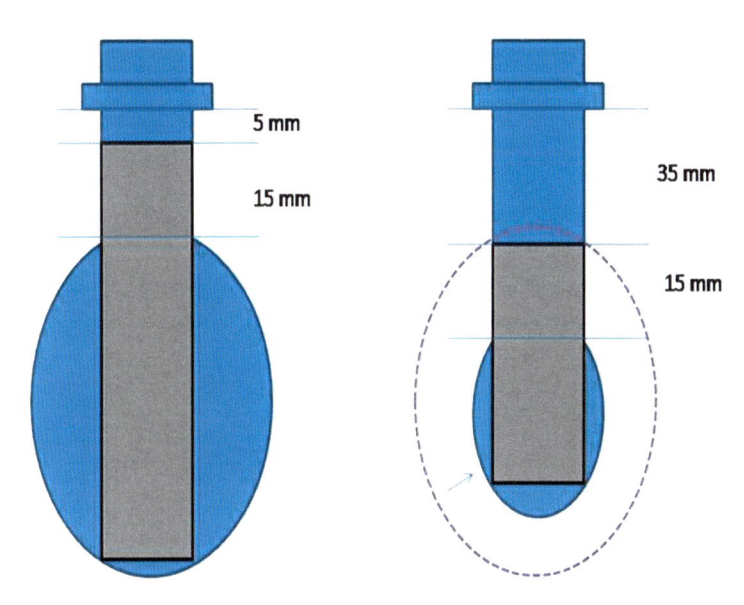

FIG. 4 A diagram demonstrating the theory of device migration in the presence of a regressing aneurysm. If the length of the seal is maintained in the presence of a regressing aneurysm this could be actual migration as opposed to aortic elongation or pseudomigration.

ta rather than caudal migration of the stent-graft. In their series of patients treated with the Aneurx graft they identified patients with little or no reduction in the length of the seal and yet increase in the distance of the stent-graft from the renal arteries. The argument seems valid that if the increased distance from the renal arteries was due to migration then the length of the seal should reduce. If such is not the case then aortic elongation may have occurred.

An additional possibility (Fig. 4) when the length of seal is maintained but the distance between the graft and renal arteries has increased might be that the aneurysm sac has regressed and the neck length has therefore increased. In this circumstance true migration may have occurred despite the length of seal being maintained. It is well known that migration may occur in the presence of a shrinking aneurysm and there are hemodynamic reasons that may explain this. The longitudinal displacement force is dependent on the pressure gradient between the stent-graft and the aneurysm sac. If the aneurysm is reducing in size and depressurized then the pressure gradient is high and the displacement forces also consequently high. This theory supports the clinical observation which is made during surveillance after EVAR when migration is detected despite aneurysm regression and this migration may lead to late proximal type 1 endoleak and rupture in a shrinking aneurysm.

The work of Litwinski et al. [4] is important and introduces the possibility of pseudo-migration when interpreting surveillance CT scans. It also emphasizes the relationship between migration and residual seal zone which is relevant both in diagnosis and management of stent-graft migration.

CT scanning after thoracic EVAR allows the assessment of migration with respect to proximal and distal aortic reference points. The proximal reference point will be a patent aortic arch branch and the distal reference point the celiac axis if patent. O'Neill et al. [5] have elegantly demonstrated the importance of using 3D analysis in this typically tortuous anatomy and showed considerable advantage to using a technique of semi-automated centerline of flow measurement. Aortic elongation was also observed in their study and they recommend calculation of the total aortic length between the proximal and distal reference points to determine if elongation has occurred as this will potentially explain apparent endograft migration in a small number of cases.

Migration may be detected at ultrasound or be inferred by surrogate markers of possible migration. Ultrasound is not suitable for the surveillance of thoracic aneurysms but is now increasingly used as an alternative test to CT scanning in the surveillance of abdominal stent-grafts. Migration may be assessed with reference to a fixed aortic reference point such as the SMA which is more reliably seen than the renal arteries. Migration is diagnosed if the distance from the SMA to the top of the stent-graft increases in excess of an arbitrary threshold which reflects the likely measurement error. Migration must also be considered when a graft-related endoleak is observed or if there is reduced limb blood flow. Graft distortion may be secondary to migration and this is the reason that altered limb blood flow must prompt a search for stent-graft migration.

Ultrasound is not the optimal test for the assessment of migration and is used in surveillance primarily to measure the sac diameter and detect endoleak. Ultrasound is therefore combined with plain radiography in surveillance. Plain radiographs performed according to a standardized protocol [6] are a good test for migration and component separation. Currently migration is typically assessed with reference to non-aortic landmarks such as the vertebral bodies. It is possible that implanted aortic markers may be used in future to further improve the accuracy of the plain radiographic assessment of migration [7].

When significant migration is detected at ultrasound or on plain radiographs then it is our practice to perform a multi-slice CT scan to confirm the diagnosis, exclude the possibility of pseudo-migration as described above and to quantify the residual seal zone to guide management.

Prevalence

Varying approaches to the detection of migration are likely to explain much of the different reported rates of migration of thoracic and abdominal endografts. The reported migration rates of thoracic grafts varies from 0%-30% [5]. Different fixation mechanisms are used for abdominal grafts and this is likely to partly explain the different rates of migration with different devices; however, even with the same device there are widely varying reported migration rates: 0.0%-21.0% for the Aneurx graft, 2.0%-17.5% for the Talent graft and 1.9%-8.2% for the Zenith graft (Table).

There have been a small number of reports of apparent cranial migration of the proximal portion of infra-renal stent-grafts [21]. The typical scenario is that a completion angiogram is performed demonstrating patent renal arteries. A delayed investigation reveals renal artery occlusion and therefore proximal migration of the stent-graft is assumed. The report from Katzen et al. [21] bases this on a catheter angiogram without CT confirmation.

It should be noted that significant renal artery coverage with fabric may be present and yet not impair flow immediately after deployment. Unless the image intensifier is aligned optimally with the renal ostia, typically using cranial and oblique angulation, then the operating team may be unaware of this partial renal coverage. When these renal arteries occlude in a delayed manner, as it may happen, then it is possible for an erroneous conclusion of proximal stent-graft migration to be made. Unless comparative high quality CT datasets are available at different time points to clearly show movement in relation to aortic reference points, then it is our opinion that the inference of cranial stent-graft migration solely based on delayed renal artery thrombosis is likely to be inaccurate.

Fenestrated grafts incorporate the renal and other visceral arteries in the seal zone and therefore caudal migration of the proximal sealing stent could result in catastrophic visceral artery occlu-

Table INCIDENCE OF DEVICE MIGRATION BY ENDOGRAFT

Device/study	First author [ref.]	N	Follow-up, mo	Definition (mm)	Migration (%)
AneuRx	Zarins [8]	190	12	NA	6.0
	Cao [9]	113	28	≥10	15.0
	Conners [10]	49	24	≥5	20.4
	Sternbergh [11]	81	26	≥5	8.6
	Tonnessen [12]	77	39	≥10	18.2
Talent	Lee [13]	40	17	≥10	17.5
	Criado [14]	240	13.5	≥5	2.0
	Ouriel [15]	39	12	≥10	0.0
	England [16]	38	24	≥10	15.8
Zenith	Greenberg [17]	301	14	≥5	2.7
	Ouriel [15]	144	12	≥10	8.2
	Sternbergh [18]	261	12	≥5	2.3
	Tonnessen [12]	53	30.8	≥5	7.5
Excluder	Kibbe [19]	235	24	NA	1.0
	Ouriel [15]	25	12	>10	0.0
EUROSTAR	Mohan [20]	2862	1-6 years	>5	3.5

NA: not available

sion. The Zenith fenestrated graft is based on a composite body design and the fenestrated proximal component is tubular. The distal component incorporates the graft bifurcation where the largest forces act [22] and this design is intended to minimize the risk of caudal migration of the proximal component. The bifurcated distal component, subjected to the longitudinal distraction force, may migrate caudally (Fig. 5) and adequate overlap is needed to allow for this potential distraction. The renal stents contribute to the stability of the proximal component and experimental data record a significant increase in the pullout force of a fenestrated graft compared to a standard device [23]. In our series of 52 fenestrated cases we have not seen significant migration of the proximal graft although we have seen minor migration in one case consistent with barb engagement.

Causative factors

Graft deployment is within the direct control of the operator. Freedom from migration will be aided by optimal implantation. Ultimately this depends on the stent-graft delivery system, experience of the operator and real-time image guidance. The attachments sites must be adequately profiled to allow maximum engagement of the endograft. Typically for infra-renal grafts this involves cranial and oblique angulation for the proximal landing zones and caudal and oblique angulation at the iliac landing zones.

Aortic neck dilatation has been identified as a risk factor for migration by many authors. Following EVAR, up to one third of patients will experience proximal neck dilatation whilst the prevalence for device migration is much lower. It is notoriously difficult to predict patients who will experience proximal neck dilatation and subsequent migration. Late neck dilatation following EVAR is a major cause of concern because of the potential loss of a proximal attachment site seal. Significant neck dilatation should be taken into consideration when outlining the surveillance programme for a particular patient even in the absence of any adverse events. Surveillance intervals should be kept under regular review as initial neck expansion may plateau over time [24]. A contributing factor to neck dilatation is the radial force from the stent-

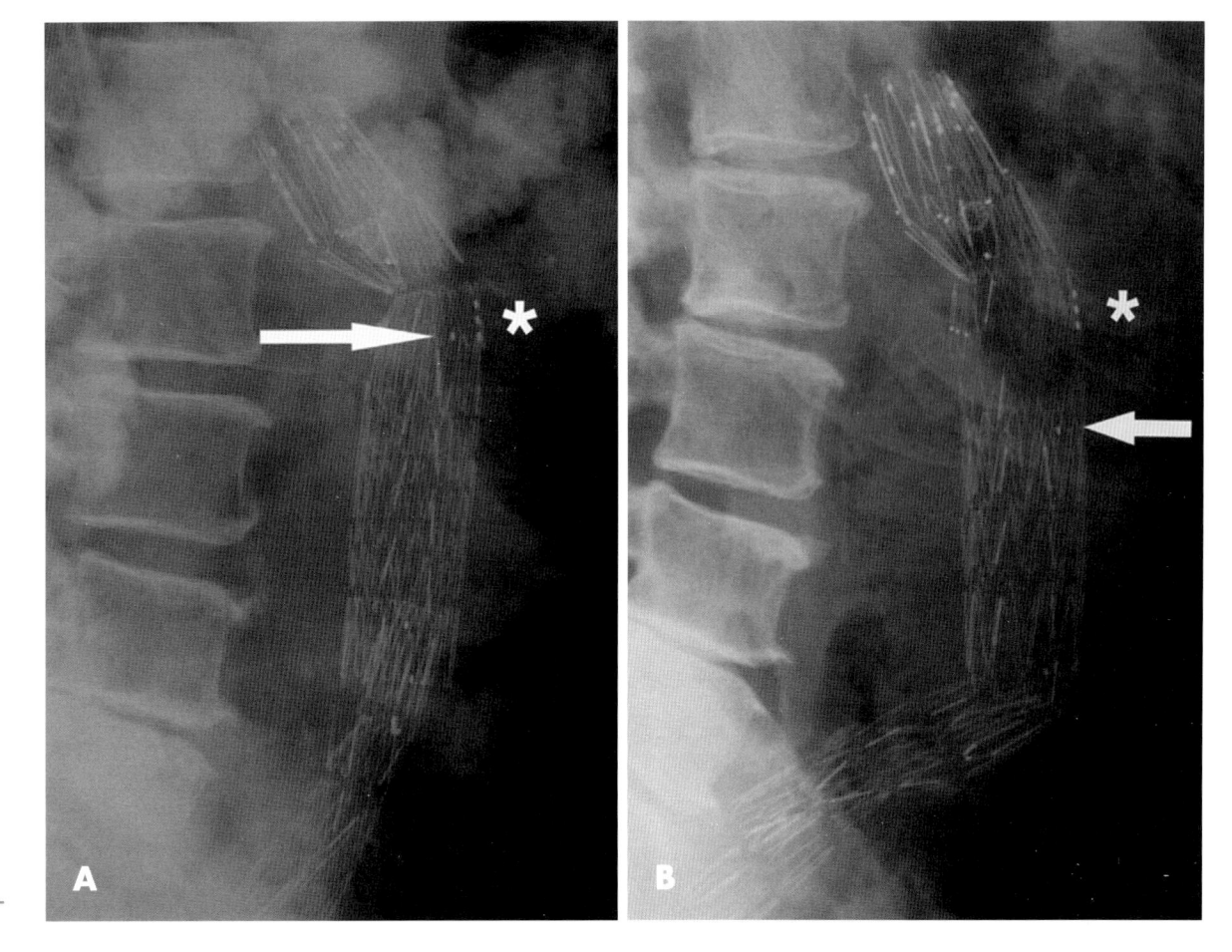

FIG. 5 Lateral abdominal radiographs demonstrating a distal bifurcated component separation of a fenestrated Zenith endograft. The proximal portion of the distal component (arrow) has moved caudally (B).

graft, this may vary between devices and is certainly affected by the degree of stent-graft oversizing.

Currently most stent-graft manufacturers recommend stent-graft oversizing from between 10% to 20%. Careful selection of the appropriate proximal stent-graft diameter is essential in order to provide both a seal and prevention of a proximal type I endoleak. The oversizing of stent-grafts must be used with caution as oversizing beyond 20% has been associated with a greater rate of proximal neck dilatation which in turn can lead to device migration. In the US Zenith multicenter trial, stent-graft oversizing greater than 30% was the only significant predictor of migration at 12-months [18].

The individual design of stent-grafts may play a significant role in the prevention of device migration. As stated previously there are a number of specific design features on stent-grafts which are aimed at preventing device migration. These include radial force stents, hooks and barbs, and longitudinal columnar support. Research using cadaveric aortas [25] has demonstrated differences in the forces needed to displace stent-grafts with hooks or barbs against stent-grafts without. This invitro work by Malina et al. [25] identified that by adding hooks and barbs to stent-graft devices the fixation of the device could be increased tenfold. Early clinical experience using hooks and barbs (Ancure device) yielded relatively high migration rates (>50%) but with improvements in device technology and stent-graft implantation expertise the incidence fell considerably [26]. The Zenith stent-graft subsequently has an accepted low migration rate, however, this has not been found to be significantly better than other stent-grafts systems which do not utilise hooks and barbs [15,27]. As stated previously these studies are limited in mean follow-up period, migration definition and assessment methodology. In the UK EVAR trial [27] the definition of migration was not recorded and made by the individual centres and not a core lab.

Most EVAR preoperative imaging protocols rely on contrast-enhanced CT angiography (CTA) with three dimensional post-processing for sizing the endograft and planning the procedure. The resulting images are static and may not fully demonstrate the degree of aortic conformational changes during the cardiac cycle. With current high-speed CT scanners the time taken to scan the aneurysm neck is only a fraction of the cardiac cycle and therefore the images could be acquired during diastole (minimum diameter) or systole (maximum diameter), or somewhere in between. Following work by van Herwaarden et al. [28] there may be significant changes within the aortic neck during the cardiac cycle which may lead to improper endograft sizing, with subsequent graft migration, intermittent type I endoleaks, and poor patient outcome. Herwaarden et al. [28] stressed the need to consider the role of dynamic imaging tools in the assessment of preoperative aortic dynamics like high-resolution ECG-gated cine magnetic resonance angiography (MRA).

There are also questions about the influence of aortic neck thombus and calcification as a risk factor for migration. Severe calcification of the aortic neck may restrict the hooks and barbs engaging in the aortic wall and thus reduce the effectiveness of this in protecting the device from the downward pulsatile force of blood. Alternatively a calcified aortic neck may restrict the tendency of the neck to dilate and provide further protection from migration. The benefit or risk of having a calcified aortic neck in preventing migration needs further investigation. Similarly little is known about the effect of neck thrombus on the stability of the device. The majority of interventionalists are cautious about deploying a stent-graft in a thrombus lined neck in view of the likelihood of endoleak or embolus. Consequently it may be difficult to ascertain the influence of this variable on migration.

Along with overlap, neck angulation has been linked with migration. Increasing incidences of migration have been associated with increasing degrees of aortic neck angulation. Both Albertini et al. [29] and Sternbergh et al. [11] confirmed an association between graft neck angulation and migration.

The importance of the distal seal zones has received relatively little attention in its ability to prevent migration. Heikkinen et al. [30] were first to report on the potential importance of iliac fixation; in their study migration was identified in 10% of patients and all were found to have suboptimal iliac fixation on the post-implantation CT. Iliac fixation in this study was categorized according to fixation length and distance from the common iliac bifurcation. This study failed to take into consideration the common iliac artery diameters, presence of calcification, tortuosity and other potentially influential factors. More recently a publication by Benharash et al. [31] found that suprarenal and infrarenal stent-graft devices may rely heavily on iliac fixation to maintain positional stability.

Component separation

In modular stent-graft systems there is the potential for individual components to separate. Zarins [1] emphasises the need to assess movement of stent-graft components as well as assessing the proximal and distal margins of the stent-graft. Component separation in the majority of cases is operator dependant and due to inadequate junctional overlap between stent-graft components. Component separation was originally a relatively early occurring complication which was more prevalent in first generation endografts. Even today radiological surveillance either by plain film or CT is essential in order to identify junctional component separation. A junction separation (Fig. 6) can lead to a type III endoleak and subsequently require secondary reintervention with either a bridging stent-graft or more infrequently an aorto-uniiliac conversion [31].

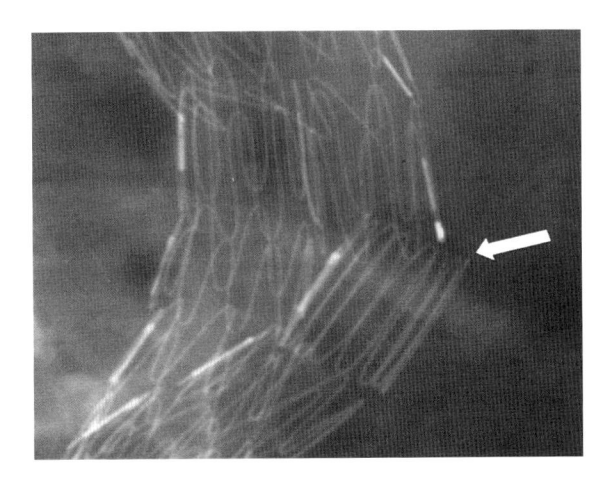

FIG. 6 Lateral abdominal radiograph demonstrating a junctional separation of a Zenith endograft (arrow).

There is in addition the possibility of the metallic components of the endograft to fracture and separate. For the covered portions of the stent-graft the fabric will provide some resistance against the fractured component moving. However, if there is a fracture of bare portions of the stent-graft e.g. bare suprarenal struts, there can be separation from the main body of the device (Fig. 7).

Treatment

The management of migration can be conservative, endovascular or surgical and depends on many factors including the extent of migration, stent-graft device implanted, fitness of the patient and local skills available.

Not all migration will produce clinical sequelae or require secondary reintervention. There is the potential for an endograft to migrate caudally and stabilize without failing into the aneurysm sac and subsequently losing its seal. More often migration can lead to seal failure and endoleak and therefore requires secondary intervention. Using data from the EUROSTAR registry Hobo et al. [32] reported that 1.5% of patients required a secondary procedure as a result of migration. Data from the more recent UK EVAR trial supports this whereby 2.3% of patients required a secondary interventional procedure as a consequence of migration.

It is not uncommon to see a very small amount of caudal migration of the Zenith graft due to engagement of the downward pointing barbs (Fig. 8). The migration distance for this engagement to occur is typically 3-5 mm. The barbs should remain downward pointing after engagement and the fixation force at this point should be much higher. We are happy to manage this conservatively in a surveillance programme as the mechanism is understood and further migration is not expected.

If a graft without barbs migrates then it is possible that the distraction force has exceeded a constant fixation force and the level of concern should be higher in this circumstance. Review of the original infra-renal neck anatomy will sometimes indicate that the stent-graft has settled into a more stable position in a neck that has varying caliber. We have seen some cases of caudal migration of the proximal stents of endografts without barbs into a new position after which no further migration occurs.

If there has been minor migration, which we elect to treat conservatively, then we will increase the frequency of surveillance to 6-monthly review until either the endograft can be shown to have a new stable position or until intervention is mandated because of progressive migration.

The endovascular management of caudal migration of the proximal endograft usually involves proximal cuff extension (Fig. 9). If an endograft without barbs has migrated then it is logical to extend proximally with a cuff that has a greater pull-out force by incorporating barbs. These can be dif-

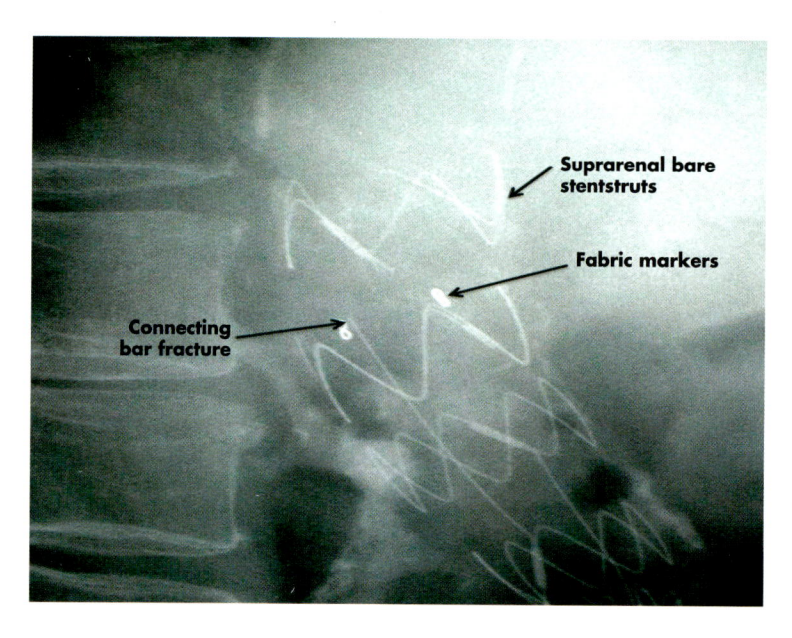

FIG. 7 Lateral abdominal radiograph 24-months following implantation of a Talent stent-graft. There is a connecting bar fracture with separation of the suprarenal component of the stent-graft and caudal migration of the main body of the endograft.

ficult procedures if the original device had a short body and it is important to ensure optimal overlap of the cuff with the body of the original device otherwise the original endograft may continue to migrate caudally and dislocate from the proximal cuff. Surveillance imaging after such an intervention must include assessment for this.

Proximal extension with a fenestrated cuff may be required if there is an inadequate seal zone in the infra-renal segment. Although fenestrated endografts are now widely used, it must be remembered that working within the confines of a pre-existing endograft makes the deployment of a cuff extension difficult. This is largely because of the risk of not having sufficient rotational control of the fenestrated graft which is required to safely position the fenestrations in relation to the target vessels.

Percutaneous suturing devices are now being devised to try and stabilize migrating devices but it is too early in their evolution to know if these will be effective. Cranial migration at the iliac attachment sites can be managed by extension with another endovascular graft either to the lower common iliac if there is a suitable landing zone or with extension to the external iliac. Migration leading to device failure may also be managed with open surgical conversion. There has also been a report of laparoscopic surgical conversion with removal of the original endograft [33].

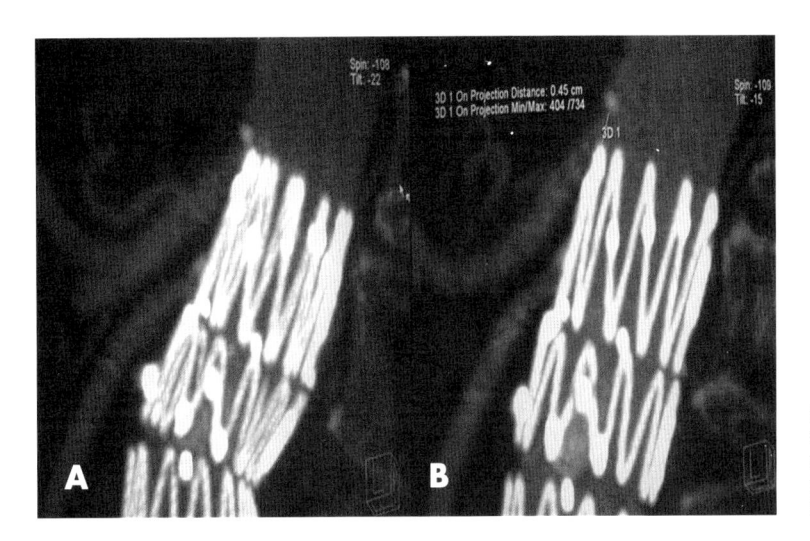

FIG. 8 Follow-up CT reformatted images demonstrating barb engagement of a Zenith endograft. There is 4.5mm of caudal device movement which represents the barbs engaging in the aortic wall.

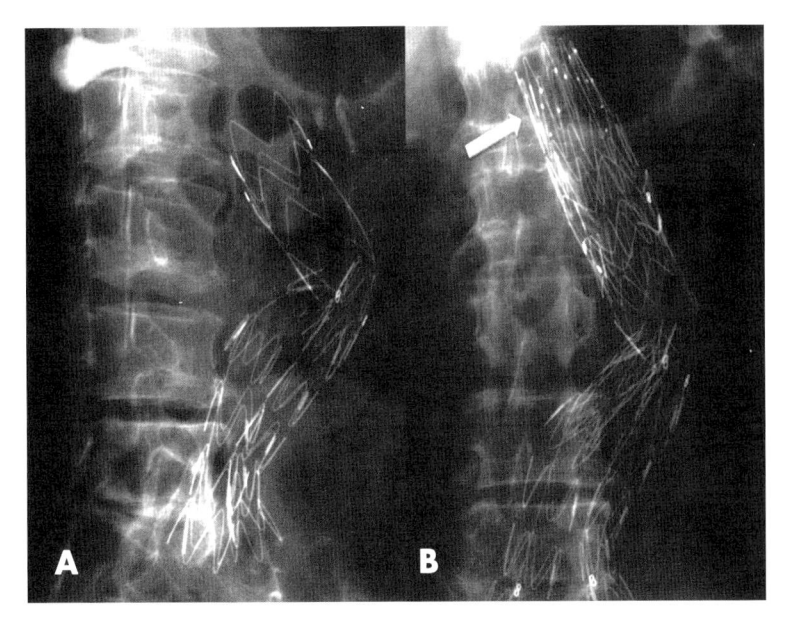

FIG. 9 There has been proximal migration of a Talent stent-graft (A). A Zenith proximal cuff (arrow) has been implanted to prevent further migration and proximal type I endoleak.

Prevention

Migration rates should be reduced by careful case selection and precise stent-graft deployment. Precise deployment ensures maximum engagement of the potential aortic, iliac and graft overlap zones. Despite good case selection and optimal deployment, we know that migration will still occur and stent-graft improvements are necessary to further reduce this problem.

Significant migration of the proximal sealing stent is an uncommon problem due to supra-renal fixation with barbed anchor stents. Cranial migration of the distal sealing stents continues to be a cause of problems and the addition of cranially angled barbs to engage in the wall of the iliac artery is worthy of consideration by manufacturers. Endovascular stapling is another potential means of arresting or preventing migration.

Hypertension was shown to be a risk factor for migration in the EUROSTAR database [20] and the blood pressure is a major contributor to the in vivo distraction force. Good control of hypertension in the post-operative phase after EVAR is not only an essential component of best medical therapy but may also help to prevent migration.

REFERENCES

1. Zarins CK. Stent-graft migration: how do we know when we have it and what is its significance? *J Endovasc Ther* 2004; 11: 364-365.
2. Chaikof EL, Blankensteijn JD, Harris PL et al. Ad Hoc Committee for Standardized Reporting Practices in Vascular Surgery of The Society for Vascular Surgery/American Association for Vascular Surgery. Reporting standards for endovascular aortic aneurysm repair. *J Vasc Surg* 2002; 35: 1048-1060.
3. Greenberg RK, Turc A, Haulon S et al. Stent-graft migration: a reappraisal of analysis methods and proposed revised definition. *J Endovasc Ther* 2004; 11: 353-363.
4. Litwinski RA, Donayre CE, Chow SL et al. The role of aortic neck dilation and elongation in the etiology of stent graft migration after endovascular abdominal aortic aneurysm repair with a passive fixation device. *J Vasc Surg* 2006; 44: 1176-1181.
5. O'Neill S, Greenberg RK, Resch T et al. An evaluation of centerline of flow measurement techniques to assess migration after thoracic endovascular aneurysm repair. *J Vasc Surg* 2006; 43: 1103-1110.
6. Murphy M, Hodgson R, Harris P et al. Plain radiographic surveillance of abdominal aortic stent-grafts: the Liverpool/Perth protocol. *J Endovasc Ther* 2003 ;10:911-912.
7. Koning O, Oudegeest O, Valstar E et al. Roentgen stereophotogrammetric analysis: an accurate tool to assess stent-graft migration. *J Endovasc Ther* 2006; 13: 468-475.
8. Zarins CK, White RA, Schwarten D et al. AneuRx stent graft versus open surgical repair of abdominal aortic aneurysms: multicenter prospective clinical trial. *J Vasc Surg* 1999; 29: 292-305.
9. Cao P, Verzini F, Zannetti S et al. Device migration after endoluminal abdominal aortic aneurysm repair: analysis of 113 cases with a minimum follow-up period of 2 years. *J Vasc Surg* 2002; 35: 229-235.
10. Conners MS 3rd, Sternbergh WC 3rd, Carter G et al. Endograft migration one to four years after endovascular abdominal aortic aneurysm repair with the AneuRx device: a cautionary note. *J Vasc Surg* 2002; 36: 476-484.
11. Sternbergh WC 3rd, Carter G, York JW et al. Aortic neck angulation predicts adverse outcome with endovascular abdominal aortic aneurysm repair. *J Vasc Surg* 2002; 35: 482-486.
12. Tonnessen BH, Sternbergh WC 3rd et al. Mid- and long-term device migration after endovascular abdominal aortic aneurysm repair: a comparison of AneuRx and Zenith endografts. *J Vasc Surg* 2005; 42: 392-400.
13. Lee JT, Lee J, Aziz I et al. Stent-graft migration following endovascular repair of aneurysms with large proximal necks: anatomical risk factors and clinical sequelae. *J Endovasc Ther* 2002; 9: 652-664.
14. Criado FJ, Fairman RM, Becker GJ et al. Talent LPS AAA stent graft: results of a pivotal clinical trial. *J Vasc Surg* 2003; 37: 709-715.
15. Ouriel K, Clair DG, Greenberg RK et al. Endovascular repair of abdominal aortic aneurysms: device-specific outcome. *J Vasc Surg* 2003; 37: 991-998.
16. England A, Butterfield JS, Jones N et al. Device migration after endovascular abdominal aortic aneurysm repair: experience with a Talent stent-graft. *J Vasc Interv Radiol* 2004; 15: 1399-1405.
17. Greenberg RK, Lawrence-Brown M, Bhandari G et al. An update of the Zenith endovascular graft for abdominal aortic aneurysms: initial implantation and mid-term follow-up data. *J Vasc Surg* 2001; 33(S2): S157-S164.
18. Sternbergh WC 3rd, Money SR, Greenberg RK et al. Influence of endograft oversizing on device migration, endoleak, aneurysm shrinkage, and aortic neck dilatation: results from the Zenith Multicenter Trial. *J Vasc Surg* 2004; 39: 20-26.
19. Kibbe MR, Matsumura JS; Excluder Investigators. The Gore Excluder US multi-center trial: analysis of adverse events at 2 years. *Semin Vasc Surg* 2003; 16: 144-150.
20. Mohan IV, Harris PL, Van Marrewijk CJ et al. Factors and forces influencing stent-graft migration after endovascular aortic aneurysm repair. *J Endovasc Ther* 2002; 9: 748-755.
21. Katzen B, MacLean A, Katzman H. Retrograde migration of an abdominal aortic aneurysm endograft leading to postoperative renal failure. *J Vasc Surg* 2005; 42: 784-787.
22. Howell BA, Kim T, Cheer A et al. Computational fluid dynamics within bifurcated abdominal aortic stent-grafts. *J Endovasc Ther* 2007; 14: 138-143.

23. Zhou SS, How TV, Vallabhaneni S et al. Comparison of the fixation strength of standard and fenestrated stent-grafts for endovascular abdominal aortic aneurysm repair. *J Endovasc Ther* 2007; 14: 168-175.

24. May J, White G, Yu W et al. A prospective study of anatomico-pathological changes in abdominal aortic aneurysms following endoluminal repair: is the aneurysmal process reversed? *Eur J Vasc Endovasc Surg* 1996; 12: 11-17.

25. Malina M, Lindblad B, Ivancev K et al. Endovascular AAA exclusion: will stents with hooks and barbs prevent stent-graft migration? *J Endovasc Surg* 1998; 5: 310-317.

26. Alric P, Hinchliffe R, Wenham P et al. Lessons learned from the long-term follow-up of a first-generation aortic stent graft. *J Vasc Surg* 2003; 37: 367-373.

27. Brown L, Greenhalgh R, Kwong G et al. Secondary interventions and mortality following endovascular aortic aneurysm repair: device-specific results from the UK EVAR trials. *Eur J Vasc Endovasc Surg* 2007; 34: 281-290.

28. van Herwaarden JA, Bartels LW, Muhs BE et al. Dynamic magnetic resonance angiography of the aneurysm neck: conformational changes during the cardiac cycle with possible consequences for endograft sizing and future design. *J Vasc Surg* 2006; 44: 22-28.

29. Albertini J, Kalliafas S, Travis S et al. Anatomical risk factors for proximal perigraft endoleak and graft migration following endovascular repair of abdominal aortic aneurysms. *Eur J Vasc Endovasc Surg* 2000; 19: 308-312.

30. Heikkinen MA, Alsac JM, Arko FR et al. The importance of iliac fixation in prevention of stent graft migration. *J Vasc Surg* 2006; 43: 1130-1137.

31. Benharash P, Lee JT, Abilez OJ et al. Iliac fixation inhibits migration of both suprarenal and infrarenal aortic endografts. *J Vasc Surg* 2007; 45: 250-257.

32. Hobo R, Buth J; EUROSTAR collaborators. Secondary interventions following endovascular abdominal aortic aneurysm repair using current endografts. A EUROSTAR report. *J Vasc Surg* 2006; 43: 896-902.

33. Lin J, Kolvenbach R, Wassiljew S et al. Totally laparoscopic explantation of migrated stent graft after endovascular aneurysm repair: a report of two cases. *J Vasc Surg* 2005; 41: 885-888.

THE RISK OF SPINAL CORD ISCHEMIA DURING THORACIC AND ABDOMINAL AORTIC ENDOGRAFTING

ROBERTO CHIESA, GERMANO MELISSANO, LUCA BERTOGLIO
MASSIMILIANO MARIA MARROCCO-TRISCHITTA, EFREM CIVILINI
YAMUME TSHOMBA, FABIO MASSIMO CALLIARI
ENRICO MARIA MARONE, GILIOLA CALORI

The pathophysiology of spinal cord ischemia (SCI), a most dreaded complication, is still poorly understood. The introduction of endovascular treatment with stent-grafts for the thoracic aorta (TEVAR) has significantly reduced the morbidity associated with thoracotomy and aortic cross clamping, but has it also reduced the incidence of SCI? Can the peculiar features of SCI after TEVAR help us to better understand its underlying mechanisms?

We believe that the clinical setting of TEVAR provides an opportunity to improve the knowledge of this devastating complication, since it removes the background noise of the effect of aortic cross-clamping and intercostal arteries reimplantation.

The aim of this study is to prospectively evaluate the incidence and characteristics of SCI in 206 consecutive patients submitted to TEVAR at our Institution between 1999 and 2007.

Patients and methods

We conducted an analysis of data prospectively collected on a computerized database of 206 consecutive patients (176 men, mean age 68.6±10.8 years) undergoing TEVAR at our Institution between January 1999 and April 2007. The results of the first 103 cases of this series have been previously reported [1]. Etiology included atherosclerotic aneurysm in 166 cases, type B dissection in 21, penetrating ulcer/intramural hematoma in 7, pseudoaneurysm in 6, trauma in 3 and different causes in other 3.

According to Ishimaru's classification [2], the proximal aortic landing zones involved were: Zone 0 in 15 cases, Zone 1 in 13, Zone 2 in 42, Zone 3 in 67 and Zone 4 in 69. In 17 patients, the distal landing zone was located below the celiac axis and therefore defined as thoraco-abdominal aortic pathology. Thirty-six patients had previous infrarenal aorta open repair that was performed sincronously to TEVAR in 4 cases; 17 patients had previous open or endovascular repair of TAA.

We implanted several different commercially available stent-grafts: 55 Excluder TAG, old and new device (WL Gore and Associates, Inc, Flagstaff, Ariz), 11 Endofit (Endomed, Phoenix, Ariz), 9 Talent and Vailant (Medtronic, Santa Rosa, Calif), 126 Zenith TX1 and TX2 (Cook Inc, Bloomington, Ind) and 5 Relay (Bolton Medical España S.L.U., Barcelona, Spain).

Diagnostic work-up to assess the feasibility of TEVAR, sizing of the stent-grafts and implant strategy was determined preoperatively, preferably with 16 or 64-Row Multislice Computed Tomography with multiplanar reconstructions. Since June 2005, localization of the Adamkiewicz artery or arteria radicularis magna (ARM) and its segmental supplier was assessed with the same preoperative computed tomography and with magnetic resonance angiography. Data analysis is currently in progress. All the procedures were performed in the operating room, using a portable digital C-arm image intensifier with road-mapping capabilities. Intra-operative transesophageal echocardiography was used in 31 patients including all cases of aortic dissection. The procedures were performed under general anesthesia in 139 cases, epidural or subaracnoid anesthesia in 50, and local anesthesia in 17. CSF drainage was instituted in 27 selected patients; indications were an aneurysm involving intercostal arteries between T8 and L1, the required coverage of a descending thoracic aortic segment ≥15 cm and, since 2005, previous AAA repair [3]. The drainage was inserted postoperatively in all the 11 patients that developed SCI-related deficits.

In 180 cases (87.4%) the common femoral artery, exposed through an inguinal incision, was used as access vessel. A direct arterial puncture without a conduit for an aorto-iliac approach was used in 21 cases (10.2%) and in 5 patients (2.4%) the device was inserted through an infra-renal aortic graft during combined surgery for synchronous AAA.

TEVAR for Zone 0 and 1 or for thoraco-abdominal aorta cases was accomplished with an associated supra-aortic or visceral vessel debranching as previously reported [4,5]. In case of aortic arch involvement (Zone 0, 1 and 2), intentional overstenting of the left subclavian artery (LSA) was performed in 50 cases. In 20 cases (2 cases of Zone 0, 4 cases of Zone 1, 14 cases of Zone 2), we performed a revascularization of the LSA. The latter was deemed necessary when LSA supplied coronary circulation through a left internal thoracic artery-to-left anterior descending coronary artery bypass grafting, when the controlateral vertebral artery was inadequate, in young patients, left handed professionals or to improve spinal cord collateral circulation (since 2005) in cases of previous abdominal aortic surgery.

All patients were evaluated with post-procedural contrast CT scan and then followed-up by means of clinical evaluation and aortic imaging at 1, 6 and 12 months, and yearly thereafter. Angiograms were obtained in selected cases (i.e. endoleaks).

Patients were stratified and results described according to the reporting standards for endovascular aortic repair [6]. Different types of endoleak were classified according to contrast CT scan findings [7].

SCI was assessed by an independent neurologist and graded according to the Modified Tarlov Scale. Paraplegia or paraparesis observed immediately or upon awakening were defined as immediate. Deficit occurring after a period of normal neurologic function were classified as delayed. We investigated the role of the following factors as possible predictors of spinal cord ischemia: demographic factors classified according to Society of Vascular Surgery Suggested Reporting Standards, peri-operative cardiac risk index according to the Goldman revised cardiac risk index (RCRI), previous abdominal or thoracic aorta surgery, etiology, proximal aortic landing zone, intentional coverage of left subclavian artery without revascularization, coverage of critical intercostals arteries (T8 to L1), preoperative CSF drainage, length and type of device used, intraoperative and postoperative lowest mean arterial pressure < 70 mmHg.

Data are shown as number (%) for categorical variables or as median, 1st quartile and 3rd quartile (Q1-Q3) and mean for continuous variables, as they did not show a gaussian distribution. Comparisons of categorical variables among different classes of patients have been performed by means of the Chi-square test or the Fisher exact test. Continuous variables have been compared by the Mann-Whitney test or Kruskal-Wallis test. Univariate and multivariate analyses were conducted for risks factors associated to spinal cord ischemia and odds ratio and 95% confidence limits (95% C.I.) are shown. Analyzes were performed using SAS 8.02 software (SAS Institute Inc, Cary, NC-USA) and SPSS/PC+ 15.0 statistical software (SPSS, Inc, Chicago, III) for Windows (Microsoft, Redmond, Wash).

Results

Overall, a primary technical success was achieved in 195/206 cases (94.7%). One patient died intra-operatively [8]. Ten patients (4.9%) had a residual type IA endoleak that was left untreated because the aortic proximal neck was deemed inadequate for further endovascular procedures.

An initial (30 day) clinical success was obtained in 185/206 cases (89.8%) with a mortality rate of 5.3%. Causes of death included: intra-operative graft migration in 1 case, stroke in 3 cases, multi-organ embolization in 1 case, multiple organ failure in 4 cases, bleeding and acute respiratory failure in 1 case each. One patient was electively submitted to a successful surgical conversion 2 weeks after the procedure because of a total collapse of the graft.

SCI was recorded in 13/206 cases (6.3%): 4 cases were immediate and more severe and 9 cases had a delayed onset (up to 35 days after the procedure). Among patients with immediate SCI, 2 died in-hospital, 1 had a partial recovery and 1 did not improve. Among those with delayed SCI, after CSF drainage, steroids administration and arterial pressure pharmacologic adjustment, 6 patients recovered completely, 2 had a partial improvement and one case did not improve (Table I).

At a mean follow-up of 11±8 months 1 patient who suffered from a delayed moderate SCI that

Table I — PRINCIPAL CHARACTERISTICS OF PATIENTS WITH SPINAL CORD ISCHEMIA

Case	Zone	Previous aortic surgery	Preoperative CSFD	Onset (days)	Tarlov at onset	Tarlov at discharge	Outcome
#1	3	No	No	Immediate	0	4	Discharged
#2	4	No	No	Immediate	0	1	Late death (3 m.)
#3	4	Previous AAA	No	Immediate	0	0	In-hospital death
#4	2	Previous AAA	No	Immediate	0	0	In-hospital death
#5	3	Previous AAA	Yes	Immediate	3	4	Discharged
#6	TAAA	Previous TAAA	No	Delayed (3)	3	5	Discharged
#7	4	Pervious AAA	No	Delayed (2)	2	5	Discharged
#8	4	No	No	Delayed (1)	1	5	Discharged
#9	2	No	No	Delayed (4)	4	5	Late death (9 m)
#10	3	AAA syncronous	No	Delayed (1)	4	5	Discharged
#11	3	Untreated AAA	Yes	Delayed (2)	3	3	Discharged
#12	3	No	No	Delayed (41)	0	5	Discharged
#13	4	No	No	Delayed (3)	3	4	Discharged

CSFD: cerebrospinal fluid drainage

completely resolved, died of pneumonia 9 months after the procedure and 1 patient with immediate severe and improved SCI, died three months later of sepsis following urinary infection.

Patients demographics and risks factors, cardiac risk index, etiology, proximal aortic landing zone, intentional coverage of left subclavian artery without revascularization, coverage of critical intercostals arteries (T8 to L1), preoperative CSF drainage and length and type of device used were not found to be related to SCI.

Univariate analyses showed peri-operative lowest mean arterial pressure < 70 mmHg (p=0.002) and previous AAA surgery (p=0.004) to significantly predict the occurrence of paraplegia. Multivariate analysis also identified peri-operative lowest mean arterial pressure < 70 mmHg [p<0.0001] (odds ratio = 39.038; 95% CI 8.907-171.107) and previous AAA surgery [p=0.0380] (odds ratio = 4.894; 95% CI 1.092-21.940) as independent risk factors (Table II).

Discussion

Despite the improvements in the surgical and anesthesiological techniques, SCI remains a terrible complication that may arise after open and endovascular surgery of the thoracic and thoracoabdominal aorta in a significant number of cases [9-11].

The pathophysiology of SCI is definitely multifactorial but is still ill defined, and many concepts, summarized in Table III, are linked to SCI from both clinical and preclinical studies.

Due to its relatively inaccessible location, the knowledge of the vascular anatomy of the spinal cord is still not totally clear and relies on a rather limited number of studies that use post-mortem angiography, micro-angiography and dye injection techniques. Most studies are limited to the arteries and refer to subjects without aortic pathology. Moreover, the literature does not provide a nomenclature uniformity, bringing even more confusion to an already complex topic. Only recently, the advances of CT and MR techniques are allowing a better knowledge of the in-vivo anatomic pattern of individual patients [12].

The superficial arteries to the spinal cord include two systems (Fig. 1):
A) The longitudinal arterial trunks (anastomotic channels between ascending – smaller – and descending branches of neighboring radicular arteries):
- Anterior spinal artery (single)
- Posterior or Posterolateral spinal arteries (double)

B) The Perimedullary vascular network or Pial Plexus.

The input to these arteries includes the vertebral arteries, a variable number of segmental vessels originating from the intercostal and lumbar arteries and the hypogastric arteries.

Spinal cord perfusion greatly depends on a collateral circulation that has a large anatomic variability. This explains the lack of consequence of intercostal artery exclusion during stent-graft deployment and the low incidence of paraplegia (2%) reported in the series from Griepp et al. [10] with no intercostal arteries reattachment. Coselli et al. [13] also stressed the value of the "simple clamping" technique with outstanding results. Unfortunately not many centers have been able to duplicate these encouraging results. While the "collateral network" may guarantee adequate vascularization in many instances, this may not always be the case.

During open surgery, the extension and length of aortic cross clamping also play a key role in the development of SCI; paraplegia is usually immediate and severe and CSF drainage, while effective as a prophylactic adjunct, is in fact of limited use once the deficit has occurred. Other authors pointed out the role of blood volume redistribution and hemodynamic response to aortic cross-clamping [14,15]. Many factors are altered by the anesthesiological management which is therefore also pivotal in the prevention of paraplegia. The adequacy of collateral circulation, however, does have a role in some instances: delayed and incomplete paresis may occur and CSF drainage may be effective in their treatment [9]. With TEVAR there is no aortic cross clamping, no reimplantation of intercostal arteries and no steal from the network, therefore several important factors are removed from the equation. However, this setting does have differences with the open procedure. First, the extent of segmental artery sacrifice is greater since it includes not only the length of the aneurysm but also that of the proximal and distal landing zones (Fig. 2). Second, the moderate passive hypothermia that is employed during open surgery is not obtained. Third, CSF drainage which is used

Table II ANALYSIS OF RISK FACTORS FOR SPINAL CORD ISCHEMIA

Risks factors	No Paraplegia (%)	Paraplegia (%)	P
Overall	193	13	
Male	164 (85)	12 (92.3)	
Age (years)	69.0±10.2	72.4±5.5	NS
Cardiac risk index			
I	131 (67.9)	7 (53.8)	NS
II	37 (19.2)	2 (15.4)	NS
III	23 (11.9)	3 (23.1)	NS
IV	2 (1.0)	1 (7.7)	NS
Hypertension			
0 (diastolic < 90 mmHg)	75 (38.9)	4 (30.8)	NS
1 (easily controlled, single drugs)	52 (26.9)	4 (30.8)	NS
2 (requires 2 drugs)	42 (21.8)	3 (23.1)	NS
3 (> 2 drugs or uncontrolled)	25 (13)	2 (15.4)	NS
Diabetes			
0 (none)	130 (67.4)	5 (38.5)	NS
1 (adult onset, diet controlled)	45 (23.3)	8 (61.5)	NS
2 (adult onset, oral medication-controlled)	8 (4.1)	0	NS
3 (adult onset, insulin controlled)	6 (3.1)	0	NS
4 (juvenile onset)	4 (2.1)	0	NS
Smoking			
0 (none; abstinence > 10 yrs)	91 (47.2)	7 (53.8)	NS
1 (none; abstinence 1-10 yrs)	65 (33.7)	3 (23.1)	NS
2 (< 1 pack/day or abstinence >1 yrs)	26 (13.5)	3 (23.1)	NS
3 (current 1 > pack / day)	11 (5.7)	0	NS
Hyperlipemia			
0 (within normal limits for age)	127 (65.8)	5 (38.5)	NS
1 (mild elevation, diet controlled)	16 (8.3)	3 (23.1)	NS
2 (types II, III, or IV, strict diet control)	27 (14.0)	3 (23.1)	NS
3 (requires drug control)	23 (11.9)	2 (15.4)	NS
Pulmonary status *			
0	110 (57)	4 (30.8)	NS
1	39 (20.2)	6 (46.2)	NS
2	31 (16.1)	3 (23.1)	NS
3	13 (6.7)	0	NS
ASA score			
1	0	0	NS
2	20 (10.4)	0	NS
3	130 (67.4)	10 (76.9)	NS
4	43 (22.3)	3 (23.1)	NS
5	0	0	NS

Table II ANALYSIS OF RISK FACTORS FOR SPINAL CORD ISCHEMIA

Risks factors	No Paraplegia (%)	Paraplegia (%)	P
Renal status ‡			
0	145 (75.1)	8 (61.5)	
1	37 (19.2)	4 (30.8)	
2	9 (4.7)	1 (7.7)	
3	2 (1.0)	0	
Thoracic pathology			
Atherosclerotic aneurysm	154 (79.8)	12 (92.3%)	NS
Post-traumatic aortic rupture,	3 (1.6)	0	NS
Aortic type B dissection	20 (10.4)	1 (7.7)	NS
Penetrating ulcer/intramural haematoma	7 (3.6)	0	NS
Pseudoaneurysm	6 (3.1)	0	NS
Others	3 (1.6)	0	NS
Previous AAA surgery	31 (16.1)	5 (38.5)	=0.0036
Previous TAA surgery	16 (8.3)	1 (7.7)	NS
Proximal landing zone			
Zone 0	15 (7.8)	0	NS
Zone 1	13 (6.7)	0	NS
Zone 2	40 (20.7)	2 (15.4)	NS
Zone 3	59 (30.6)	5 (38.5)	NS
Zone 4	50 (25.9)	5 (38.5)	NS
TAAA	16 (8.3)	1 (7.7)	NS
Intentional coverage of LSA without revascularization	49 (25.4)	1 (7.7)	NS
Coverage of critical intercostals arteries (T8 to L1)	68 (35.2)	4 (30.8)	NS
Preoperative CSFD	25 (13.0)	2 (15.4)	NS
Device used			
Excluder TAG	54 (28)	1 (7.7)	NS
Endofit	11 (5.7)	0	NS
Talent and Vailant	8 (4.1)	1 (7.7)	NS
Zenith TX1 and TX2	116 (60.1)	10 (76.9)	NS
Relay	4 (2.1)	1 (7.7)	NS
Length of thoracic coverage	165±38 mm	170±30 mm	NS
Intra-operative and postoperative lowest MAP < 70 mmHg	12 (6.2)	9 (69.2)	<0.0001

* Pulmonary status: 0: asymptomatic, normal chest X-ray, pulmonary function test (PFT) 20% of predicted; 1: asymptomatic or mild dyspnea on exertion, mild X-ray parenchymal changes, PFT65 to 80% of predicted; 2: between 1 and 3; 3: vital capacity less than 1.85 L, FEV less than 35% of predicted, maximal voluntary ventilation less than 28 L/min or less than 50% of predicted, PCO greater than 45 mmHg, supplemental oxygen use necessary or pulmonary hypertension.

‡ Renal status: 0: no known renal disease, serum creatinine <1.5 mg/dL, creatinine clearance greater than 50 mL/min; 1: creatinine 1.5-3.0 mg/dL, clearance 30-50 mL/min; 2: creatinine 3.0-6.0 mg/dL, clearance 15-30 mL/min; 3: creatinine >6.0 mg/dL, clearance <15 mL/min or on dialysis or with transplant.

Table III	CONCEPTS THAT ARE LINKED TO SCI FROM BOTH CLINICAL AND EXPERIMENTAL LITERATURE	
	Concept	Consensus
	Influenced by time of aortic cross-clamping	+++
	Influenced by aortic region involved	+++
	Influenced by extent of aorta involved	+++
	Very rare after chronic thrombosis of intercostal aa.	+++
	Distal perfusion	++
	Spinal fluid drainage (prevention)	+++
	Spinal fluid drainage (treatment)	++
	Avoid steal	++
	Reattachment of intercostal arteries	++
	Preoperative location of ARM (Angio)	+
	Evoked potentials	+

routinely during open surgery, is instituted only in selected cases in most series. Fourth, thrombosis of the excluded sac may not be immediate and some collateral circulation between intercostal arteries could be present (i.e. type II endoleak).

How can our observations, and particularly the differences with post-surgical SCI, help us to better understand the phenomenon?

1. Relationship with hypotension: most of our cases of SCI have been associated with hypotension, even if temporary or only mild or moderate. This suggests that perfusion relies on smaller vessels with greater resistance, or that edema produces an extrinsic compression on the vessels, even more increasing resistances. This would also explain the beneficial effect of CSF drainage.

2. Delayed onset: in many cases, the deficit occurred days to weeks after the procedure, sometimes also related to hypotension (in one case related to thoracotomy). The onset, however, was always sudden. We can assume that some branches thrombosed late, making the collateral network insufficient. Moreover, complete thrombosis of the aneurismal sac could interrupt collateral pathways that are still present in the sac (type II endoleak).

3. Previous AAA or aorto-iliac surgery: during TEVAR, the adequacy of collateral pathways represents the corner stone of the etiology of SCI. Lumbar arteries that originate from the infrarenal aorta and both internal iliac arteries provide significant collaterals that may be thrombosed due to the presence of aneurysmatic disease or ligated during previous surgery. This clearly emerged as a significant risk factor in our data analysis.

All the factors that decrease the efficacy of the collateral network to the spinal cord, such as systemic hypotension, CSF hypertension, and thrombosis of collaterals, may induce paraplegia even hours or days after the procedure. However, if treated timely, symptoms may improve or resolve in a rather astonishing way. Interestingly, in our study we observed a case of delayed paraplegia in a patient who underwent a right pulmonary resection for cancer through a right thoracotomy 41 days after TEVAR. This patient experienced SCI one day after the pulmonary intervention during a hypotensive episode and he was successfully treated with CSFD. After one year the patient underwent open repair of AAA and experienced another SCI two days after intervention that completely reverted after CSFD.

Thoracic endografts, and particularly those of the earlier generation, are associated with specific technical complications. Older stent-grafts were not firmly anchored to the delivery systems and the wind-socket or parachute effect during deployment of the stent graft mandated a period of asystole or profound hypotension to allow safe and precise deployment. Nowadays technical improvements in the stent-graft and delivery systems of many manufacturers allow safe and precise deployment with normal systemic pressure. Maintaining an adequate intra and postoperative systemic pressure is crucial to prevent paraplegia. An errant deployment may result in a period of aortic occlusion comparable to surgical cross-clamping, and restoration of aortic patency after deployment completion may cause a spinal cord reperfusion injury [16]. Also, endoluminal maneuvers entail the risk of intercostal arteries and/or visceral organs embolization.

If possible, trying to avoid coverage of the ARM with the stent-graft may indeed have a role in preventing paraplegia. Kawaharada et al. [17], among 71 patients with pre-operative visualization of the

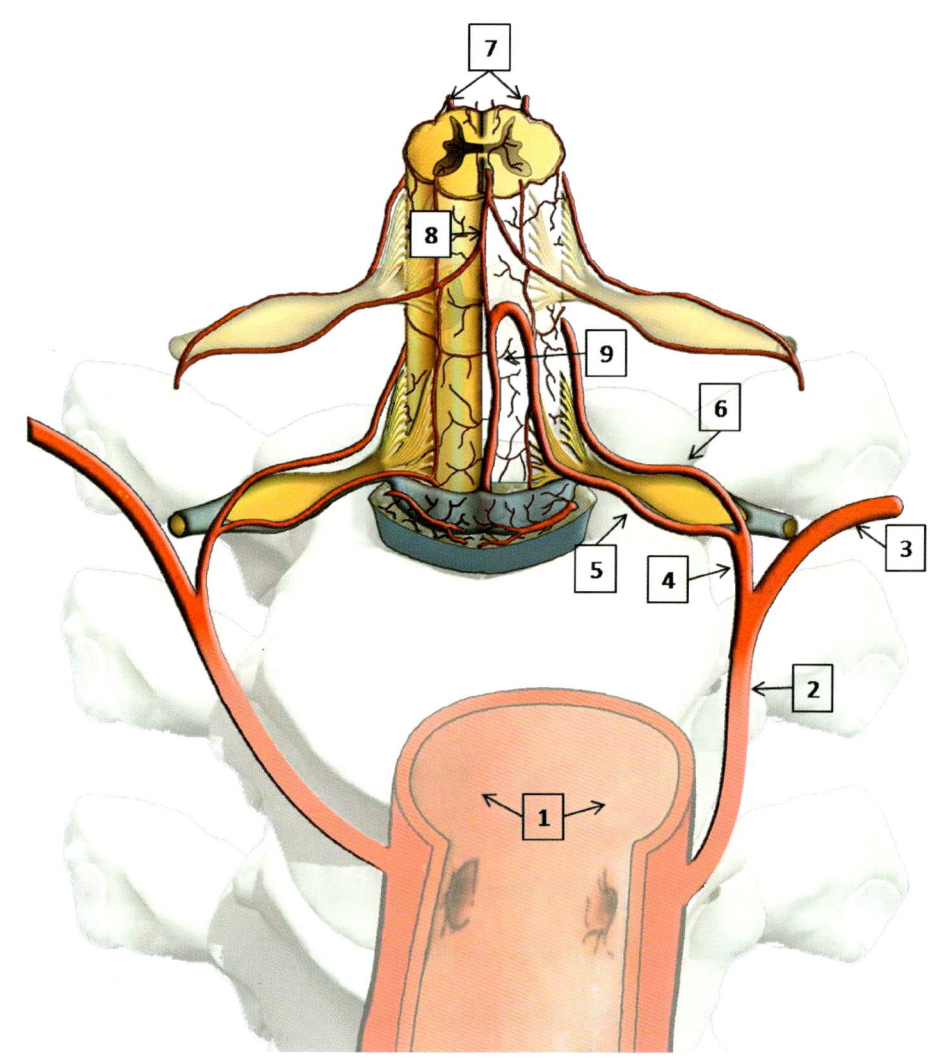

FIG. 1 Schematic view of spinal cord supply. From the aorta arises segmental posterior intercostal arteries (2) that provides a vertebral branch (3) and the nervomedullary artery (4). The nervomedullary arteries (4) divide into constant branches that supply the ventral or dorsolateral surface of the medulla called the anterior (5) and posterior (6) radicular artery respectively. The anterior radicular artery provides one anterior spinal artery (8) and the posterior radicular artery provides two posterolateral spinal artery (7). One of the anterior radicular artery is always distinctly dominant in caliber and is therefore termed the great radicular artery by Adamkiewicz (9).

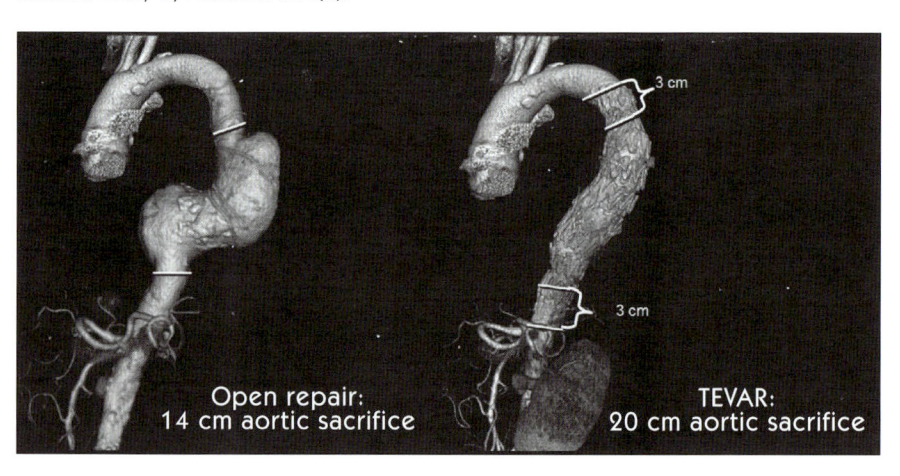

FIG. 2 The extent of segmental aortic sacrifice is greater with TEVAR since it includes not only the length of the aneurysm and but also the proximal and distal landing zones.

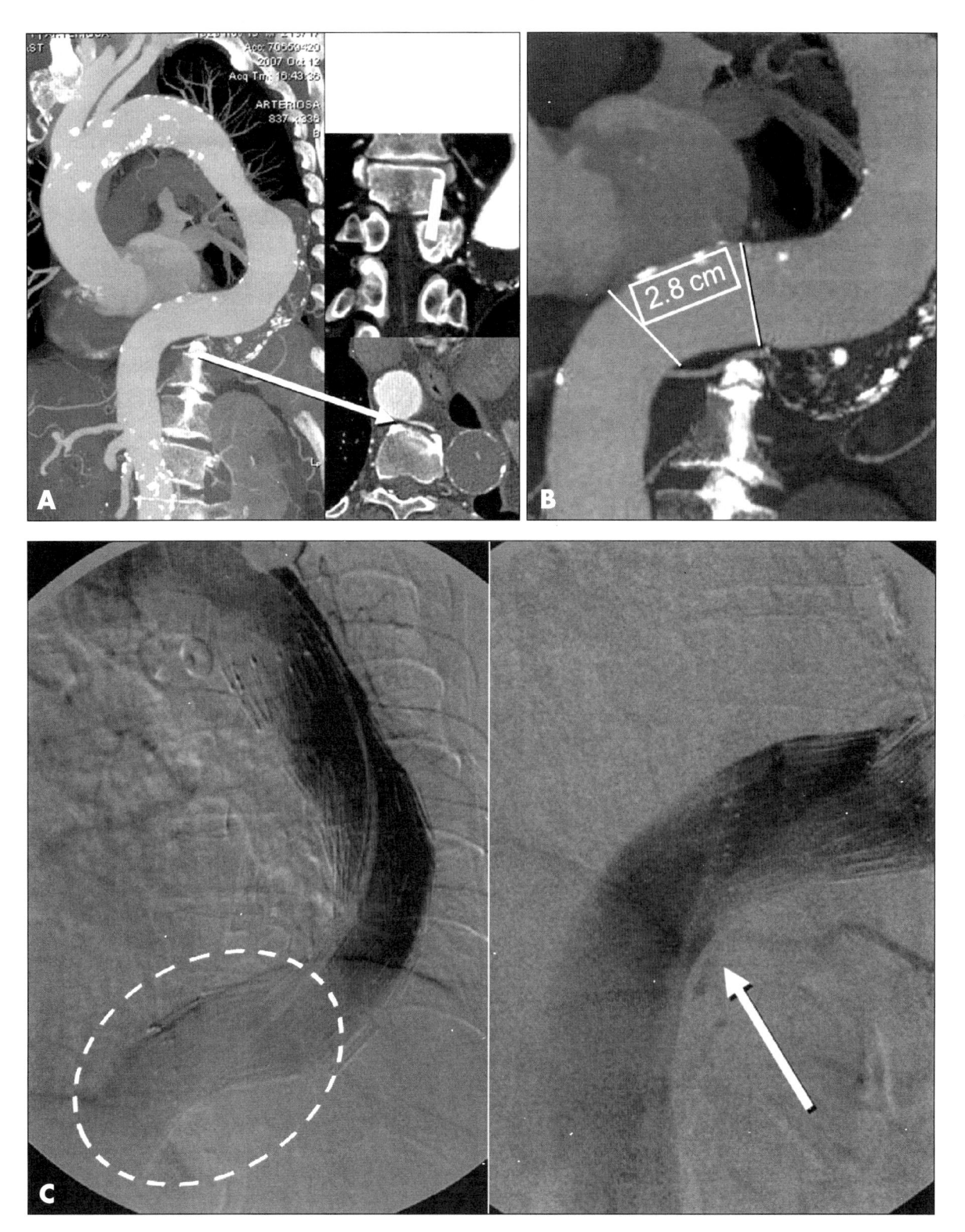

FIG. 3 A - Preoperative CT scan reconstruction of a descending thoracic aneurysm and identification of an intercostal artery feeder of the anterior spinal artery. B - The critical intercostal artery originate 2.8 cm below the distal end of the aneurysm. C - Intraoperative angiogram shows successful exclusion of the descending thoracic aneurysm with preservation of the critical intercostal artery.

ARM, reported a 9.1% incidence of paraplegia in the subgroup which had occlusion of the intercostal artery feeder to ARM due to the stent-graft versus a 0% in the subgroup that did not require coverage of the critical intercostal artery. As a consequence of this and their personal experience that focus on the strong relationship between postoperative SCI and ARM coverage, Kieffer et al. [18] referred systematically to open surgery patients in whom pre-operative arteriography revealed the emergency of the ARM from within the aneurysm [Fig. 3]. Intentional overstenting of the LSA with selective indication to revascularization have been proposed by several authors [4,19] with few adverse events reported (cerebrovascular accident, subclavian steal syndrome). However, this issue is still debated. The data from the Talent Thoracic Retrospective Registry [20] demonstrated that occlusion of the left subclavian artery without previous revascularization was significantly associated to stroke (p=0.004) but not to SCI. The only factors significantly associated to SCI was a length of covered aorta greater than 20 cm (p=0.001). Recently, the data from EUROSTAR registry [21] demonstrated an independent correlation with SCI and four factors: left subclavian artery covering without revascularization (p=0.027, OR=3.9), renal failure (p=0.02, OR=3.6), concomitant open abdominal aortic surgery (p=0.37, OR=5.5) and a number of used stentgrafts ≥ 3 (p=0.041, OR=3.4).

Routine insertion centers CSF drainage has not been used in most center, including ours, due to the risks related to its use, the requirement of postoperative care, monitoring and horizontal bed rest, and the discomfort associated with its institution in patients treated under loco-regional anesthesia. Also, paraplegia is not exceedingly common in many series. The amount of CSF to be drained and duration of drainage are not standardized. While there is not enough evidence to suggest a routine use of CSF drainage during TEVAR, it is absolutely clear that its timely use together with systemic blood pressure optimization and steroids use have the potential to improve or even cure SCI symptoms after TEVAR.

In conclusion, in this series most cases of SCI were delayed and related to hypotension or previous AAA. They are clearly treatable by different means that concur to improve indirect spinal perfusion through collateral circulation. The nature and prognosis of SCI after TEVAR suggest that it may be related to impaired collateral circulation to the spinal cord in patients in whom feeders of the ARM is either covered by the stent-graft or not present preoperatively. SCI should be managed promptly and aggressively due to its reversibility. Ongoing technical improvements of non-invasive diagnostic modalities will provide an in-vivo preoperative assessment of spinal cord vascular network allowing a safe planning of thoracic aorta stent-graft repair.

REFERENCES

1. Chiesa R, Melissano G, Marrocco-Trischitta MM et al. Spinal cord ischemia after elective stent-graft repair of the thoracic aorta. *J Vasc Surg* 2005; 42: 11-17.
2. Mitchell RS, Ishimaru S, Ehrlich MP et al. First International Summit on Thoracic Aortic Endografting: roundtable on thoracic aortic dissection as an indication for endografting. *J Endovasc Ther* 2002; 9: 98–105.
3. Baril DT, Carroccio A, Ellozy SH et al. Endovascular thoracic aortic repair and previous or concomitant abdominal aortic repair: is the increased risk of spinal cord ischemia real? *Ann Vasc Surg* 2006; 20: 188-194.
4. Melissano G, Civilini E, Bertoglio L et al. Results of endografting of the aortic arch in different landing zones. *Eur J Vasc Endovasc Surg* 2007; 33: 561-566.
5. Chiesa R, Tshomba Y, Melissano G et al. Hybrid approach to thoracoabdominal aortic aneurysms in patients with prior aortic surgery. *J Vasc Surg* 2007; 45: 1128-1135.
6. Chaikof EL, Blankensteijn JD, Harris PL et al; Ad Hoc Committee for Standardized Reporting Practices in Vascular Surgery of The Society for Vascular Surgery/American Association for Vascular Surgery. Reporting standards for endovascular aortic aneurysm repair. *J Vasc Surg* 2002; 35: 1048-1060.
7. Parmer SS, Carpenter JP, Stavropoulos SW et al. Endoleaks after endovascular repair of thoracic aortic aneurysms. *J Vasc Surg* 2006; 44: 447-452.
8. Melissano G, Tshomba Y, Civilini E et al. Disappointing results with a new commercially available thoracic endograft. *J Vasc Surg* 2004; 39: 124-130.
9. Wong DR, Coselli JS, Amerman K et al. Delayed spinal cord deficits after thoracoabdominal aortic aneurysm repair. *Ann Thorac Surg* 2007; 83: 1345-1355.
10. Griepp RB, Griepp EB. Spinal cord perfusion and protection during descending thoracic and thoracoabdominal aortic surgery: the collateral network concept. *Ann Thorac Surg* 2007; 83: S865-869.
11. Conrad MF, Crawford RS, Davison JK et al. Thoracoabdominal aneurysm repair: a 20-year perspective. *Ann Thorac Surg* 2007; 83: S856-61.
12. Nijenhuis RJ, Jacobs MJ, Jaspers K et al. Comparison of magnetic resonance with computed tomography angiography for preoperative localization of the Adamkiewicz artery in thoracoabdominal aortic aneurysm patients. *J Vasc Surg* 2007; 45: 677-685.

13. Coselli JS, LeMaire SA, Conklin LD et al. Left heart bypass during descending thoracic aortic aneurysm repair does not reduce the incidence of paraplegia. *Ann Thorac Surg* 2004; 77: 1298-1303.

14. Gelman S, Khazaeli MB, Orr R et al. Blood volume redistribution during cross-clamping of the descending aorta. *Anesth Analg* 1994; 78: 219-224.

15. Kawanishi Y, Okada K, Matsumori M et al. Influence of perioperative hemodynamics on spinal cord ischemia in thoracoabdominal aortic repair. *Ann Thorac Surg* 2007; 84: 488-492.

16. Kasirajan K, Dolmatch B, Ouriel K et al. Delayed onset of ascending paralysis after thoracic aortic stent graft deployment. *J Vasc Surg* 2000; 31: 196-199.

17. Kawaharada N, Morishita K, Kurimoto Y et al. Spinal cord ischemia after elective endovascular stent-graft repair of the thoracic aorta. *Eur J Cardiothorac Surg* 2007; 31: 998-1003.

18. Kieffer E, Chiche L. Descending thoracic aortic aneurysms: open repair or stent-grafting? In: Branchereau A, Jacobs M (eds). Open surgery versus endovascular procedures. Oxford: Paris Consultant, 2007: pp 105-113.

19. Gorich J, Asquan Y, Seifarth H et al. Initial experience with intentional stent-graft coverage of the subclavian artery during endovascular thoracic aortic repairs. *J Endovasc Ther* 2002;9 Suppl 2:II39-43.

20. Fattori R, Nienaber CA, Rousseau H et al. Talent Thoracic Retrospective Registry. Results of endovascular repair of the thoracic aorta with the Talent Thoracic stent graft: the Talent Thoracic Retrospective Registry. *J Thorac Cardiovasc Surg* 2006; 132: 332-339.

21. Buth J, Harris PL, Hobo R et al. Neurologic complications associated with endovascular repair of thoracic aortic pathology: incidence and risk factors. A study from the European Collaborators on stent graft techniques for aortic aneurysm repair (Eurostar Registry). *J Vasc Surg* 2007, in press.

11

ENDOVASCULAR REPAIR OF AORTIC ARCH ANEURYSMS

TIMOTHY CHUTER

The aortic arch is curved, compliant, mobile, wide, far from the femoral arteries and close to the heart. All these features complicate the endovascular aneurysm repair in the aortic arch, but none more so than the presence of its branches, which supply an organ, the brain, with little tolerance for ischemia. Endovascular repair must exclude the aortic arch from the circulation, while maintaining uninterrupted flow to these branches. Various techniques of endovascular repair achieve this goal in different ways. One approach is to provide the supra-aortic trunks with an alternative source of blood through surgical bypass from a remote location, thereby "debranching" the arch [1-3]. Another approach is to supply each branch of the aortic arch through a branch of the stent graft [4-6]. Aneurysms that are close to, but not involving, the origins of the supra-aortic trunks are only slightly less problematic. In such cases, one can maintain branch artery flow through a hole (fenestration) in the fabric of the stent graft [7], or through a stent alongside the primary stent graft [8,9]. These techniques are not mutually exclusive; they can be combined in various ways. Whatever the challenges of endovascular repair, all these techniques of branch preservation are greatly facilitated by the accessibility of the carotid and subclavian arteries in the root of the neck.

Stenting of the supra-aortic trunks

A short stent can be used to push the margin of a misplaced stent graft down the aorta, thereby uncovering the orifice of an otherwise occluded subclavian or carotid artery. A slightly longer stent can be used to treat more extensive branch artery encroachment by pushing the stent graft in a trans-axial direction away from the wall of the aorta, thereby maintaining a channel from the margin of the stent graft to the orifice of the artery in ques-

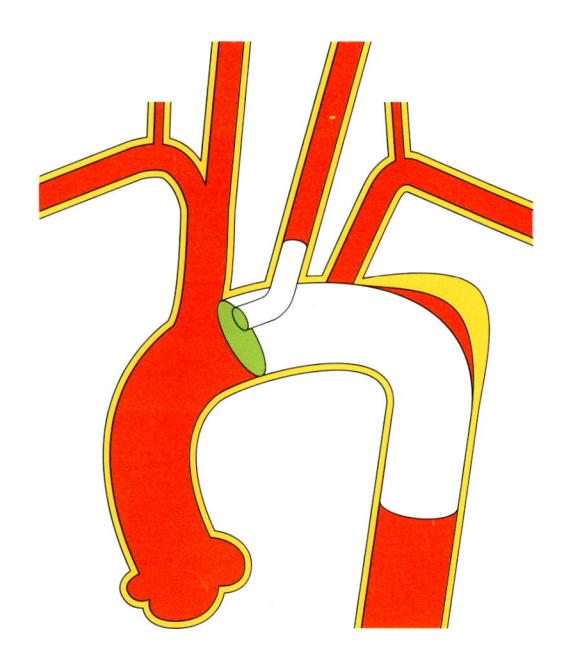

FIG. 1 A stent, or covered stent, extends from the branch lumen to the proximal end of the stent graft to form a "chimney", "snorkel", or "double-barrel stent graft", which preserves a route of flow into the stented supra-aortic trunk.

tion. (Fig. 1). This use of a branch artery stent, or covered stent, has been described variously as a "chimney" [9], a "snorkel", or one barrel of a "double-barreled stent graft" [8]. It appears that many authors first used the approach to restore flow rapidly to an inadvertently covered artery, and then applied it electively to treat aneurysms that encroached on the distal aortic arch. The approach has been used alone, or in combination with bypass, to secure inflow to the subclavian, carotid and innominate arteries.

At its best, the combination of a branch artery stent and an aortic stent graft functions as a form of branched stent graft, excluding the affected aortic segment while maintaining branch artery flow. Yet, however much the prosthetic lumens conform to one another, each retains an essentially circular cross-section and side-by-side they can never fully occupy the aorta. The gap between them always represents a potential route for type I endoleak. This should be borne in mind when planning the endovascular repair of an arch aneurysm. The longitudinal channels at one either side of the branch artery stent run around the *outer* curvature of the arch, and the risk of endoleak is least when the aneurysm is confined to the *inner* curvature, or when there is a rim of non-dilated aorta distal to the orifice of the branch artery.

The branch artery stent technique has several advantages over fenestration, stent graft branching, or aortic debranching. First, all the components are readily available. The application may be off label, but there are none of the regulatory hurdles and delays that are an unavoidable part of customized stent graft manufacture. Second, the additional stent, or covered stent, can be inserted only when needed. If the primary stent graft deploys at the intended location and there are no signs of branch artery impingment or endoleak, the branch artery can be left unstented. Third, once access to the branch artery has been obtained, the implantation of a stent is a rapid and reliable way to restore flow. Fourth, the insertion of a branch artery stent is arguably less invasive than surgical bypass, especially in the case of an innominate stent, which replaces AKA bypass from the ascending aorta.

Fenestration

Like a branch artery stent (double-barrel stent graft, snorkel, or chimney), a fenestrated stent graft depends on direct apposition between the wall of the stent graft and the wall of the aorta for the prevention of type I endoleak. When the aneurysm involves the area around the orifice of the corresponding supra-aortic trunk, and there is a gap between the stent graft and the aortic wall, the fenestration will become a route of leakage into the aneurysm. Leakage at this site can be treated by adding a covered stent to turn the fenestrated stent graft into a form of branched stent graft, but this is unlikely to be a durable solution. The balloon expanded branch is a fragile object, subject to plastic deformation. It is probably not well suited to use in such a mobile segment of the aorta.

Despite a huge worldwide experience with fenestrated stent graft implantation in cases of juxtarenal aneurysm, the technique is not likely to be applied so often in the aortic arch where the size, curvature, distance from the femoral arteries, and risk of embolism complicate the instrumentation and manipulation of a partially deployed stent graft.

In-situ fenestration dispenses with the need for both customized manufacture and precise alignment (Figs. 2 A-C). The technique employs small sharp wires, needles and cutting balloons to perforate the wall of the fully deployed stent graft. Potential problems include: the effect of fenestration on the long-term durability of the surrounding

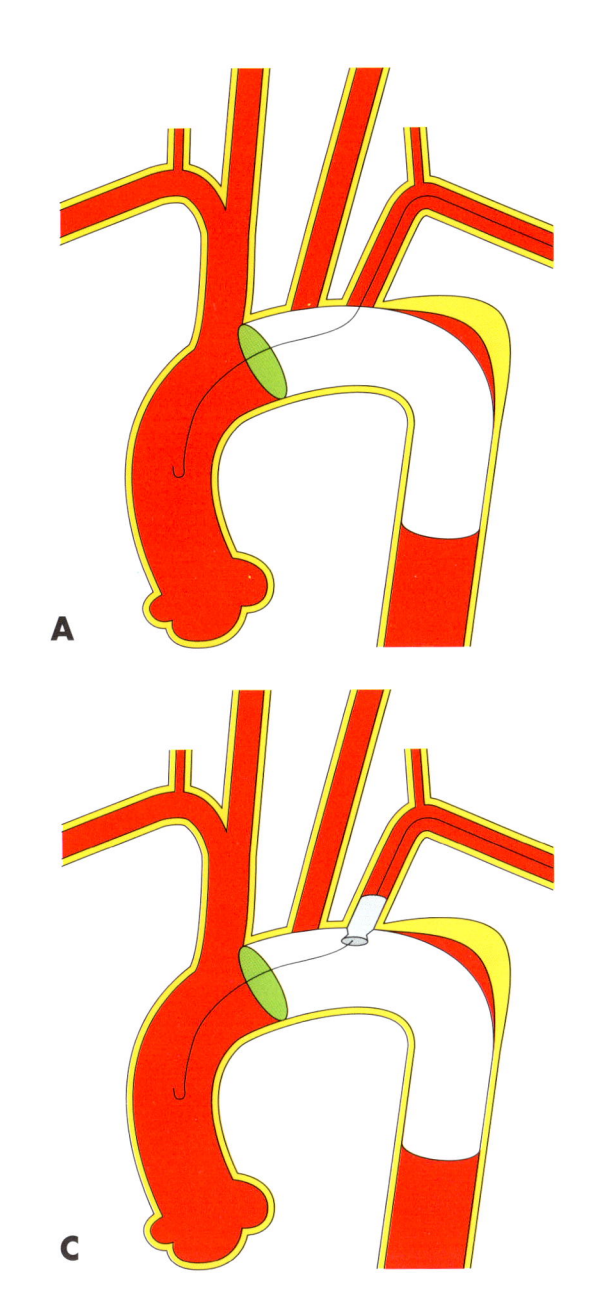

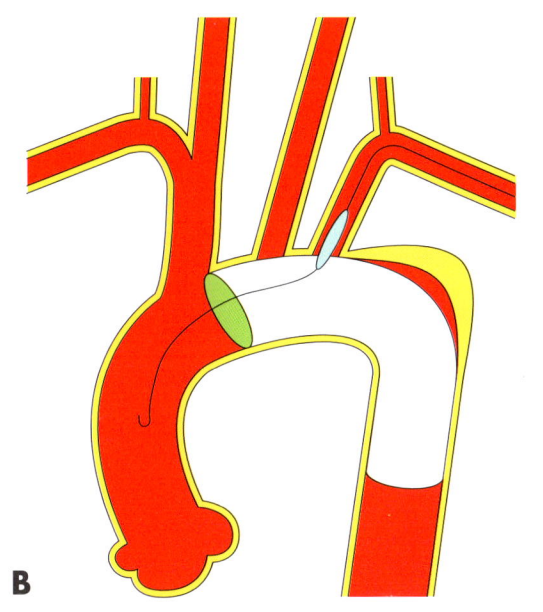

FIG. 2 A - In the first stage of this in-situ fenestration technique [7], the back end of a coronary guidewire is forced through the fabric of the stent graft. B - The hole (fenestration) is then enlarged using first a needle, then a large cutting balloon. C - The hole is stented to maintain its position and patency.

graft, and the potential for hypoperfusion of the brain during the interval between stent graft insertion and the re-establishment of flow into covered supra-aortic trunks.

Debranching

The most commonly practiced form of debranching is a bypass between the left carotid and subclavian arteries in cases of descending thoracic aortic repair [1]. The resultant increase in the length of the proximal implantation site varies with the distance between these arterial orifices, but even a small amount of lengthening can help achieve the proper orientation, attachment and seal, especially in cases of severe angulation. The only absolute indications for left subclavian artery preservation are the presence of a dominant left vertebral artery, and the presence of a left internal mammary bypass to a coronary artery. Left upper extremity claudication is uncommon and easily addressed if, and when, it occurs [10]. However, routine left subclavian occlusion is no longer the norm [11]. For one thing, the left subclavian artery is being increasingly recognized as a source of collateral flow to the spinal cord. Endovascular repair of the distal descending thoracic aorta, and prior repair of the abdominal aorta, are relative indications for carotid-subclavian bypass to maintain subclavian artery flow, and mitigate the increased the risk of paraplegia [12,13].

More extensive distal arch involvement calls for more extensive debranching of the supra-aortic trunks. With each additional bypass the source of blood moves proximally. Since the only source of flow proximal to the innominate artery is the ascending aorta, innominate involvement necessitates median sternotomy and aortic clamping, or partial clamping, for complete supra-aortic debranching. The risks of aorta-based debranching depend on the patient's comorbidity, surgical history, and the state of the aorta.

Branched stent grafts

Experience with conventional endovascular repair of the descending thoracic aorta shows that long operations, and repeated instrumentation of the aortic arch are associated with elevated stroke rates, especially in the presence of ascending and arch aortic disease. One might therefore expect stroke to be a common complication of the more complex forms of endovascular repair in and around the aortic arch. Although there are, as yet, too few cases of complex endovascular arch repair (branches or fenestrations) to test this assumption, it is clear than unibody branched stent grafts are more complicated than modular branched stent grafts, and multiple branches are more complicated than single branches. Until we have more data, both are to be avoided for fear of causing embolic stroke.

This line of thinking, together with the findings of in-vitro experiments [14], led us to perform endovascular repair of true arch aneurysms using a bifurcated stent graft with one branch to the lower body and one branch to a supra-aortic trunk (Figs. 3 A-C). In this approach, blood is distributed to the other supra-aortic trunks through a series of bypass grafts. The resulting technique combines branched stent graft insertion and aortic debranching. The goal is to keep the endovascular part quick and easy. The supra-aortic branch requires no additional endovascualr instrumentation because it lies along the line of stent graft insertion through the right subclavian, right carotid, or left subclavian arteries. This route of stent graft insertion is short and straight, which simplifies stent graft orientation, positioning and deployment. The distal aortic branch is added in usual modular fashion to an attachment site on the primary stent graft. The selective catheterization of the attachment site might be difficult and dangerous were the target not so wide.

The bifurcated approach works best when the ascending aorta is long and narrow, and the right carotid artery is wide. If the ascending aorta is wide and the carotid artery narrow, the bifurcated stent graft delivery system has to pass through a conduit to the subclavian, or innominate arteries. Once the bifurcated stent graft is in place, the conduit is generally converted into an extra-anatomic bypass grafts, as part of the cervical distribution network. Right-sided routes stent graft insertion requires the ascending aorta to be long enough to accommodate the trunk and short wide branch of the bifurcated stent graft, which may not be the case, especially when the patient has undergone prior aorto-coronary bypass. Aneurysm of the innominate artery is another contraindication to right-sided insertion, for lack of a suitable implantation site for the long ascending branch of the stent graft. In such cases, left-sided access through the left subclavian artery increases the available space at the expense of reducing the diameter of the supra-aortic branch. In such cases, it may be necessary to provide an additional inflow to the brachiocephalic circulation through an additional branch to the left carotid (Figs. 4 A-D), or innominate (Fig. 5) arteries. This additional instrumentation possibly increases the risk of stroke, but locating the branch attachment site (cuff) well proximal to the corresponding supra-aortic trunk helps to keep the catheterization as simple as possible.

Conclusion

Endovascular repair of the aortic arch is becoming a viable alternative to the conventional surgical repair, especially in the presence of a reoperative field or serious cardiopulmonary comorbidity. In cases of extensive arch involvement the only completely endovascular technique involves the implantation of a branched stent graft. Our preferred approach minimizes the risks of the endovascular portion of the repair by combining transcervical implantation of a bifurcated stent graft with extra-anatomic bypass in the neck. Most of the current experience is in cases of arch aneurysm. Other potential applications include cases of arch dissection [6], either following surgical repair of the ascending aorta or even as primary therapy in the absence of coronary or aortic root involvement.

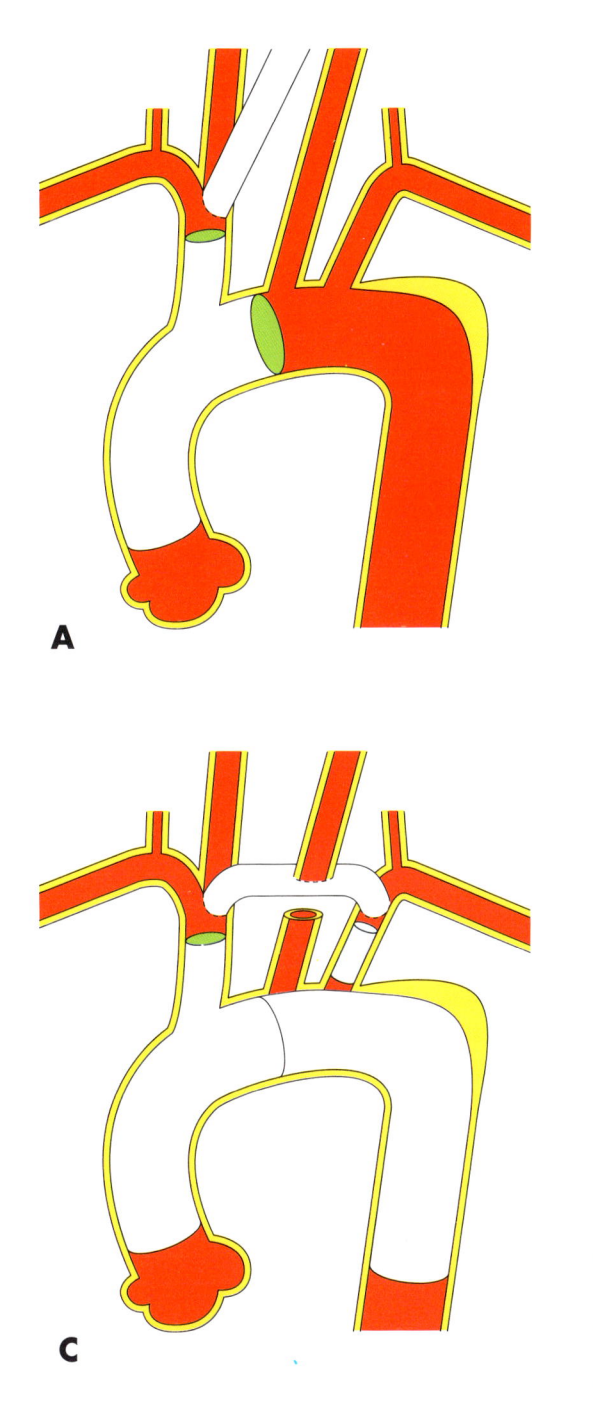

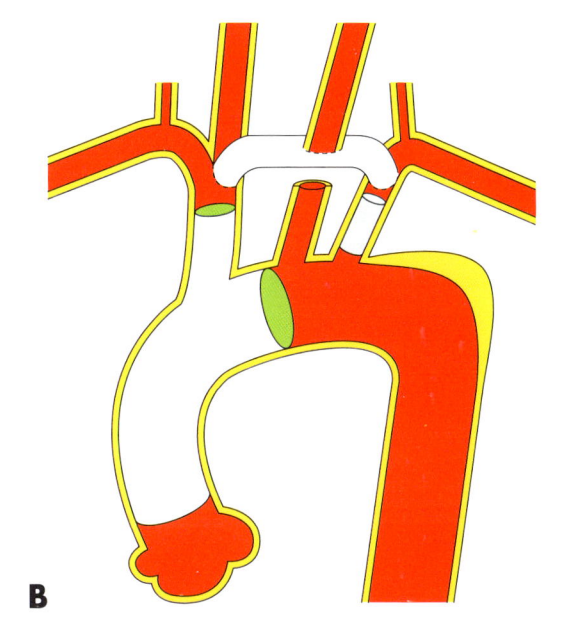

FIG. 3 A - The bifurcated ascending aortic stent graft is inserted through one of the supra-aortic trunks. B - A series of bypass grafts distribute inflow from the long limb of the bifurcated stent graft to the other supra-aortic trunks. C - An extension to the non-dilated descending thoracic aorta completes aneurysm exclusion.

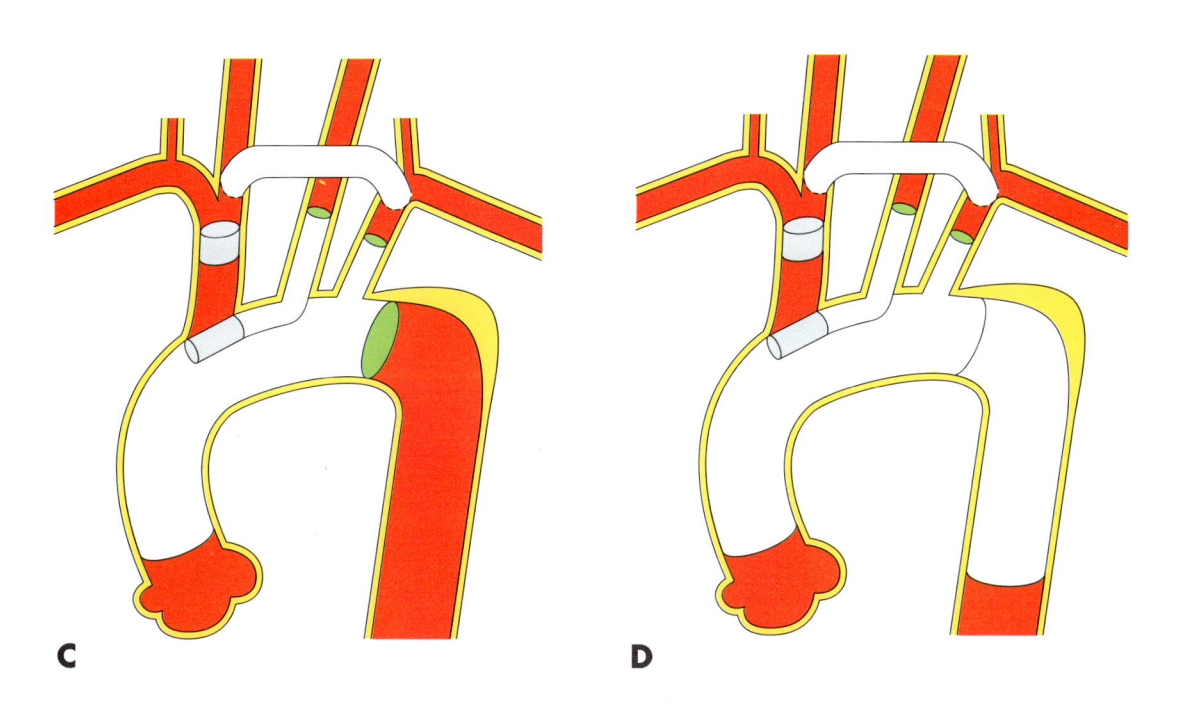

FIG. 4 A - The bifurcated aortic stent graft can also be inserted through a conduit on the left subclavian artery. B - This approach provides a convenient location for the attachment of an additional branch of the stent graft. C - The additional branch on the stent graft replaces one graft of the distribution network. D - The procedure is completed in the usual way with an extension to the descending thoracic aorta.

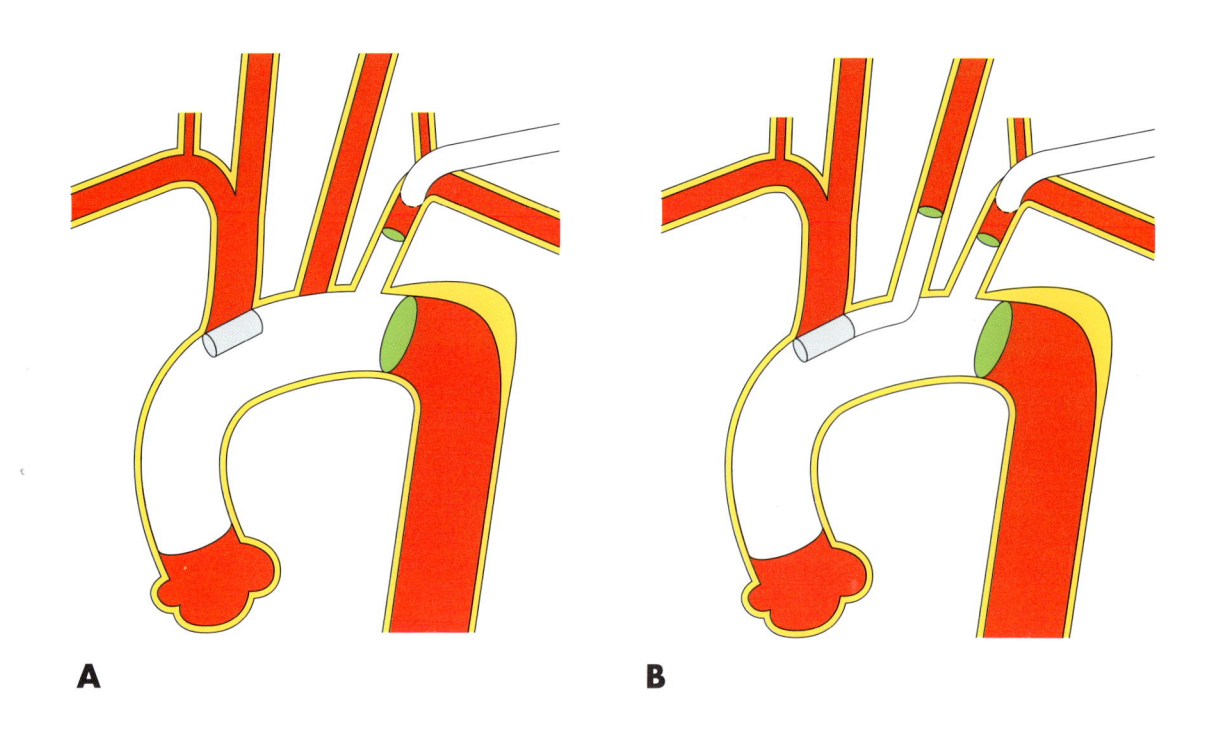

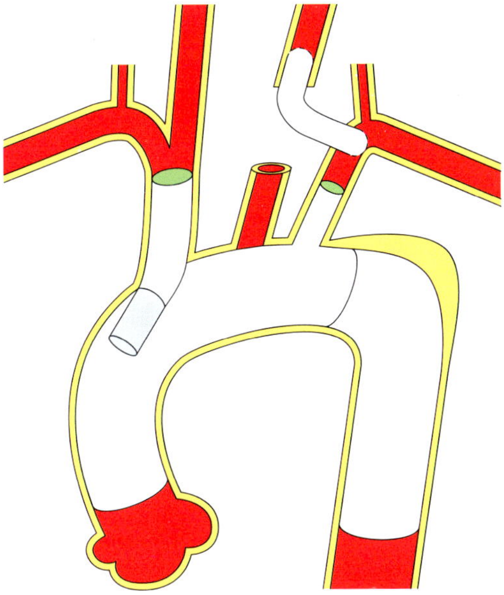

FIG. 5 In cases of left-sided stent graft insertion, the additional branch can go instead to the innominate artery.

REFERENCES

1. Criado FJ, Clark NS, Barnatan MF. Stent graft repair in the aortic arch and descending thoracic aorta: a 4-year experience. J Vasc Surg 2002; 36: 1121-1128.
2. Czerny M, Gottardi R, Zimpfer D et al. Mid-term results of supraaortic transpositions for extended endovascular repair of aortic arch pathologies. Eur J Cardiovasc Surg 2007; 31: 623-627.
3. Bergeron P, Mangialardi N, Costa P et al. Great vessel management for endovascular exclusion of aortic arch aneurysms and dissections. Eur J Vasc Endovasc Surg 2006; 32: 38-45.
4. Saito N, Kimura T, Odashiro K et al. Feasibility of the Inoue single-branched stent-graft implantation for thoracic aortic aneurysm or dissection involving the left subclavian artery: short-to-medium-term results in 17 patients. J Vasc Surg 2005; 41: 206-212.
5. Chuter TA, Schneider DB, Reilly LM et al. Modular branched stent graft for endovascular repair of aortic arch aneurysm and dissection. J Vasc Surg 2003; 38: 859-863.
6. Verhoeven EL. Endovascular reconstruction of aortic arch by modified bifurcated stent graft for Stanford type A dissection. Asian J Surg 2007; 30: 296-297.
7. Mc Williams RG, Murphy M, Hartley D et al. In situ stent-graft fenestration to preserve the left subclavian artery. J Endovasc Ther 2004; 11: 170-174.
8. Hiramoto JS, Schneider DB, Reilly LM et al. A double-barrel stent-graft for endovascular repair of the aortic arch. J Endovasc Ther 2006; 13: 72-76.
9. Criado FJ. Chimney grafts and bare stents: aortic branch preservation revisited. J Endovasc Ther 2007;14: 823-824.
10. Gorich J, Asquan Y, Seifarth H et al. Initial experience with intentional stent-graft coverage of the subclavian artery during endovascuclar thoracic aortic repairs. J Endovasc Ther 2002; 9 Suppl2: II39-43.
11. Peterson BG, Eskandari MK, Gleason TG et al. Utility of left subclavian artery revascularization in association with endoluminal repair of acute and chronic thoracic aortic pahtology. J Vasc Surg 2006; 43: 433-439.
12. Morales JP, Taylor PR, Bell RE et al. Neurological complications following endoluminal repair of thoracic aortic disease. Cardiovasc Intervent Radiol 2007; 30: 833-839.
13. Sullivan TM, Sundt TM 3rd. Complications of thoracic aortic endografts: spinal cord ischemia and stroke. J Vasc Surg 2006; 43 Suppl A: 85A-88A.
14. Chuter TA, Buck DG, Schneider DB et al. Development of a branched stent-graft for endovascular repair of aortic arch aneurysms. J Endovasc Ther 2003; 10: 940-945.

BRANCHED AND FENESTRATED ENDOGRAFTS: TECHNOLOGY, PLANNING PROCESS AND IMPLANTATION TECHNIQUE

STÉPHAN HAULON, RICHARD AZZAOUI, ELIXÈNE JEAN-BAPTISTE
TOMMASO DONATI, PIERVITO D'ELIA, SÉBASTIEN AMIOT
JONATHAN SOBOCINSKI, MOHAMAD KOUSSA

Successful endovascular repair of abdominal aortic aneurysms (AAA) requires undilated proximal (infrarenal neck) and distal landing zones (common or external iliac arteries). A range of approved endografts are available to exclude such aneurysms. Recent multicentric prospective randomized trials have demonstrated a short and midterm decrease in aneurysm-related deaths of the endovascular technique compared to open surgery [1-4]. These results have induced an overall increase in the rate of endovascular repair of AAA. Patients with more complex aortic aneurysms, involving the visceral vessels (juxta, para and thoraco-abdominal aneurysms) or both common iliac arteries, have an increased peri-operative morbidity and mortality after open repair compared to AAA [5,6]. These patients could potentially benefit from an endovascular approach. Branched and fenestrated endografts have been developed to address this endovascular challenge [7-14]. The chapter written by Roy Greenberg et al. will focus on the data already available to evaluate these new endovascular procedures. We will describe the available technology, the planning process and the implantation technique.

Branched and fenestrated endografts

The only CE approved fenestrated and branched endograft are manufactured by Cook Inc. (Bloomington, Indiana, USA). The former device has been designed to treat abdominal aneurysm with short necks (4 to 15 mm) and the latter to treat common iliac aneurysms with no distal neck. In addition, a wide range of custom-endografts combining fenestrations and branches can be manufactured to match most aortic aneurysms complex anatomy. The general concept can be summarized as follows:
- the proximal and distal sealing zones of the endograft will be positioned over healthy arterial segment (>20 mm).
- Any ostium (visceral or internal iliac = target vessels) covered by the fabric of the endograft will be perfused by a balloon-expandable stent-graft through a fenestration if the distance between the deployed endograft and the origin of the target vessel is less than 10 mm. When this distance is larger than 10 mm the target vessels are perfused through branches. The bridging stent-graft in the latter setting can be balloon-expandable or self-expandable.
- The anatomy of the target vessel will also have an impact on the endograft design. When the angulation between the aorta and the target vessel is less than 60°, selective catheterization of this vessel through a fenestration can be challenging from a femoral access. In this setting, the diameter of the aortic endograft can ultimately be reduced to add a branch that will facilitate the access to the target vessel from a brachial approach.
- It is mandatory to design large overlap segments between the various aortic endografts and between the bridging stent-grafts and the fenestrations or branches. More specifically, the bridging stent-graft implanted through a fenestration will protrude (4-5 mm) in the aortic endograft lumen. Subsequently, the aortic extremity of the stent-graft will be flared (like a rivet) to ensure a perfect seal at the level of the fenestration. The latter is now always manufactured "reinforced" with a nitinol ring sutured to its perimeter.

The endograft design to exclude most juxta, para and type IV thoraco-abdominal aneurysms is a 3-component system. A proximal tubular endograft is customized with fenestrations to match the patient specific orientation of the visceral vessels. A bifurcated endograft is subsequently implanted inside the tubular component with an optimal 3-stent overlap. The addition of a limb extension usually completes the implant (Fig. 1). The fenestrations incorporated in the proximal tubular component can be *small* (diameter between 6 to 8 mm, located at a minimum of 15 mm from the top of the fabric), *large* (diameter between 8 and 12 mm, located at a minimum of 10 mm from the top of the fabric), or *scallop* (hemi ovals, 6 to 12 mm in height and 10 mm large, located at the most proximal portion of the fabric). The lumen of the small fenestrations is placed between stent struts of the aortic endograft to allow the implantation of a balloon expandable stent within the target vessel. A strut from the aortic endograft will often cross the lumen of large fenestrations, and thus not permit fixation of the fenestrations with an additional stent. A scallop for the superior mesenteric artery (SMA) and 2 small fenestrations for the renal arteries is the standard or most frequent association of fenestrations in the setting of a juxta-renal aneurysm. However, in specific settings, different fenestration combinations will be designed:
- (a) if the SMA origin is located less than 3 mm from the origin of the most proximal renal artery, the scallop will be replaced by a large fenestration;
- (b) if one or both renals are located more than 10 mm from the origin of the aneurysm, a scallop could be preferred to perfuse the highest or both renal arteries;
- when (a) and (b) are present, 2 scallops can perfuse both the SMA and the highest renal artery. For manufacturing purpose, the origin of the 2 arteries have to be more than 30° apart. A small fenestration will perfuse the lowest renal artery.

The proximal tubular component is fixed to the aortic wall by the barbs located on the proximal uncovered stent (10 or 12 depending on diameter). The radial force of the balloon expandable stents (or stent-grafts) implanted through the fenestrations will also secure the endograft's position. The downward force exerted by the aortic flow on the endograft bifurcation is only supported by the bifurcated body. The risk of migration of the proximal tubular endograft is therefore limited and thus relieves the stress on the renal stents. The bifurcated endograft is likely to migrate downstream. To avoid a disconnection, we previously stated that a

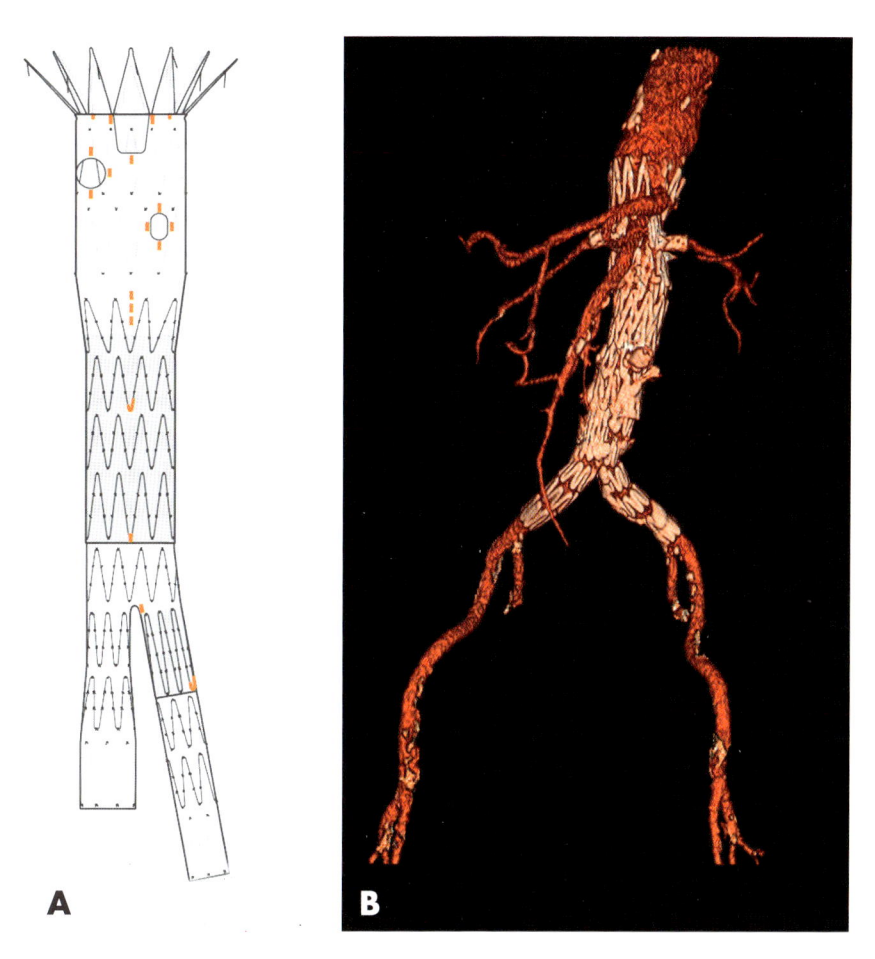

FIG. 1 Illustration (A) and post operative (B) images of a fenestrated endograft. The fenestrations (scallop fenestration for the superior mesenteric artery [SMA] and small fenestrations for the renal arteries) are positioned on the proximal tubular component. The overlap between the tubular and the bifurcated endografts is > 3 stents (grey area on the illustration). Radio opaque gold markers (yellow markers on figure A) are placed around the fenestrations.

minimum 3-stent overlap between both endografts was mandatory. The distal diameter of the tubular component is usually 22 mm whereas the proximal diameter of the bifurcated component is 24 mm. This slender oversizing will prevent from type III endoleaks but will not limit the distal migration of the bifurcated body until it seats on the aortic bifurcation.

The fenestrated endografts have only been CE approved for AAA with short necks. The endografts described in the next chapters are custom made devices (CMD) for compassionate use.

In the setting of pararenal and type IV thoracoabdominal aneurysms, the sealing zone will be located above the origin of the SMA. Small fenestrations will perfuse the renal arteries, a large strut free fenestration the SMA, and a scallop or a second large strut free fenestration the celiac trunk.

In the absence of major aortic angulation (>90°), patients with type I, II and III thoraco-abdominal aneurysms are potential candidates for an endovascular repair. The choice between a fenestration and a branch to perfuse the visceral arteries in the aneurysm sac has been previously described and primarily depends on the anatomy of these vessels and the diameter of the aortic lumen (Fig. 2). It is crucial to assess the anatomy of the aortic arch when a branch has been designed. Obviously, because of the high embolic stroke risk, a bovine arch with a "shaggy" wall cannot be considered as a possible remote access to a branch. A theoretical limit to the use of branches is the need to diminish the aortic endograft diameter to incorporate the side branches (Fig. 3). Similarly and in addition to

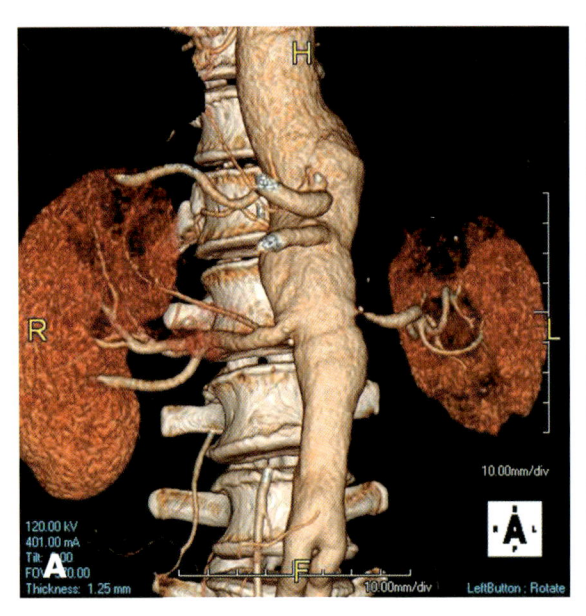

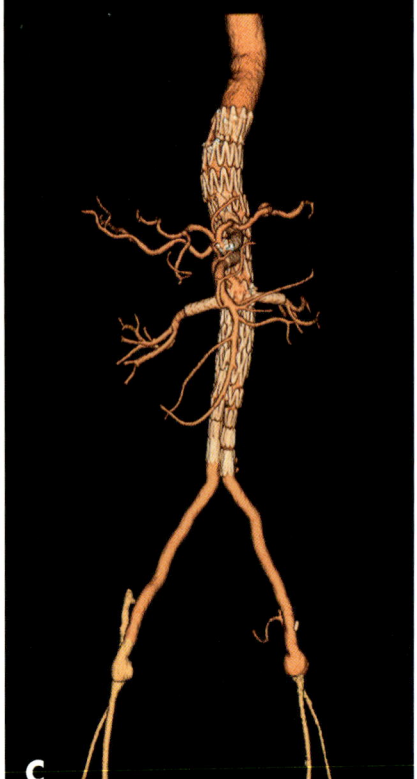

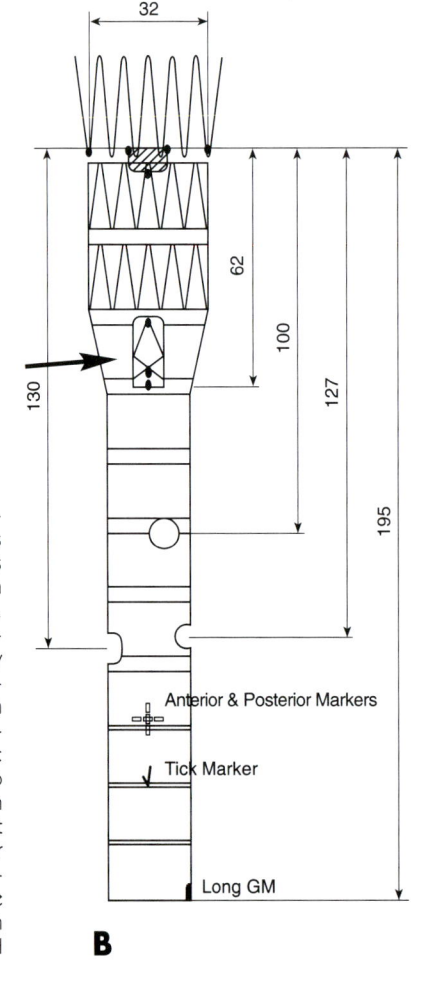

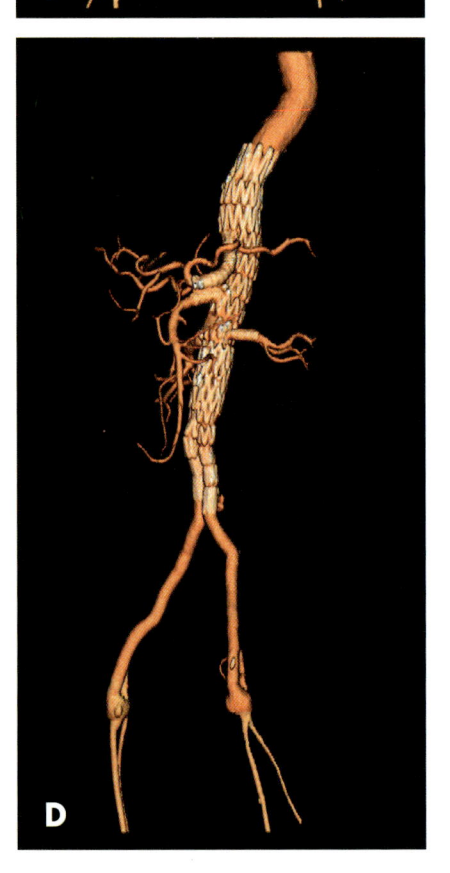

FIG. 2 A - A type 3 thoracoabdominal aneurysm is depicted above a previous aortobifemoral bypass on the preoperative CT scan. The diameter of this aneurysm enlarges significantly above the SMA. The endograft was designed with a branch (red arrow on figure B) to perfuse the celiac trunk and 3 fenestrations to perfuse the SMA and both renal arteries. The post operative CT scan anterior (C) and lateral (D) VRT reconstructions confirms the exclusion of the aneurysm sac and the patency of all 4 visceral arteries.

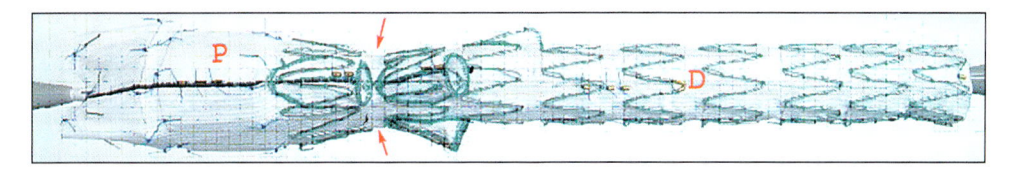

FIG. 3 This endograft was designed with 4 branches to perfuse the visceral arteries. The proximal diameter (P) of the endogaft narrows (red arrows) at the level of the branches to provide space between the endograft and the aortic wall to implant the bridging stents.

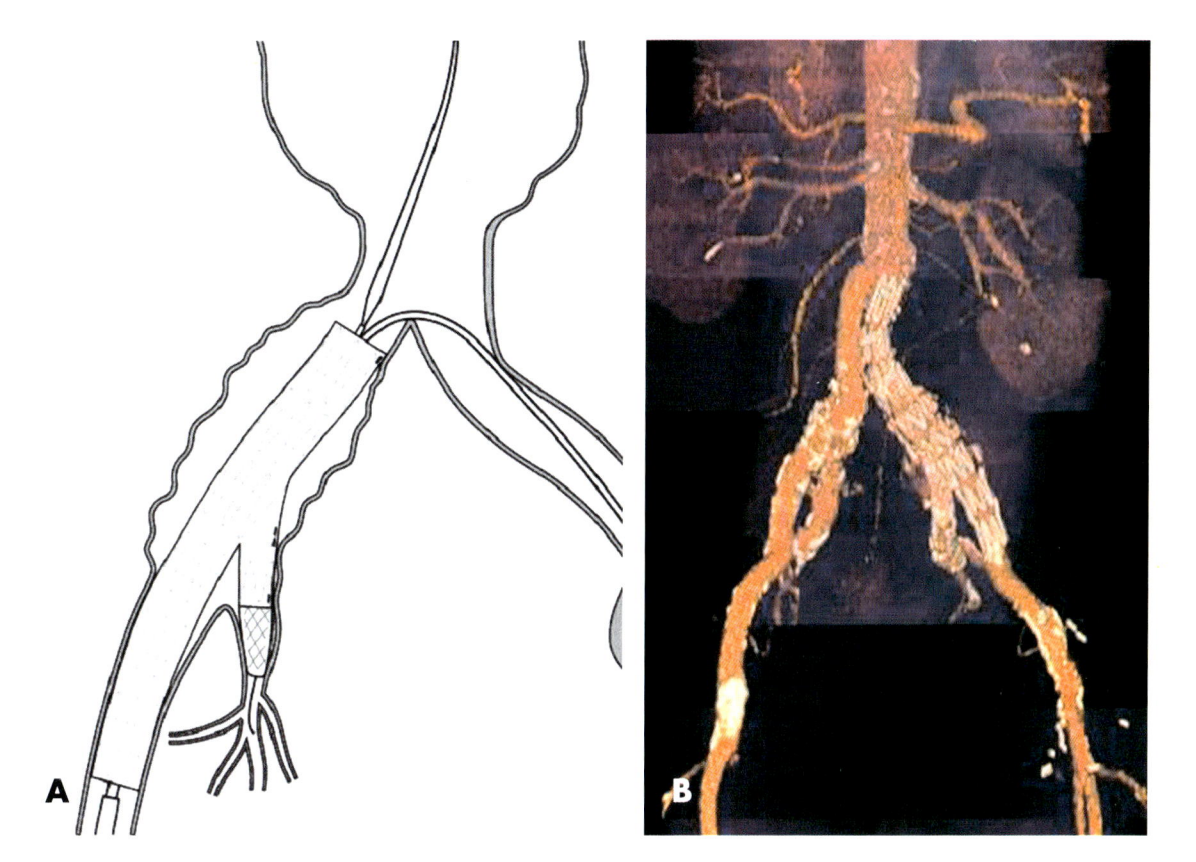

FIG. 4 A - The internal iliac artery is accessed from a contralateral femoral approach. A bridging stent graft is then advanced above the aortic bifurcation and implanted. This manoeuvre is not possible when the iliac aneurysm is located below an aorto-bi-iliac bypass (B). In this latter setting, the internal iliac is catheterized and the stent graft advanced from a brachial access.

bifurcations, the aortic flow will apply a downward force on a tapered endograft, thus creating a potential migration risk that would result in branch kinking and occlusion. These theoretical risks have not yet been observed with this specific endograft design. Defenders of this latter design will advocate the easy target vessel access from above and the potentially more stable branch/mating stent-graft association compared to the fenestration/mating stent-graft association over time (less material fatigue issues).

Endovascular repair of grade IIC AAA (bilateral common iliac artery aneurysms) can be achieved with a specific branched iliac limb. Two versions are available. The former has a helical internal iliac branch (8 mm diameter, 20 mm long) that runs lateral and posterior (helical path). Another version, the Zenith Bifurcated Iliac Sidebranch (ZBIS), has a more conventional downward bifurcation (also 8 mm diameter, 8 mm long). Both devices (Fig. 4) are placed in a 20Fr sheath delivery system and fixed proximally and distally with trigger wires. A

4Fr catheter and 0.035" Starter wire are preloaded into the side branch of the graft. The catheter and guide wire passes along the external aspect of the distal segment of the device, through the branch and out the proximal segment.

To appropriately select the target IIA for the branch endograft, tight atherosclerosis stenosis of the origin of the IIA and extensive aneurysmal disease of the IIA have to be excluded. The diameter of the common iliac artery bifurcation has to be > 18 mm to avoid any compression of the IIA branch or compression of the origin of the IIA by the delivery system positioned in the iliac axis. If compression of the helical branch is depicted or suspected, a complementary balloon expandable stent with a high radial force has to be implanted in the branch to guarantee durable patency.

Preoperative imaging

Designing an infrarenal endograft is a relatively simple procedure, requiring preoperative length and diameter measurements. Designing a device which will accommodate the aortic branches is more complex. Critical end organs depend on blood flow through the fenestrations or branches of the endograft. Inappropriate orientation of the visceral branches and fenestrations will preclude successful endovascular repair. Essential information needed for preoperative assessment of aortic aneurysms includes the relationship of the aneurysm to the aortic branches, the degree of iliac arterial involvement with the aneurysm, the presence of other coexisting iliac arterial or aortic aneurysms, the presence of supernumerary or aberrant aortic branches and the presence of coexistent iliac arterial occlusive disease.

Thus, high resolution spiral computed tomography (CT) scans (0.75 mm reconstructions) and 3D workstations are mandatory for designing complex aortic endografts. While the pathology is evident on the axial images, the angiographic quality of the reformations allows rapid identification of the vascular abnormality. On currently available 3D workstations, there are four principle visualization techniques: multiplanar (axial, sagittal and coronal) reformation (MPR); curved planar reformation (CPR); maximum intensity projection (MIP), and 3D volume rendering (VR). The overall aortic morphology is first analyzed on the color VR images. Multiplanar reconstructions are then performed to depict proximal and distal sealing zones. MPR and MIP reconstructions are also performed to depict intercostal arteries location and patency. Curved planar reconstruction (CPR) assesses the true cross-sectional diameters and is mandatory to accurately assess lengths in a curved aorta. CPR is performed following an automated vessel centerline extraction between two points subsequently selected proximal and distal to the aneurysm. Various vessel view layout are then required to analyze diameters and lengths in support of an accurate endograft design. Primarily, the following measures are performed:
1) true sealing zones cross-sectional diameters;
2) total length of aorta to be covered by the endograft;
3) length between the ostium of each target vessels;
4) diameters of the aortic lumen at the level of the target vessels;
5) diameter and "clock position" of the origin of each target vessel.

Procedure description

PARARENAL AND TAA ANEURYSM

Open or percutaneous access is required to both common femoral arteries. When necessary (i.e. in the setting of severe external iliac stenosis), access to the common iliac arteries is performed. On one side, the main body of the graft is introduced and on the contralateral side, a 20 or 24Fr sheath is inserted over a stiff wire. The tip of this sheath will be positioned just above the aortic bifurcation. The stiff wire is retrieved, and three or four 5Fr sheaths are introduced through the valve of the large sheath. An angiography catheter is advanced over a guide wire through one 5Fr sheath to a suitable position in the aorta (above the target vessels). Under fluoroscopy the fenestrations, branches and the associated markers are recognized and the orientation of the main body of the device is checked. On the ipsilateral side, a stiff guide wire is advanced to the level of the aortic arch. The fenestrated/branched body is inserted over this stiff wire to the required position so that the appropriate fenestrations are correctly aligned with their matching target vessels (checked by repeated angiographies with small volumes of contrast). The outer sheath of the delivery system is withdrawn. The diameter reducing ties restrain the endograft partially. It can therefore still be rotated, advanced or pulled back as necessary. Through a contralateral 5Fr sheath, access to the lumen of the endograft is obtained. A side branch access sheath is then advanced on this wire and catheterization of a target vessel through its appropriate fenestration performed. The access sheath is then advanced into the vessel over a stiff wire. The maneuver is repeated for each target vessel and its fenestration. Appropriate covered stents are advanced through the access sheaths into the target vessels. When the endograft's design includes one or more branches, a hydrophilic wire is then advanced in the branch-preloaded catheter until it is in the descending thoracic aorta. A 7 or 8Fr sheath is also positioned into the descending aorta from a brachial artery. A snare is advanced through this sheath to capture the wire from the preloaded catheter, to create through and through access from the groin to the brachial artery. Over this wire, the brachial sheath is advanced into the endograft and ultimately into the side branch. The target vessel is then selectively catheterized. When a stiff wire has been positioned in the target vessel, the through and through wire is retrieved. This latter maneuver is necessary to advance the brachial sheath and subsequently the bridging stent-graft into the target vessel. A 7Fr sheath is required when a balloon-expandable bridging stent-graft is implanted, and a 9Fr sheath in the setting of a self-expandable bridging stent-graft.

Once the stent-grafts are all positioned in their target vessels, the diameter reducing ties of the endograft are released. If a proximal uncovered fixation stent has been designed on top of the fenestrated/branched endograft, it is deployed at this stage. For each target vessel, the C-arm tube is oriented tangential to the fenestration. The bridging stent is positioned with 3-4 mm protruding in the aorta and expanded once the access sheath has been withdrawn. The aortic extremity of the bridging stent is the flared with a 12 mm-diameter 2 cm-long balloon.

The fenestrated/branched component is then connected to other aortic components as planned, being careful not to dislodge or disrupt the existing device, or the fenestration stents.

Common iliac aneurysms

Both common femoral arteries are exposed. The delivery system is advanced over a stiff wire into the iliac axis ipsilateral to the target IIA artery. The distal end of the branch (visualized by specific gold markers) is positioned approximately 5 mm above the origin of the internal iliac artery. The outer sheath of the delivery system is withdrawn to expose the branch limb, leaving the distal end constrained within the sheath in the external iliac artery. The preloaded wire is advanced into the distal aorta and snared from the contralateral femoral artery. This provides through-and-through access from the contralateral common femoral artery to the ipsilateral one. A 10Fr sheath is advanced over this wire from the contralateral groin, over the aortic bifurcation, into the proximal segment of the device and finally into the sidebranch. An angled catheter (vertebral or cobra) is introduced into this sheath to selectively catheterize the internal iliac artery with a guidewire. The guidewire is then exchanged for a stiffer wire. The mating component (self expanding or balloon expandable stent-graft) is advanced over the stiff wire into the desired position. The mating device is oversized by 5%-10% with respect to the target internal iliac artery. Once the mating graft is deployed and appropriately ballooned, the remainder of the external iliac limb is deployed. The component is then mated to the remainder of a Zenith graft with a limb extension.

Advancing a large introducer sheath over the aortic bifurcation is the major technical challenge during this procedure. It is usually not a concern in the setting of a native aneurysmal aorto-iliac bifurcation. On the contrary, in the setting of a narrow and calcified bifurcation, or the presence of an aorto-bi-iliac prosthetic bypass snaring the preloaded catheter and gaining access to the branch from the left brachial artery is recommended.

Conclusion

Endovascular exclusion of complex aortic aneurysms with fenestrated and branched endografts is now performed in many academic centers throughout the world. Training experienced endovascular therapists to implant these endografts is not a challenge. Device planning remains probably the most difficult part of the procedure. Dedicated planning training programs are therefore developed.

Mid-term results of endovascular complex aortic repairs are favorable compared to open surgery in high risk patients. Long-term results will be necessary to evaluate specific complications such as migration, material fatigue and component separation that can result in loss of visceral branches.

REFERENCES

1. Greenhalgh RM, Brown LC, Kwong GP et al. EVAR trial participants. Comparison of endovascular aneurysm repair with open repair in patients with abdominal aortic aneurysm (EVAR trial 1), 30-day operative mortality results: randomised controlled trial. *Lancet* 2004; 364: 843-848.
2. Prinssen M, Verhoeven EL, Buth J et al. Dutch Randomized Endovascular Aneurysm Management (DREAM) Trial Group. A randomized trial comparing conventional and endovascular repair of abdominal aortic aneurysms. *N Engl J Med* 2004; 351: 1607-1618.
3. Blankensteijn J, de Jong S, Prinssen M et al. Two-year outcomes after conventional or endovascular repair of abdominal aortic aneurysms. *N Engl J Med* 2005; 352: 2398-2405.
4. Anonymous. EVAR Trial participants. Endovascular aneurysm repair versus open repair in patient with abdominal aortic aneurysms (EVAR 1): randomized controlled trial. *Lancet* 2005; 365: 2179-2186.
5. Cambria RP, Clouse WD, Davison JK et al. Thoracoabdominal aneurysm repair: results with 337 operations performed over a 15-year interval. *Ann Surg* 2002; 236: 471-479.
6. Coselli JS. Thoracoabdominal aortic aneurysms: experience with 372 patients. *J Card Surg* 1994; 9: 638-647.
7. Greenberg RK, Haulon S, Lyden SP et al. The endovascular management of juxtarenal aneurysms with fenestrated endovascular grafting. *J Vasc Surg* 2004; 39: 279-287.
8. Greenberg RK, Haulon S, O'Neill S et al. Primary Endovascular Repair of Juxtarenal Aneurysms With Fenestrated Endovascular Grafting. *Eur J Vasc Endovasc Surg* 2004; 27: 484-491.
9. Scurr JR, Brennan JA, Gilling-Smith GL et al. Fenestrated endovascular repair for juxtarenal aortic aneurysm. *Br J Surg* 2008; 95: 326-332.
10. Ziegler P, Avgerinos ED, Umscheid T et al. Fenestrated endografting for aortic aneurysm repair: a 7-year experience. *J Endovasc Ther* 2007; 14: 609-618.
11. O'Neill S, Greenberg RK, Haddad F et al. A prospective analysis of fenestrated endovascular grafting: intermediate terms outcomes. *Eur J Vasc Endovasc Surg* 2006; 32: 115-123.
12. Greenberg RK, West K, Pfaff K et al. Beyond the aortic bifurcation: branched endovascular grafts for thoracoabdominal and aortoiliac aneurysms. *J Vasc Surg* 2006; 43: 879-886.
13. Chuter TA, Rapp JH, Hiramoto JS et al. Endovascular treatment of thoracoabdominal aortic aneurysms. *J Vasc Surg* 2008; 47: 6-16.
14. Haulon S, Greenberg RK, Pfaff K et al. Branched grafting for aortoiliac aneurysms. *Eur J Vasc Endovasc Surg* 2007; 33: 567-574.

FENESTRATED AND BRANCHED ENDOGRAFTS: CURRENT RESULTS

TARA MASTRACCI, ROY GREENBERG, COLETTA VIDMAR

Thoraco-abdominal aortic aneurysm (TAAA) is a complex disease that usually presents with anatomic variations requiring a treatment tailored to both the patient anatomy, and underlying comorbidities. Advancements in branched and fenestrated devices make endovascular TAAA repair a possibility, and have evolved since the early experience reported in 1999 [1,2]. In order to refine both the technology of graft design and accommodate the learning curve of physicians as they approach this broadening field, the methods of innovators have been to initiate their experience with branched devices for the hypogastric artery. In this light, success may be rewarded by the absence of hip claudication, while failure of the branched procedure simply relegates the patient to the current standard of care, which is internal iliac embolization followed by stentgraft exclusion. Following the development of expertise with branched procedures, more complex visceral branches were constructed. Over time, directional branches have been combined with fenestrated procedures to offer a variety of devices and options for patients with complex aortic pathology and frequently without other options. In this chapter, we will present the systematic experience at the Cleveland Clinic Foundation of placing branched or fenestrated grafts into different aortic distributions, and the outcomes associated with each.

Basic considerations

Before describing the details of our experience, it is important to note that early work has dealt with high risk individuals who have no other surgical options, which is reflective of the initial paucity of evidence as to the durability of repair and the desire of early innovators to proceed with caution. As technical aspects of this technique have evolved, the indications have been extended to somewhat healthier patients with difficult anatomic problems. However, we all recognize that the ultimate success of these technologies rests in the long-term device performance. Thus extended follow-up studies that are properly controlled or randomized will help to define the place of these procedures in patients with aortic disease.

Imaging is an integral component to the development and design of all endovascular devices. Prior to undertaking fenestrated or branched endografting, it is important to obtain high resolution computed tomography (CT) scans of the entire aorta to assess for concomitant pathology in other aortic distributions, and to allow for the careful interrogation of the anatomy to facilitate graft design. The use of post-processing software to manipulate DICOM data in three dimensions, and create center lumen of flow projections has been essential to the creation of devices that fit the patient's anatomy and can be successfully deployed. It has also allowed for the careful investigation to identify vessels that may be unfavorable for endovascular repair. This includes severe angulation, extensive thrombus, and the presence of occlusive disease in the access vessels. Although none of these factors are absolute contraindications, they do increase the risk of the procedure and should be carefully identified preoperatively.

Branched grafts for common iliac aneurysms

Hypogastric branched devices are intended to preserve antegrade flow into the internal iliac artery, replacing the technique of coil embolization and stentgraft exclusion. The primary complication avoided is that of buttock or hip claudication. Expertise with these devices is readily applicable to similar branched devices used to treat proximal anatomy. The preservation of antegrade internal iliac flow appears to be clinically important in patients with more extensive proximal disease, as it likely serves as a collateral bed for the anterior spinal artery.

A multicenter prospective analysis of patients undergoing implantation of branched endografts into the internal iliac artery was reported in the European Journal of Vascular and Endovascular Surgery in 2007 [3]. The study was conducted from 2003 to 2006 and involved five hospitals globally which enrolled patients who were considered to be high risk for open surgical repair and had common iliac artery (CIA) aneurysms greater than 20 mm. The

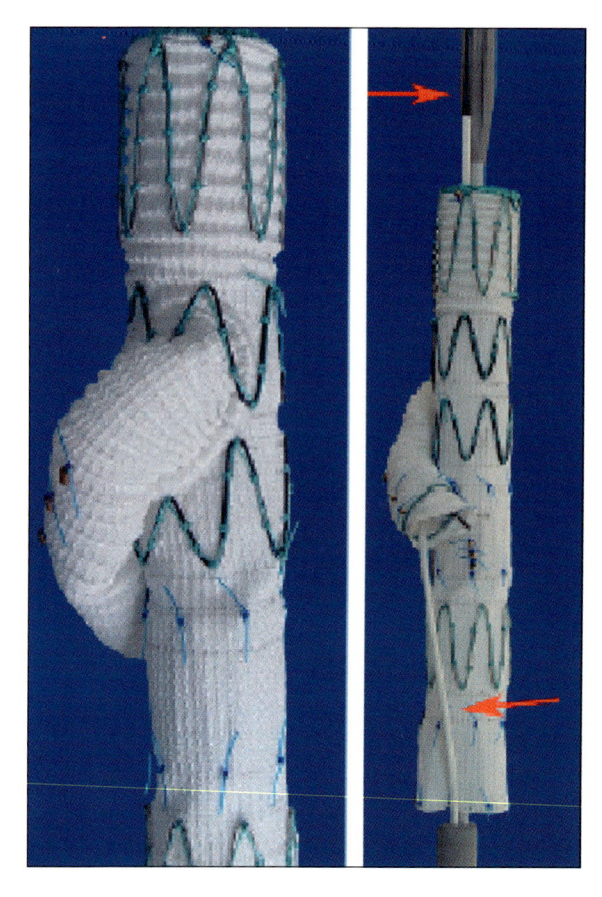

FIG. 1 Ex-vivo images of Iliac branched graft. Red arrows illustrate preloaded catheter and wire. (Reprinted with permission, Haulon S, Devos P, Willoteaux S et al. Risk factors of early and late complications in patients undergoing endovascular aneurysm repair. Eur J Vasc Endovasc Surg 2003; 25: 118-124 [3]).

devices were 12 mm stent grafts with an internal iliac helical limb in the left or right orientation, as previously described (Fig. 1). Anatomic eligibility was assessed using a high resolution preoperative spiral CT scan, and device sizing was performed using post processing software (TeraRecon Inc) and center lumen of flow measurements. Measurement and device sizing were performed by a physician with expertise in the device. Presence of other aneurysms in the visceral, infrarenal or thoracic distribution did not exclude the patient from inclusion in the trial. Implantation was performed by endovascular specialists who underwent training in the specific protocol for this device (Fig. 2). Follow-up was conducted at 1, 6, 12 and 24 months, and included clinical visits and contrast, high resolution CT scans which were analyzed using the same post processing software to determine device

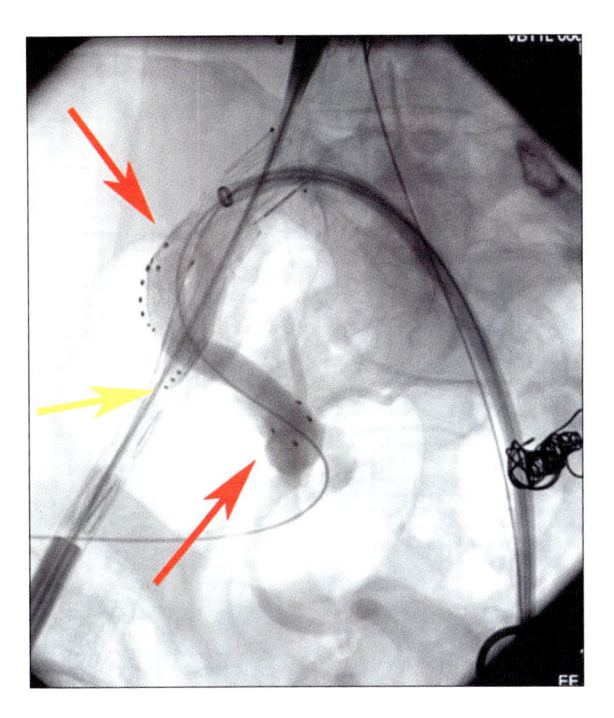

FIG. 2 Angiographic image of the deployed internal iliac branch graft. A 12F Balkin sheath is within the tubular section immediately proximal to the branch. A Rosen wire has been passed into the distal internal iliac circulation. The red arrows denote the margins of the 10 mm x 60 mm Fluency graft, while the yellow arrow notes the position of the three distal markers that are intended to be placed immediately above the internal iliac origin. *(Reprinted with permission, Haulon S, Devos P, Willoteaux S et al. Risk factors of early and late complications in patients undergoing endovascular aneurysm repair. Eur J Vasc Endovasc Surg 2003; 25: 118-124 [3]).*

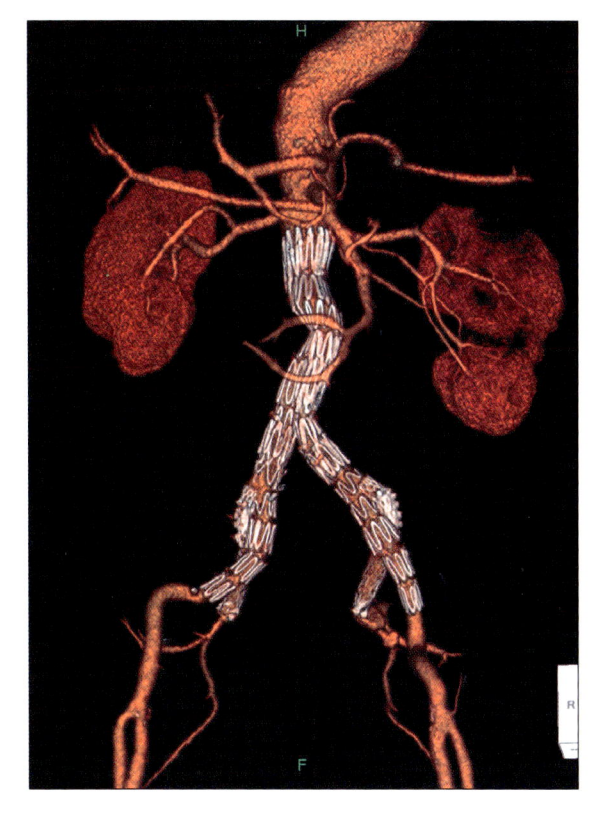

FIG. 3 Post procedural CT scan demonstrating the versatility of the device. In this image, both internal iliacs were treated with helical branches. *(Reprinted with permission, Haulon S, Devos P, Willoteaux S et al. Risk factors of early and late complications in patients undergoing endovascular aneurysm repair. Eur J Vasc Endovasc Surg 2003; 25: 118-124 [3]).*

patency and placement. Clinical outcomes including perioperative mortality and complications, and other endovascular outcomes were reported in accordance with the most recent reporting standards. Buttock claudication was an outcome of particular interest, determined a *priori*.

After 3 years of enrollment, 51 patients (90% male) were enrolled, with a mean age of 72 years (range 56-86 years), and a mean follow-up of 14.2 months. The maximum diameter of the common iliac artery was 38 mm (range 23-78 mm) and abdominal aorta was 56 mm (range 32-89 mm), including 4 patients with isolated common iliac aneurysms. Bilateral iliac aneurysms were present in 80% of patients (41/52) but only one patient had bilateral devices placed (Fig. 3). The proximal device used was a Zenith Trifab in 61% of patients and a Zenith branched or fenestrated device to treat more proximal aortic pathology in 33%. The remaining repairs included and aorto-uni-iliac device (2%) and other devices (4%). Technical success was achieved in 94% of patients, with no conversions to open surgery, and no aneurysm related mortality. During the follow-up period, 7 patients died of non-aneurysm related causes. No branch vessel occlusions occurred after 30 days. Aneurysm treatment was also successful, as CIA aneurysm shrinkage was observed in 42% of patients at 6 months, and 81% of patients at 12 months, with no aneurysm growth demonstrated in any patient during the follow-up period. Furthermore, there were no type I or III endoleaks observed in the perioperative or follow up period. In 2 patients, contralateral iliac limbs thrombosed due to tortuous external iliac arteries, and in 1 patient, a branched limb thrombosed 1 week after the branch itself occluded. Thus, all limb thrombosis occurred in the setting of an occluded internal iliac artery. All such cases were successfully treated with thrombolytic therapy, without reocclusion of the limbs during follow-up. There were no cases of colonic or spinal cord ischemia in the follow up period. The contralateral internal iliac artery was embolized and excluded in all but one of the patients with bilateral common iliac aneurysms. The resulting claudication in the contralateral side was universal and persisted throughout the course of follow-up.

In addition to the device reported in this trial, there are other devices that have been utilized. Publications from centers of excellence such as Malmo Sweden, Frankfurt and Muenster, as well as from Australia describe similar results with sister devices [4-6]. At this point, devices are commercially available in most places, but remain investigational in the United States.

Fenestrated endografts for juxtarenal aneurysms

The treatment of juxtarenal aneurysms is the next degree of complexity for branched and fenestrated grafts. Our experience with fenestrated devices was conducted as a prospective study designed to determine the feasibility and outcome of endovascular repair of juxtarenal aneurysms [7]. Our most recent publication included 119 patients (82% male, mean age 75 +/- 7 years) between 2001 and 2005 who were considered high risk for open repair, but also had contraindications to conventional infrarenal stenting. These patients underwent preoperative high resolution CT scans which were used to design fenestrated devices incorporating the visceral vessels into the design. The aim was to extend the sealing zone into the visceral segment of the aorta, thereby both increasing the number of patients who would be eligible for endovascular repair, and the distance of normal caliber aorta included in the sealing zone to prevent type I endoleaks. Patients found eligible for inclusion in the trial were implanted with a Zenith fenestrated device (Fig. 4), and had protocolized follow up at 1, 6, 12 months, and yearly thereafter, which included routine ultrasonography, plain films and CT scans.

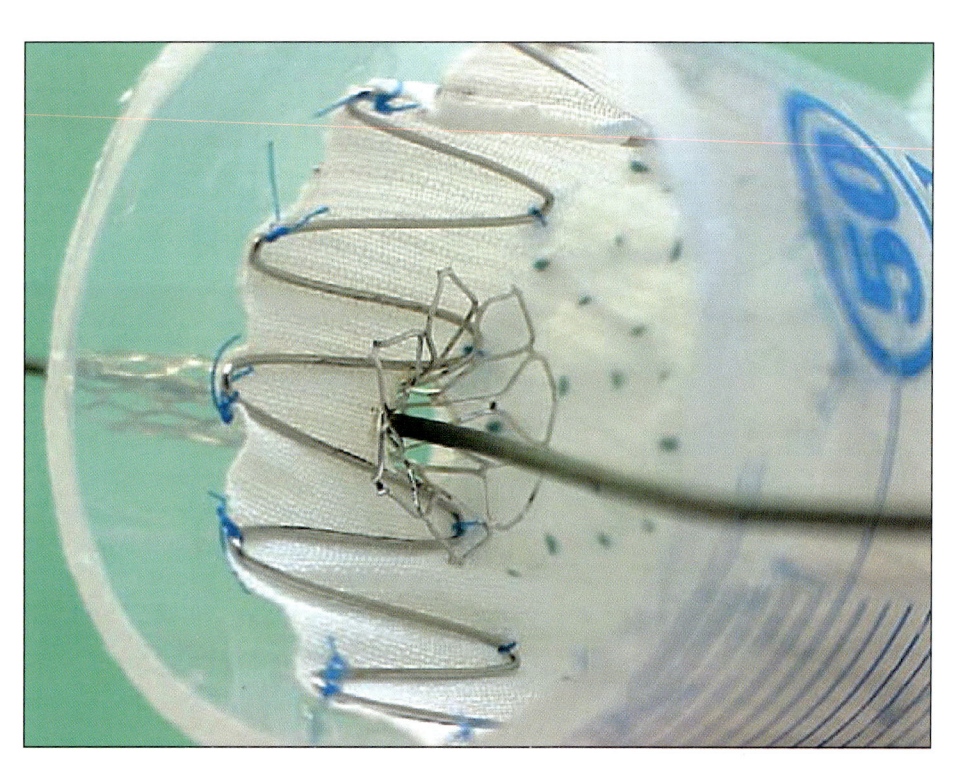

FIG. 4 Magnified image of an ex-vivo deployment of the Zenith Fenestrated Device, with an uncovered stent flared in the single fenestration. The aortic portion of the uncovered stent was initially flared with a 10 mm balloon and subsequently with a latex compliant balloon. (Reprinted with permission, O'Neill S, Greenberg RK, Haddad F et al. A prospective analysis of fenestrated endovascular grafting: intermediate-term outcomes. Eur J Vasc Endovasc Surg 2006; 32: 115-123 [7]).

Postoperative studies were performed to determine device migration, the presence of endoleaks, interval size in aneurysm diameter and other postoperative complications in accordance with the most current endovascular reporting standards. Patients were also monitored for interval change in renal function (assessed by serum creatinine increased to greater than 2 mg/dL or a rise of >30% from baseline levels).

After a mean follow up of 19 months (range 0-48), the results of fenestrated endografting in high risk patients are quite favorable. Aneurysms treated in this series had a mean proximal neck diameter of 26±3.5 mm (range 17-34) with a length of 8 mm ± 4 mm (range 3-18). All prostheses were successfully implanted, and technical success was excellent. Of all branch vessels in the intended repairs, only one renal artery was not successfully catheterized and stented at the time of the original procedure. Ancillary devices were required intraoperatively in some of the cases, including a Palmaz stent deployed below the renal arteries in 19% (23/119) of patients, balloon expandable stents at the junction of the fenestrated and bifurcated component in 12% (14/119) of patients, and self expanding stents into tortuous iliac limbs in 5.9% (7/119) of patients. Extension grafts were required to treat modular joint leaks in 1.7% (2/119) of patients. This aggressive correction of endoleaks at the time of original procedure, as well as aggressive reintervention for the 30 endoleaks found on post-discharge imaging resulted in a very low rate of late type I endoleak. The mortality in this series is depicted in Fig. 5: one patient died secondary to sepsis from aspiration pneumonia within 30 days of surgery, following a fenestrated graft placement with extra-anatomic bypass to the internal iliac artery to preserve pelvic flow. A total of 15 patients died within the subsequent follow up period. Aneurysm sac shrinkage of more than 5 mm was noted in 51% of patients at 6 months (40/78), 79% of patients at 12 months (41/52) and 77% of patients at 2 years (23/30). Impaired renal function (creatinine >1.2 mg/dL) was present in 42% of patients (45/119) prior to repair, and during the follow up period, 30 patients (25%) developed an increase in serum creatinine of >30%. This was also the subject of a specific review resulting in a publication detailing renal artery issues [8]. Visceral vessel compromise was manifest as 10 renal artery occlusions, 12 renal artery stenoses and 1 superior mesenteric artery stenosis. The later patient presented with postprandial abdominal pain within 30 days of the procedure. The cause of this was noted to be fabric from an unstented fenestration partially obstructing the superior mesenteric artery (SMA), and was treated to resolution with stent placement into the SMA.

Several groups have published results with fenestrated endografts. A recent meta-analysis included about 500 patients, with results similar to these [9]. A prospective study is underway in the United States, and the devices remain commercially available elsewhere in the world.

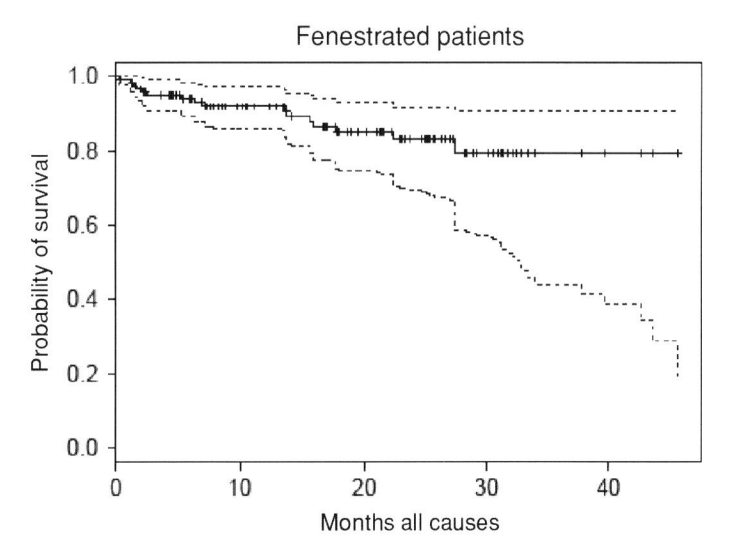

FIG. 5 Kaplan-Meier estimate of the survival function for all-cause mortality, with pointwise 95% confidence limits. (Reprinted with permission, O'Neill S, Greenberg RK, Haddad F et al. A prospective analysis of fenestrated endovascular grafting: intermediate-term outcomes. Eur J Vasc Endovasc Surg 2006; 32: 115-123 [7]).

Thoraco-abdominal branched grafting

The treatment of aneurysms involving the visceral segment is daunting for both open and endovascular interventions. Considerable morbidity and mortality has been demonstrated in many open surgical series, and the need for a less invasive, durable option is palpable. We reported our first 73 patients with thoraco-abdominal aneurysms treated with branched devices in 2007 in the Journal of Thoracic and Cardiovascular Surgery, following a publication of the same series earlier on in the Journal of Vascular Surgery [10,11]. The patients were considered high-risk for open surgical repair, 76% were male, and had a mean age of 75 years. Their comorbidities were marked, including 19% on supplemental home oxygen, 26% with chronic renal insufficiency, and 29% with prior aortic repairs. Overall, there were 45 patients with type IV thoracoabdominal aneurysms, and 28 patients with type I, II or III aneurysms. The mean aneurysm size in the study was 71 mm.

The devices employed were all variants of the Zenith device (Fig. 6). Reinforced fenestrations were mated with balloon expandable stentgrafts, and directional branches were coupled with self-expanding stentgrafts. Proximal fixation was accomplished with a TX2P device, while distal fixation occurred within the iliac arteries or the body of a previously placed aortic graft. The procedures were all done in an operating room with a fixed imaging system.

Technical success, defined as device deployment with all intended branched intact, survival through 24 hours, and the absence of a type I or III endoleak was achieved in 93% of the patients. One patient died as a result of an myocardial infarction within 24 hours of the procedure. His procedure was complicated by the need for an iliac conduit in addition to an iliac artery endarterectomy. There was a single patient where access into the celiac branch was not possible. A secondary procedure was performed on the patient three days later, and the celiac artery was successfully cannulated and incorporated into the repair with a stentgraft. Unsuccessful access to 1 of 2 renal arteries occurred in three patients, resulting in worsening renal function in two of the three cases.

The morbidity of the procedure, although likely lower than an open surgical cohort, was still significant. There were 2 cases of paraplegia, both of which required tracheostomies, and ultimately expired between the 1 and 6 month follow-up visits. One patients required hemodialysis (also a spinal cord ischemia patient), and 5 patients had persistent elevations of their serum creatinine, but did

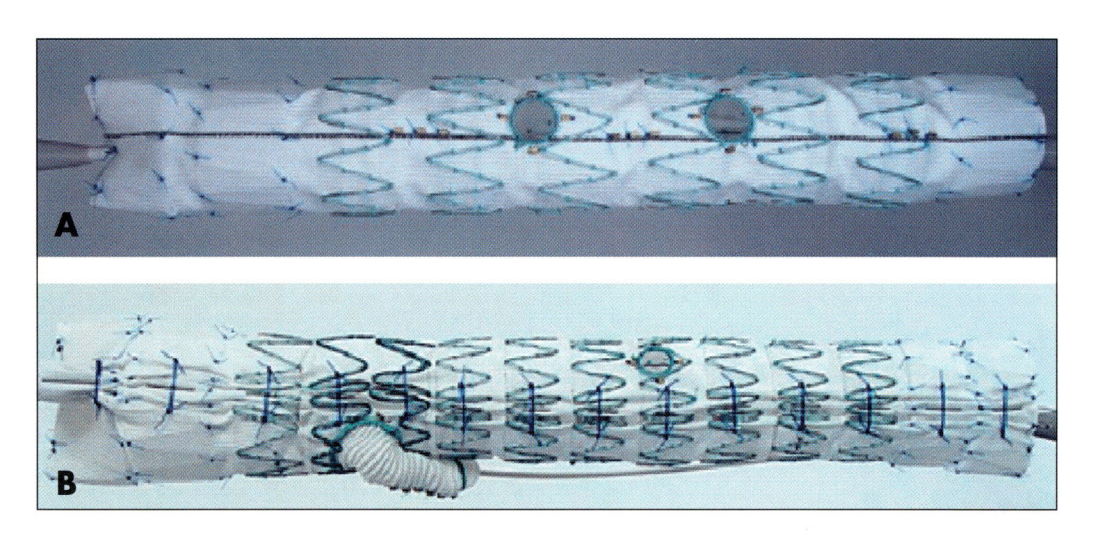

FIG. 6 Cook Zenith Branched and Fenestrated Devices. Main body device tethered to delivery system demonstrated branch fenestrations for the (A) celiac and superior mesenteric arteries and (B) helical branch in antegrade orientation for the celiac artery (posterior view) and a reinforced fenestration for the left renal vein. (Reprinted with permission, Roselli EE, Greenberg RK, Pfaff K et al. Endovascular treatment of thoracoabdominal aortic aneurysms. J Thorac Cardiovasc Surg 2007; 133: 1474-1482 [10]).

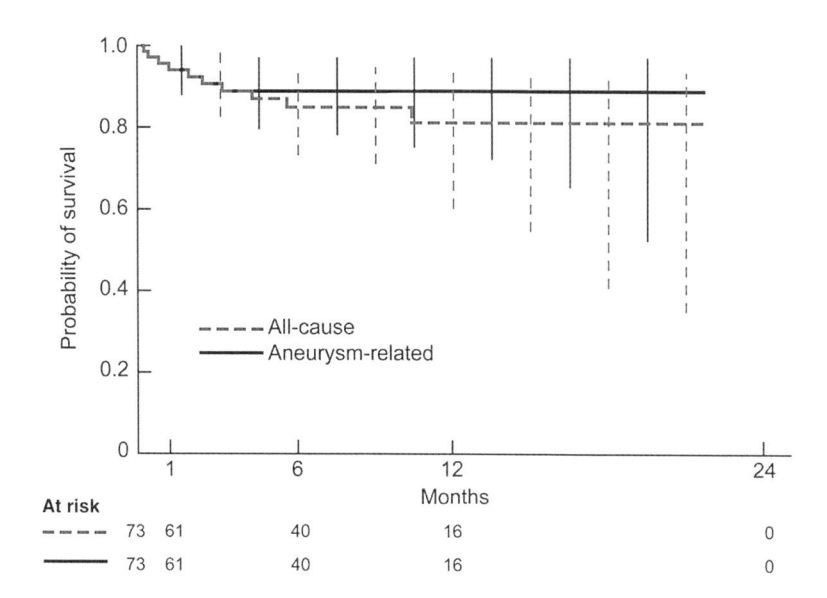

FIG. 7 Kaplan-Meier estimate of the survival function for freedom from all-cause mortality (black line) and aneurysm related mortality (grey line) with 95% confidence limits. (Reprinted with Permission, Roselli EE, Greenberg RK, Pfaff K et al. Endovascular treatment of thoracoabdominal aortic aneurysms. J Thorac Cardiovasc Surg 2007; 133: 1474-1482 [10]).

not require any dialysis. There were 4 patients who had myocardial infarctions, all of which occurred in the setting of normal cardiac functional studies (stress testing). Interestingly, the 10 patients with reversible cardiac ischemia on physiologic cardiac testing had no cardiac adverse events. Prior to hospital discharge, 11% of patients had endoleaks, 7 of which (type I and III endoleaks) were treated with secondary interventions. There were 7 patients with type II endoleaks of which 2 were treated, 2 resolved, and the remainder were followed.

Survival through one year for this high risk group was 85% (Fig. 7). Since that time, we now have 184 patients enrolled in this study and continue to revise the implant, procedure, and sizing protocols. However, our comfort with the ability to achieve an acceptable result has increased dramatically, and now would consider endovascular grafting for thoraco-abdominal aneurysms in otherwise healthy patients a reasonable option (Fig. 8).

Automating measurement for TAAA device design

At the present time, repair of TAAA using endovascular technology is a process that requires meticulous measurement and inside knowledge of graft engineering and design to achieve successful clinical outcomes. The experience accrued by a few individuals in the field is very difficult to replicate, which means that the widespread availability of these devices is not a current reality. However, because a majority of the error can come in the planning stages of the procedure, creation of an automated process to measure and design the grafts may expand the feasibility of the technique and decrease the time intensive process of measurement and graft design.

Collecting aortic dimensions for the purposes of graft design requires a software that allows for the segmentation of the aorta from surrounding tissue, and then calculation of both longitudinal and rotational relationships of the vessels, commonly using center lumen of flow projections of the intended treatment area. The judgment of the user is as important as the accuracy of the quantitative measurements in terms of the success of the final design, so creation of an automated process would also have to include "rules" that mimic the rationale used by the individual expert. The goal of automation of this process is to find the balance that will increase precision, but allow for sufficient user input that the critical areas of judgment remain.

Our group has developed a patient specific mathematical model based on DICOM CT data to create geometric analysis of aortic dimensions in an efficient and reproducible way [12]. This algorithm has been applied to 15 patients selected at random from a larger population of 350 patients

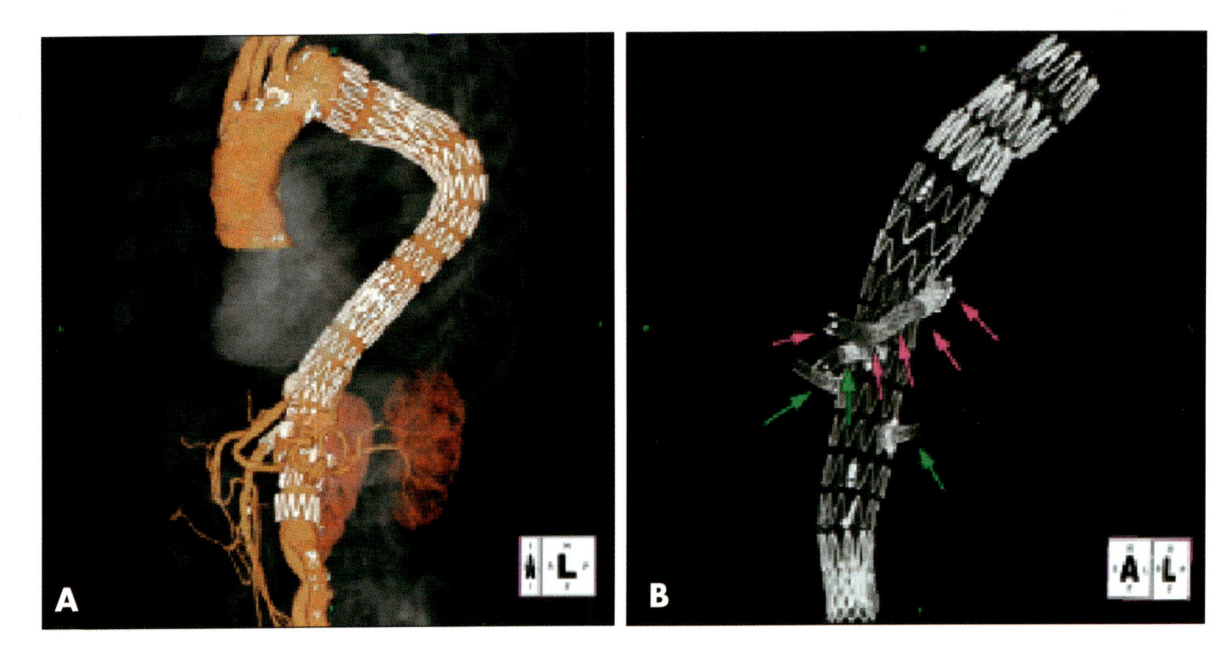

FIG. 8 Completion CT scans post procedure. A - Arterial contrast phase reconstruction of a type II TAAA after repair with a 4-branch reinforced fenestrated device. B - Noncontrast images reconstructed to demonstrate the in-vivo appearance of a stent graft used to treat type III thoraco-abdominal aneurysm using composite device design with a helical celiac branch (purple arrows) and 3 reinforced fenestrated branches (green arrows). (Reprinted with Permission, Roselli EE, Greenberg RK, Pfaff K, et al. Endovascular treatment of thoracoabdominal aortic aneurysms. J Thorac Cardiovasc Surg 2007; 133: 1474-1482 [10]).

with thoraco-abdominal aneurysms who underwent high resolution preoperative CT scan. The computer generated measurements for both longitudinal and rotational relationships were compared with measurements generated by a blinded investigator with expertise in measurement of thoraco-abdominal aneurysms, using TeraRecon Aquarius workstation. For the automated process, there are seven steps to sizing using this algorithm that include segmentation, definition of the aortic wall and calculation of the distance of each voxel within the lumen relative to this edge, 3D transformation, identification of the centerline, fitting of the segmented scan and the center lumen line, and measurement. An example of the process is illustrated in Fig. 9. Accuracy was determined by calculating the mean absolute differences for intrarenal distances and intra-renal clock position.

After completing measurements using both techniques, the mean absolute difference between the automated and manual longitudinal distance measurements for the renal arteries was 1.33 mm, and the median was 1.19 mm. The mean absolute difference between the automated and manual rotational distance was 20.1 minutes with a median of 18.0 minutes.

This work demonstrates that a mathematical algorithm can be developed to measure critical aortic dimensions of thoraco-abdominal aneurysms for the purpose of automated graft design with an acceptable degree of error compared with individual expert measurements, although more work needs to be done. Intrinsic in the measurement techniques used by both methods, however, is that the quality of the CT scan data be high. This requires appropriate contrast bolus timing, accurate scan timing in order to achieve segmentation, which is a critical step to the remainder of the process. For manually interpreted scans, the method of measurement can be adjusted or adapted, although time consuming, to account for poorly acquired images, but the automated method will not be as forgiving. Thus, the ultimate utility of this software will be determined by the quality of the CT scan data generated at the user's institution, and subsequently implant the designed graft with an acceptable rate of complication.

Future directions

The pace of development of endovascular techniques for thoraco-abdominal aneurysm repair has been increasing over the last decade. The advent

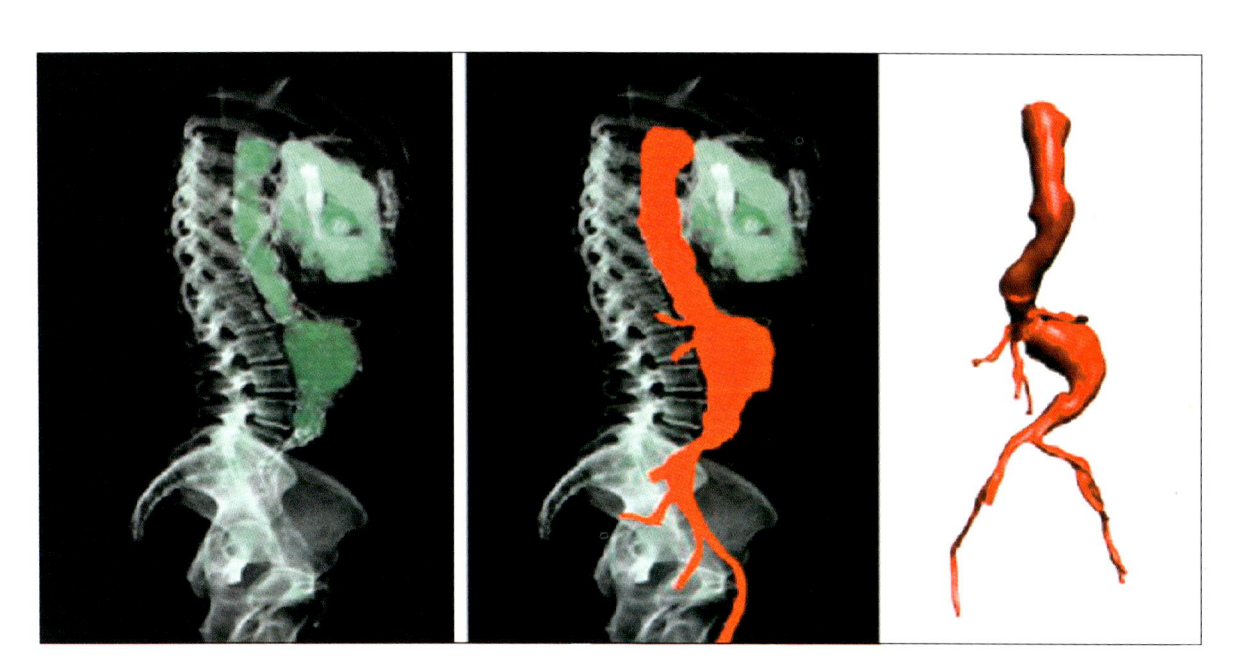

FIG. 9 Preoperative CT scan shown with analytical surfaces generated with our geometric analyses. The intensity-cropped arterial scan is shown on the left. The middle image shows the analytical surface superimposed in wireframe. The right image shows the same surface rendered with a shading model to show the complexity of the geometry. (Reprinted with Permission, IEEE Computer Graphics and Applications. Goel VR, Greenberg DP, Greenberg RK. Automated Vascular Geometric Analysis of Aortic Aneurysms, In press, 2007.)

of branched grafts and the increasing refinement of CT scan imaging are two critical advances that have contributed to the evolution. In addition to this, the development of delivery systems that are lower profile and have greater maneuverability through tortuous segments of aorta can only speed our progress towards the holy grail of total aortic replacement.

There are some sentinel aspects of endovascular therapy that require further development. The first is the assessment of individual preoperative risk. Although much has been written about the indications for endovascular intervention in patients with prohibitive risk for open repair, it is yet to be determined which patients will benefit from endovascular intervention. Scales or scoring systems proposed to date have not provided reliable estimates of perioperative or long term risk, making the development of this information critical to the success of future endovascular management of patients with high medical comorbidities.

A second area of investigation that is required is the need for the development of a device that can navigate and treat the diseases of the ascending aorta and aortic arch. The curvature of the arch, variability of the rotational alignment of the supraaortic trunks, and the anatomic limitations of the proximal ascending aorta have posed a hurdle for graft design at present, but the experience being gained with visceral devices will certainly inform the evolution of a usable arch device.

A third area of needed investigation is in the realm of aortic dissection. The majority of devices available commercially and through investigational use at this time have been developed for aneurysmal disease. Aortas involved in acute and chronic aortic dissection have their own unique characteristics that may not be treated adequately with the current technology. The next generation of aortic device may need to be disease specific in order to perform best in the highly variable anatomy of the dissected aorta.

Conclusion

The evolution of endovascular management for TAAA is continuing, and shows promise that one day the goal of total aortic replacement might be realized. Further investigation and innovation, building on the principles learned in the past 10 years, is needed to carry the field toward this ambitious goal.

REFERENCES

1. Faruqi RM, Chuter TA, Reilly LM et al. Endovascular repair of abdominal aortic aneurysm using a pararenal fenestrated stent-graft. *J Endovasc Surg* 1999; 6: 354-358.
2. Browne TF, Hartley D, Purchas S et al. A fenestrated covered suprarenal aortic stent. *Eur J Vasc Endovasc Surg* 1999; 18: 445-449.
3. Haulon S, Devos P, Willoteaux S et al. Risk factors of early and late complications in patients undergoing endovascular aneurysm repair. *Eur J Vasc Endovasc Surg* 2003; 25: 118-124.
4. Serracino-Inglott F, Bray AE, Myers P. Endovascular abdominal aortic aneurysm repair in patients with common iliac artery aneurysms–Initial experience with the Zenith bifurcated iliac side branch device. *J Vasc Surg* 2007; 46: 211-217.
5. Ziegler P, Avgerinos ED, Umscheid T et al. Branched iliac bifurcation: 6 years experience with endovascular preservation of internal iliac artery flow. *J Vasc Surg* 2007; 46: 204-210.
6. Abraham CZ, Reilly LM, Schneider DB et al. A modular multi-branched system for endovascular repair of bilateral common iliac artery aneurysms. *J Endovasc Ther* 2003; 10: 203-207.
7. O'Neill S, Greenberg RK, Haddad F et al. A prospective analysis of fenestrated endovascular grafting : intermediate-term outcomes. *Eur J Vasc Endovasc Surg* 2006; 32: 115-123.
8. Haddad F, Greenberg RK, Walker E et al. Fenestrated endovascular grafting: The renal side of the story. *J Vasc Surg* 2005; 41: 181-190.
9. Sun Z, Mwipatayi BP, Semmens JB et al. Short to midterm outcomes of fenestrated endovascular grafts in the treatment of abdominal aortic aneurysms: a systematic review. *J Endovasc Ther* 2006; 13: 747-753.
10. Roselli EE, Greenberg RK, Pfaff K et al. Endovascular treatment of thoracoabdominal aortic aneurysms. *J Thorac Cardiovasc Surg* 2007; 133: 1474-1482.
11. Greenberg RK, West K, Pfaff K et al. Beyond the aortic bifurcation: branched endovascular grafts for thoracoabdominal and aortoiliac aneurysms. *J Vasc Surg* 2006; 43: 879-886.
12. Goel VR, Greenberg DP, Greenberg RK. Automated Vascular Geometric Analysis of Aortic Aneurysms. IEEE Computer Graphics and Applications. In press, 2007.

14

DEBRANCHING PROCEDURES FOR THORACO-ABDOMINAL AORTIC ANEURYSMS

ANDREW CHOONG, NICHOLAS CHESHIRE

Open repair of thoraco-abdominal aortic aneurysms (TAAA) has a high mortality and morbidity [1,2]. These risks have persisted despite advances in operative technique (including cardiopulmonary or left heart bypass, hypothermic cardiopulmonary arrest, selective visceral perfusion, spinal cord protection) and higher standards of peri-operative care. The repair of extensive TAAA remains a formidable challenge to vascular surgeons. Despite significant advances in surgical technique and peri-operative critical care, the traditional open repair, even in the best centers in the world, is still associated with a high morbidity and mortality.

Thoracic stent-grafting is limited to the descending thoracic aorta by either the arch vessels proximally or the visceral and renal vessels distally. However, by first revascularizing and/or debranching these vessels, one can subsequently complete aneurysm exclusion by thoraco-abdominal aortic endografting. The less invasive nature of these hybrid procedures represents a viable treatment alternative to those patients that may have previously been declined an open procedure due to advanced age or comorbidities. As endovascular techniques and technology are constantly improving and evolving, the full impact of fenestrated stents and branched grafts on TAAA repair is yet to be realized. Whilst a total endovascular approach is the future of TAAA repair, hybrid surgery will always remain a robust and adaptable method of treating this complex and life-threatening disease process particularly in individuals with unfavorable anatomy.

Evolution of the hybrid repair

In 1991, Parodi et al. [3] described the deployment of the first endovascular stent-graft (EVSG) in an infrarenal abdominal aortic aneurysm. By 1994, as a direct evolutionary step, Dake et al. [4] used an EVSG for isolated descending thoracic aortic aneurysms. This use of EVSG for aortic aneurysms limited to the thoracic segment showed significant early promise. However, their use for extensive TAAA was necessarily limited by the presence of the arch vessels proximally and the visceral and renal vessels distally.

In 1999, Quinones-Baldrich et al. [5] were the first to report a combined endovascular and open surgical approach for a type IV TAAA. Previous abdominal aortic surgery and concomitant visceral artery aneurysms precluded an open repair. Retrograde visceral bypasses from a limb of a pre-existing bifurcated aortic tube graft were performed followed by TAAA stent-grafting. By revascularizing the visceral and renal branches first, total endovascular aneurysm exclusion was achieved by completion endo-grafting.

In 2003, at the Regional Vascular Unit at St Mary's Hospital, we used a similar technique of retrograde visceral/renal revascularization with completion endo-grafting for a 49 year old man with a 9 cm aneurysm of native aorta occurring between a previous infrarenal abdominal and an upper descending thoracic aortic aneurysm repair [6]. Three years later, we then reported the largest published series of these repairs describing a total of 29 attempted *visceral hybrid* procedures [7]. Our unit performs this technique in preference to an open repair for Crawford type I, II, and III TAAA, while an open approach with medial visceral rotation is used for Crawford type IV aneurysms. These repairs are particularly attractive and deemed less invasive as they avoid the need for a thoracotomy, single-lung ventilation, aortic cross clamp, left or full heart bypass as well as the extensive tissue dissection all associated with an open repair.

Visceral hybrid repair

TECHNIQUE

The patient is placed in a supine position under general and epidural anesthesia. Cerebrospinal fluid drainage is always used. We routinely use cell salvage techniques with rapid infusers available. Arterial and central venous lines, urethral catheterization and transesophageal echocardiography are all mandatory peri-operative invasive monitoring.

A mid-line laparotomy allows for adequate exposure of the abdominal aorta, the origins of the renal arteries, the celiac axis, and the superior mesenteric artery (SMA). The in-flow site for retrograde visceral bypass grafting is determined by the distal extent of aneurysmal disease and previous abdominal surgery. If a previous infrarenal repair has been undertaken, the bypass grafts are anastomosed in an end-to-side fashion to the existing graft. If an infrarenal repair is possible, this is completed first and bypass grafts are subsequently sutured as before. If the infrarenal aorta is normal an arteriotomy is performed and the bypass grafts anastomosed in an end-to-side fashion to the native aorta. If the aneurysmal disease extends to the bifurcation, one external iliac artery can provide the in-flow to the bypass grafts.

Two inverted (14 by 7 mm or 16 by 8 mm) Dacron® trouser-grafts can function as the conduits. Otherwise a single trouser-graft is used with additional side-limbs sutured in an end-to-side manner. This four-limbed "spaghetti graft" is fashioned in a bespoke way during the procedure.

The renal arteries are sequentially anastomosed in an end-to-side fashion. The two remaining graft limbs are routed along the base of the small bowel mesentery to the celiac axis and SMA in an end-to-side fashion. If Doppler signals are satisfactory in the bypass grafts (with the origins of the native vessel clamped) they are subsequently suture-ligated to prevent retrograde flow into the aneurysm sac (type II endoleak).

Following successful visceral and renal bypass a suitable access site is chosen for endovascular stent deployment. A dedicated conduit attached to the common iliac artery or the abdominal aorta is common but native vessels are also used provided they are of suitable caliber. An angiogram catheter is introduced on the contra-lateral side and the stents are deployed in a sequential fashion from the left subclavian artery through the thoracic aorta to the landing zone (Figure). Completion angiography after adjunctive procedures (extension cuff, giant Palmaz stent, balloon moulding) then confirms exclusion of the aneurysm.

OTHER EXPERIENCES OF HYBRID REPAIRS OF TAAA

Several centers around the world have published individual cases/small series (<5) of hybrid

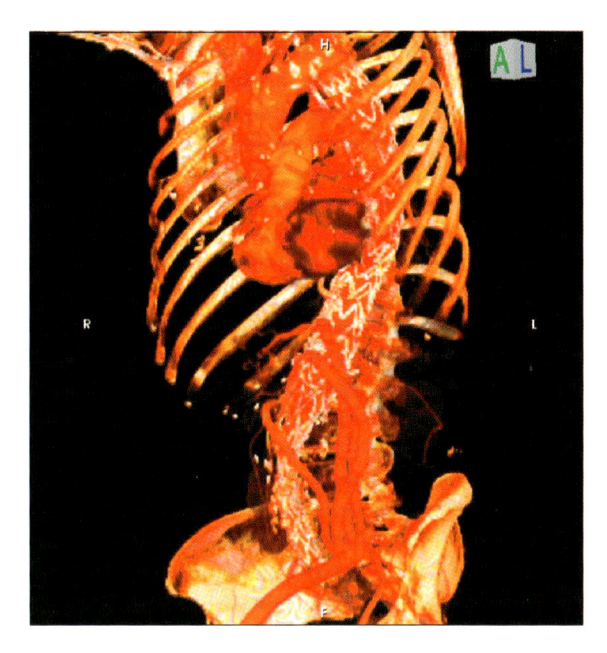

FIGURE Type III TAAA repaired with visceral hybrid procedure.

approaches to TAAA [5,6,8-23]. The results of these cases are encouraging considering the complicated nature of the TAAA disease process as well as the patients' comorbidities. Of the 30 patients in this combined series, spinal cord ischemia appeared to be rare or went unreported. Other postoperative complications were greatly reduced and intensive care stay was less than that of open TAAA surgery. Of note, no standard operative technique was employed and there was much variation in the EVSG used.

Resch et al. [24] have reported their series of 13 staged hybrid repair of TAAA. They all underwent retrograde visceral bypasses (11 ilio-visceral and 2 infrarenal aortic-visceral) as a first procedure prior to completion with EVSG. They report a 30-day mortality of 23% (3/13) for all patients. Their mean follow-up in the 10 surviving patients was 23 months (1-45) during which time a further 2 deaths were related to the hybrid repair. Two patients unfortunately suffered paraplegia and 2 further patients had transient parapetic events.

Zhou et al. [25] published their series of 31 high-risk patients undergoing hybrid approaches to TAAA. Although there were a variety of hybrid approaches used for these TAAA, 18 of these patients had aneurysms involving the visceral vessels: Crawford type I (3), III (8) and IV (7). They reported that 15 patients required iliac to celiac artery bypasses, 15 required iliac to SMA bypasses and 10 required iliac to renal artery bypass grafting. There was no incidence of stroke or paraplegia reported in their series.

Donas et al. [26] recently analyzed published data in their systematic review of "hybrid open-endovascular repairs of TAAA" (Table). Their study eligibility criteria were as follows:
1) TAAA was diagnosed on the basis of the Crawford classification, modified by Safi;
2) hybrid open-endovascular repair (visceral bypass followed by endovascular stent-graft implantation) was the intended repair strategy and was completed in all patients;
3) there had been a minimum follow-up period of 4 months;
4) diagnosis of complex TAAA had been made according to computed tomographic scans of the thorax, abdomen and pelvis;
5) at least one of the basic outcome criteria (neurological, renal, respiratory morbidity, visceral vessel patency and endoprosthesis related complications, as well as the primary technical success rate, and the total mortality rates were stated;
6) articles were excluded if TAAA repair was only by surgical or endovascular approaches alone.

Of the 13 studies identified and included in their statistical analysis, the number of patients reported totaled 58 (37 male, 21 female). The mean age of the patients was 68.8 years (range 35-80). There were 15 Crawford type I TAAA, 21 type II, 11 type III, 6 type IV and 5 type V. The mean follow-up period was 14.3 +/- 8.4 months (range 4-36). The mean aneurysm diameter was 7.15 cm (range 5-12 cm).

In this, no patient developed paraplegia or other procedure-related neurological deficits due to spinal cord injury or ischemia. Thirty-day elective and urgent mortality was 10.7% (6/55). Three patients with a ruptured TAAA who underwent a hybrid procedure died. The overall early and long-term mortality for completed procedures was 15.5% (9/58).

Advantages

The authors perceive several advantages of the visceral hybrid approach over standard, open techniques:
1) no thoracotomy:
   i. fewer pulmonary complications;
   ii. fewer cardiac arrhythmias;
   iii. less pain.

Table	Systematic review of Donas et al. [26] assessing outcome of hybrid procedures			
First author [ref.]	Year	Follow-up (months)	Number of patients	30-day mortality (number)
Quinones-Baldrich [5]	1999	6	1	0
Black [7]	2006	8	26	6
Macierewicz [8]	2000	22	1	0
Agostinelli [10]	2002	6	1	0
Saccani [11]	2002	4	3	1
Iguro [13]	2003	12	1	0
Kotsis [14]	2003	14	4	1
Flye [16]	2004	14.6	3	0
Donas [27]	2007	21	8	1
Chiesa [28]	2007	12	1	0
Lawrence-Brown [29]	2000	36	2	0
Khoury [30]	2002	21	1	0
Gawenda [31]	2007	12	6	0

2) Reduced hypothermia with subsequent reduction in:
   i. coagulopathy;
   ii. cardiovascular instability.
3) Reduced rate of spinal cord ischemia due to improved cardiovascular stability.
4) Reduced duration of mesenteric and visceral ischemia with reduction in:
   i. acidosis and associated problems;
   ii. gut bacteria translocation/sepsis;
   iii. renal failure/use of renal replacement therapy.
5) Less blood loss/reduced transfusion requirement.
6) Reduced hospital stay:
   i. Intensive therapy unit (ITU);
   ii. absolute.
7) More patients can be treated where comorbidity previously excluded them.

Disadvantages
1) Newer technique requires specialist centers with experience in the procedure;
2) long-term follow-up required for endo-grafting component;
3) still a significant physiological insult to the patient;
4) risk of paraplegia, despite better cardiovascular stability, remains theoretically high due to significant occlusion of aortic side branches particularly in extensive TAAA.

The future of TAAA repair

Although some units have reported spectacular results with the traditional open repair of TAAA [32], Rigberg et al. [33] suggest that normal 30-day mortality statistics underestimate the risk of repair of TAAA and that individual unit data is probably less useful than looking at a larger population as a whole. They identified 1 010 patients (797 elective, 213 ruptured) who underwent TAAA repair in the state of California. Mean patient ages were 70.0 (elective) and 72.1 years (ruptured). Men comprised 62% of elective and 68% of ruptured aneurysm patients, and 80% (elective) and 74% (ruptured) were white. Overall elective patient mortality was 19% at 30 days and 31% at one year. There was a steep increase in mortality with increasing age, such that elective one-year mortality increased from about 18% for patients 50 to 59 years old to 40% for patients 80 to 89 years old. The elective case 31-day to 365-day mortality ranged from 7.8% for the youngest patients to 13.5%. Mortality for ruptured cases was 48.4% at 30 days and 61.5% at 365 days, and these rates also increased with age. Clearly, any treatment modality that improves outcome in patients with TAAA is welcome and current results of the visceral hybrid repair demonstrate a clear improvement over and above some mortality and morbidity reports of the open repair.

The endovascular revolution has significantly impacted on TAAA repair and will continue to do so. Endovascular stent-grafting was integral to the development of the visceral hybrid repair, and now with the advent of fenestrated and branched graft endovascular technology, there are also wholly endovascular options available to select patients. A wholly endovascular approach is clearly the future of TAAA repair. Just as the visceral hybrid repair removed the need for thoraco-laparotomy and aortic cross clamping, a total endovascular repair even removes the need for laparotomy, intra-abdominal dissection and visceral/renal arterial clamping seen in the hybrid. Some are now questioning whether there will be a role for debranching hybrid repairs with the introduction of these newer endovascular therapies although this argument is premature.

Significant advances have been made in the total endovascular repair of TAAA. Roselli et al. [34] recently described 73 patients who underwent wholly endovascular repair of TAAA (for Crawford type I, II or III n=28 and for type IV n=45). The mean aneurysm size was 7.1 cm (range 4.5-11.3 cm). General anesthesia was used in 47% of patients and regional anesthesia in 53%. There were no conversions to open surgery and no ruptures post-treatment. Technical success was achieved in 93% of patients (68/73). Thirty-day mortality was 5.5% (4/73). Major peri-operative complications occurred in 11 (14%) patients and included paraplegia (2.7%, 2/73), new onset of dialysis (1.4%, 1/73), prolonged ventilator support (6.8%, 5/73), myocardial infarction (5.5%, 4/73), and minor hemorrhagic stroke (1.4%; 1/72). A majority of patients had no complications. Mean length of stay was 8.6 days. At follow-up, 6 deaths had occurred. There were no instances of stent migration or aneurysmal growth. From this series, it is clear that known complications of TAAA repair, either open or hybrid, are not entirely eliminated by a totally endovascular approach. However, morbidity and mortality appear to be low, relative to the high-risk population studied.

Even more recently, Chuter et al. [35] have described a similar smaller cohort of patients undergoing wholly endovascular TAAA repair. Self-expanding covered stents were used to connect the caudally directed cuffs of an aortic stent graft with the visceral branches of a TAAA in 22 patients (16 men, 6 women) with a mean age of 76±7 years. All patients were unfit for open repair, and nine had undergone prior aortic surgery. Customized aortic stent grafts were inserted through surgically exposed femoral (n=16) or iliac (n=6) arteries. Covered stents were inserted through surgically exposed brachial arteries. Spinal catheters were used for cerebrospinal fluid pressure drainage in 22 patients and for and spinal anesthesia in 11. All 22 stent grafts and all 81 branches were deployed successfully. Aortic coverage as a percentage of subclavian-to-bifurcation distance was 69% ± 20%. Mean contrast volume was 203 ml, mean blood loss was 714 ml, and mean hospital stay was 10.9 days. Two patients (9.1%) died peri-operatively: one from guide wire injury to a renal arterial branch and the other from a medication error. Serious or potentially serious complications occurred in 9 of 22 patients (41%). There was no paraplegia, renal failure, stroke, or myocardial infarction among the 20 surviving patients. Two patients (9.1%) underwent successful reintervention: one for localized intimal disruption and the other for aortic dissection, type I endoleak, and stenosis of the superior mesenteric artery. One patient has a type II endoleak. Follow-up is more than 1 month in 19 patients, over 6 months in 12, and over 12 months in 8. One branch (renal artery) occluded for a 98.75% branch patency rate at 1 month. The other 80 branches remain patent. There are no signs of stent graft migration, component separation, or fracture.

Fenestrated and branched endografts are still an emerging technology. Careful patient selection is vital, particularly for those patients with challenging aneurysmal anatomies. In addition, the costs of these new stent-grafts are prohibitive to many centers around the world who cannot afford the additional expense, despite potential patient benefits.

The future of the visceral hybrid repair of TAAA can be seen in several ways:
1) There will always be patients with challenging anatomy which renders them unsuitable for a wholly endovascular approach. In these situations, if comorbidities limit an open repair, the visceral hybrid is a robust and adaptable method of treating this complex and life-threatening disease process.
2) A great deal of pre-operative planning is required for successful wholly endovascular treatment of TAAA. Imaging, sizing and bespoke endo-graft construction all require time those symptomatic/peri-rupture patients do not have. In these cases, the visceral hybrid provides an unique way of treating TAAA, particularly if an open repair is prohibited by poor preoperative patient condition.
3) The visceral hybrid could be considered a bridging measure until fenestrated/branched EVSG technology matures to the point of established use.

Further improvement of, and access to, endovascular stent-grafts, and correct patient selection (in light of the EVAR 2 trial results [36] will probably see a reduction in the numbers of visceral hybrid procedures being performed for TAAA. Fenestrated and branched endo-grafts will be increasingly performed. However, in units that are proficient in the visceral hybrid repair, it will remain a reliable method of TAAA repair that, with the correct patient selection, can be used alongside open and endovascular approaches to TAAA repair in this challenging patient population.

REFERENCES

1. Svensson LG, Crawford ES, Hess KR et al. Dissection of the aorta and dissecting aortic aneurysms. Improving early and long-term surgical results. *Circulation* 1990; 82(5 Suppl): IV24-38.
2. Svensson LG, Crawford ES, Hess KR et al. Experience with 1509 patients undergoing thoracoabdominal aortic operations. *J Vasc Surg* 1993; 17: 357-368.
3. Parodi JC, Palmaz JC, Barone HD. Transfemoral intraluminal graft implantation for abdominal aortic aneurysms. *Ann Vasc Surg* 1991; 5: 491-499.
4. Dake MD, Miller DC, Semba CP et al. Transluminal placement of endovascular stent-grafts for the treatment of descending thoracic aortic aneurysms. *N Engl J Med* 1994; 331: 1729-1734.
5. Quinones-Baldrich WJ, Panetta TF, Vescera CL et al. Repair of type IV thoracoabdominal aneurysm with a combined endovascular and surgical approach. *J Vasc Surg* 1999; 30: 555-560.
6. Rimmer J, Wolfe JH. Type III thoracoabdominal aortic aneurysm repair: a combined surgical and endovascular approach. *Eur J Vasc Endovasc Surg* 2003; 26: 677-679.
7. Black SA, Wolfe JH, Clark M et al. Complex thoracoabdominal aortic aneurysms: endovascular exclusion with visceral revascularization. *J Vasc Surg* 2006; 43: 1081-1089.
8. Macierewicz JA, Jameel MM, Whitaker SC et al. Endovascular repair of perisplanchnic abdominal aortic aneurysm with visceral vessel transposition. *J Endovasc Ther* 2000; 7: 410-414.
9. Juvonen T, Biancari F, Ylonen K et al. Combined surgical and endovascular treatment of pseudoaneurysms of the visceral arteries and of the left iliac arteries after thoracoabdominal aortic surgery. *Eur J Vasc Endovasc Surg* 2001; 22: 275-277.
10. Agostinelli A, Saccani S, Budillon AM et al. Repair of coexistent infrarenal and thoracoabdominal aortic aneurysm: combined endovascular and open surgical procedure with visceral vessel relocation. *J Thorac Cardiovasc Surg* 2002; 124: 184-185.
11. Saccani S, Nicolini F, Beghi C et al. Thoracic aortic stents: a combined solution for complex cases. *Eur J Vasc Endovasc Surg* 2002; 24: 423-427.
12. Watanabe Y, Ishimaru S, Kawaguchi S et al. Successful endografting with simultaneous visceral artery bypass grafting for severely calcified thoracoabdominal aortic aneurysm. *J Vasc Surg* 2002; 35: 397-399.
13. Iguro Y, Yotsumoto G, Ishizaki N et al. Endovascular stent-graft repair for thoracoabdominal aneurysm after reconstruction of the superior mesenteric and celiac arteries. *J Thorac Cardiovasc Surg* 2003; 125: 956-958.
14. Kotsis T, Scharrer-Pamler R, Kapfer X et al. Treatment of thoracoabdominal aortic aneurysms with a combined endovascular and surgical approach. *Int Angiol* 2003; 22: 125-133.
15. Chiesa R, Melissano G, Civilini E et al. Two-stage combined endovascular and surgical approach for recurrent thoracoabdominal aortic aneurysm. *J Endovasc Ther* 2004; 11: 330-333.
16. Flye MW, Choi ET, Sanchez LA et al. Retrograde visceral vessel revascularization followed by endovascular aneurysm exclusion as an alternative to open surgical repair of thoracoabdominal aortic aneurysm. *J Vasc Surg* 2004; 39: 454-458.
17. Lundbom J, Hatlinghus S, Odegard A et al. Combined open and endovascular treatment of complex aortic disease. *Vascular* 2004; 12: 93-98.
18. Bonardelli S, De Lucia M, Cervi E et al. Combined endovascular and surgical approach (hybrid treatment) for management of type IV thoracoabdominal aneurysm. *Vascular* 2005; 13: 124-128.
19. Fulton JJ, Farber MA, Marston WA et al. Endovascular stent-graft repair of pararenal and type IV thoracoabdominal aortic aneurysms with adjunctive visceral reconstruction. *J Vasc Surg* 2005; 41: 191-198.

20. Gregoric ID, Gupta K, Jacobs MJ et al. Endovascular exclusion of a thoracoabdominal aortic aneurysm after retrograde visceral artery revascularization. *Tex Heart Inst J* 2005; 32: 416-420.

21. Yoshida M, Mukohara N, Shida T et al. Combined endovascular and surgical procedure for recurrent thoracoabdominal aortic aneurysm. *Ann Thorac Surg* 2006; 82: 1099-1101.

22. Ruppert V, Salewski J, Wintersperger BJ et al. Endovascular repair of thoracoabdominal aortic aneurysm with multivisceral revascularization. *J Vasc Surg* 2005; 42: 368.

23. Tachibana K, Morishita K, Kurimoto Y et al. Endovascular stent-grafting for thoracoabdominal aortic aneurysm following bypass grafting to superior mesenteric and celiac arteries: report of two cases. *Ann Thorac Cardiovasc Surg* 2005; 11: 335-338.

24. Resch TA, Greenberg RK, Lyden SP et al. Combined staged procedures for the treatment of thoracoabdominal aneurysms. *J Endovasc Ther* 2006; 13: 481-489.

25. Zhou W, Reardon M, Peden EK et al. Hybrid approach to complex thoracic aortic aneurysms in high-risk patients: surgical challenges and clinical outcomes. *J Vasc Surg* 2006; 44: 688-693.

26. Donas KP, Czerny M, Guber I et al. Hybrid Open-endovascular Repair for Thoracoabdominal Aortic Aneurysms: Current Status and Level of Evidence. *Eur J Vasc Endovasc Surg* 2007; 34: 528-533.

27. Donas KP, Schulte S, Krause E et al. Combined endovascular stent-graft repair and adjunctive visceral vessel reconstruction for complex thoracoabdominal aortic aneurysms. *Int Angiol* 2007; 26: 213-218.

28. Chiesa R, Tshomba Y, Melissano G et al. Hybrid approach to thoracoabdominal aortic aneurysms in patients with prior aortic surgery. *J Vasc Surg* 2007; 45: 1128-1135.

29. Lawrence-Brown M, Sieunarine K, van Schie G et al. Hybrid open-endoluminal technique for repair of thoracoabdominal aneurysm involving the celiac axis. *J Endovasc Ther* 2000; 7: 513-519.

30. Khoury M. Endovascular repair of recurrent thoracoabdominal aortic aneurysm. *J Endovasc Ther* 2002; 9(Suppl 2): II106-111.

31. Gawenda M, Aleksic M, Heckenkamp J et al. Hybrid-procedures for the Treatment of Thoracoabdominal Aortic Aneurysms and Dissections. *Eur J Vasc Endovasc Surg* 2007; 33: 71-77.

32. Coselli JS, Bozinovski J, LeMaire SA. Open surgical repair of 2286 thoracoabdominal aortic aneurysms. *Ann Thorac Surg* 2007; 83: S862-864.

33. Rigberg DA, McGory ML, Zingmond DS et al. Thirty-day mortality statistics underestimate the risk of repair of thoracoabdominal aortic aneurysms: a statewide experience. *J Vasc Surg* 2006; 43: 217-222.

34. Roselli EE, Greenberg RK, Pfaff K et al. Endovascular treatment of thoracoabdominal aortic aneurysms. *J Thorac Cardiovasc Surg* 2007; 133: 1474-1482.

35. Chuter TA, Rapp JH, Hiramoto JS et al. Endovascular treatment of thoracoabdominal aortic aneurysms. *J Vasc Surg* 2008; 47: 6-16.

36. Anonymous. EVAR trial participants. Endovascular aneurysm repair and outcome in patients unfit for open repair of abdominal aortic aneurysm (EVAR trial 2): randomised controlled trial. *Lancet* 2005; 365: 2187-2192.

15

ENDOVASCULAR REPAIR OF RUPTURED ABDOMINAL AORTIC ANEURYSMS

CHRISTOS KARKOS, ZORAN RANCIC, MURAT AKSOY
ALEXEI SVETLIKOV, YURIY SPIRIN

Despite improvement in intra- and postoperative care, surgical repair of ruptured abdominal aortic aneurysms (RAAAs) continues to be associated with hospital mortality rates as high as 50% and overall mortality rates as high as 90%, including deaths before hospitalization [1-4]. Although a recent meta-analysis of 50 years of RAAA repair did show a gradual reduction in peri-operative mortality, this gradual improvement in the literature may reflect reporting bias and patient selection [5]. The advent of endovascular surgery has proven beneficial to the elective treatment of abdominal aortic aneurysms (AAAs), both by reducing operative mortality and complication rates in patients with an anatomic configuration suitable to this type of surgical repair. The successful application of the endovascular approach in the elective setting has prompted a strong interest about its possible use in dealing with the longstanding challenge of a RAAA. Several centers with an expertise in performing elective endovascular repair have now published data on endovascular treatment of RAAAs, but the majority of these papers are reports of single-center experience with small number of patients [6-48]. Some of the results are promising, the reported mortality figures, however, vary widely. Therefore, there is uncertainty whether the outcome of such patients can be improved by endovascular surgery. This chapter aims at examining where things stand with regard to emergency endovascular repair of RAAAs.

Literature review

An English language literature review was undertaken through to December 2006. Only patients with true ruptures were included. A total of 28 studies were identified reporting on a total of 857 patients (Table I) [7-34].

Advantages of endovascular approach in RAAA patients

The first endovascular repair of a RAAA was described in 1994 [6], but it was some time before small series with selected patients were published. Nowadays, endovascular repair of RAAAs has become routine practice in Europe and it is increasingly performed in the United States. In certain experienced centers, in particular, the technique has evolved to be the first-line treatment option in RAAA patients [9,13,29,31,41,45]. Given that such patients have multiple comorbidities and that many present in extremis, the idea of repairing the rupture by endovascular means is appealing. Avoiding a midline laparotomy and prolonged aortic cross-clamping are unique advantages of the technique. The sudden decompression of intra-abdominal pressure associated with opening the abdomen is also avoided, and the usual accompanying decrease in blood pressure may not occur [9,41,45]. In addition, the third-space losses due to laparotomy, hypothermia, blood loss, and coagulopathy may all be minimized [9,41,45,48]. Finally, iatrogenic injuries occurring during open repair are avoided using the endovascular approach. For all the above reasons, RAAA patients may be ideal candidates for endovascular surgery.

Imaging for anatomical eligibility for endovascular repair

In conventional practice, the patient with a suspected RAAA is transferred directly to the operating theatre for emergency open repair and most surgeons would avoid radiological investigation, such as computed tomography (CT). Adam et al. [49] suggested that clinical diagnosis in experienced hands provides sufficient grounds to take patients to theatre. Of course, this policy of immediate exploratory laparotomy without confirmatory imaging may prove unnecessary in some cases - of pancreatitis, for example - and unfortunate in others, e.g. patients with cardiogenic shock. On the other hand, the penalty for obtaining a CT scan first and not taking the patient directly to theatre will be the death of some patients with RAAAs due to delay [50]. The introduction of an emergency endovascular RAAA program would require some form of imaging to determine suitability for endovascular repair. In most centers, eligibility is being assessed by contrast-enhanced CT. The majority of centers use spiral CT angiography, others, such as the Nottingham and Eindhoven groups relied initially on thin-slice axial CT without reconstructions [8,10].

Apart from confirming the suspected diagnosis of rupture, CT would provide information regarding anatomical suitability and graft configuration and sizing. However, there is concern that this may lead to unnecessary delays in transferring patients to the operating room [48,51]. The Malmö group reported a mean duration of symptoms prior to emergency endovascular repair of 12 hours compared with <1 hour for a concurrent open repair group [13]. While some will benefit from endovascular repair, in others, this intentional delay to obtain adequate anatomical information may adversely affect the outcome. A UK study in the 1980s showed that the mean survival of patients with RAAAs managed non-operatively was 8 hours after hospital admission [52]. Recently, a Leicester study investigating patients admitted to the hospital with a RAAA who did not undergo operation showed that most patients (87.5%) died more than 2 hours after hospital admission [53]. The median time from admission to death in this study was 10 hours 45 minutes. These data indicate that most patients with a RAAA who reach the hospital alive are sufficiently stable to undergo CT and to be considered for endovascular repair [54].

An alternative to this "all-comers" CT scanning policy has been proposed by the Montefiore group [9,41,45]. All patients with a presumed diagnosis of a RAAA were directly transferred to the operating room and an on-table angiography was carried out via a brachial or femoral puncture under local anesthesia. This angiogram allowed a determination of whether or not an endovascular graft repair was feasible. If not, a standard open repair was carried out. A disadvantage of this approach is that angiography will not necessarily reveal the rupture. Additionally, the accuracy of intra-operative angiogra-

Table I STUDIES REPORTING ON ENDOVASCULAR RAAA REPAIR [7-34].

First author [ref.]	Year	ER	In-hospital mortality (%)	Anesthesia (LA)	Bifurcated approach	Unstable patients	Balloon occlusion	Primary conversion to OR
Greenberg [7]	2000	3	0	0	0	2	2	0
Hinchliffe [8]	2001	20	9 (45%)	0	0	4	2	3
Veith [9]	2002	25	3 (12%)	0	0	8	8	0
Yilmaz [10]	2002	17	4 (24%)	NA	NA	12	0	0
Van Herzeele [11]	2003	9	2 (22%)	0	3	6	NA	0
Scharrer-Pamler [12]	2003	24	5 (21%)	NA	19	4	0	1
Resch [13]	2003	21	4 (19%)	12	9	5	5	NA
Lee [14]	2004	13	1 (8%)	1	13	0	0	0
May [15]	2004	3	0	NA	3	NA	NA	NA
Lombardi [16]	2004	5	0	1	4	0	0	0
Arya [17]	2004	14	3 (21%)	NA	3	0	NA	1
Gerassimidis [18]	2005	23	9 (39%)	17	14	9	0	0
Larzon [19]	2005	15	2 (13%)	2	15	11	11	1
Brandt [20]	2005	11	0	0	3	NA	NA	0
Peppelenbosch [21]	2005	35	8 (23%)	0	3	20	NA	NA
Alsac [22]	2005	17	4 (24%)	1	8	1	1	3
Hechelhammer [23]	2005	37	4 (11%)	28	35	3	3	1
Vaddineni [24]	2005	9	2 (22%)	0	9	0	0	0
Castelli [25]	2005	25	5 (20%)	0	21	7	3	0
Dalainas [26]	2006	20	8 (40%)	20	11	NA	20	0
Oranen [27]	2006	34	6 (18%)	27	NA	NA	NA	1
Greco [28]	2006	290	114 (39%)	NA	NA	36	NA	20
Visser [29]	2006	26	8 (31%)	0	24	2	NA	2
Hinchliffe [30]	2006	13	7 (54%)	0	0	5	0	2
Acosta [31]	2006	56	19 (34%)	NA	23	47	NA	NA
Peppelenbosch [32]	2006	49	17 (35%)	16	0	21	3	3
Coppi [33]	2006	33	10 (30%)	12	7	15	4	3
Franks [34]	2006	10	1 (10%)	NA	NA	3	NA	1

Only patients with true ruptures were included, whereas those who underwent emergent endovascular repair of an acute, symptomatic, non-ruptured aneurysm were excluded. Studies were also rejected if they described selected groups (such as octogenarians), or were single case reports. In case of studies reporting on duplicate clinical material, the most recent study or the larger of the two was selected.

ER: endovascular repair
LA: local anesthesia
NA: not available
OR: open repair

phy to predict aneurysm suitability and stent-graft sizing for commercially available systems has been questioned, because it will not reveal thrombus or atheroma lining the graft landing zones [38]. Nevertheless, Lindbland et al. [55] reported 3 patients in whom preoperative radiological investigations were not performed, but in whom endovascular repair was subsequently performed. The addition of intravascular ultrasound (IVUS) intraoperatively has been suggested to complement angiography in elective cases. However, it remains to be seen whether IVUS, which requires an experienced ultrasonographer on the endovascular team, would be a useful tool in RAAAs [39].

Type of anesthesia

Open repair of a RAAA requires general anesthesia. In contrast, the use of local anesthesia may be the most important factor in avoiding major hemodynamic disturbance and may account for the better chances of survival of patients undergoing emergent endovascular repair. Although the feasibility of performing endovascular repair under local anesthetic and intravenous sedation in elective cases has been demonstrated, the majority of procedures are still performed under general anesthesia [56]. Only the Zurich [23] and Thessaloniki [18] groups set out to use local anesthesia as the anesthetic technique of choice, whereas others use this selectively. Approximately one third of patients that are reported in the literature had been operated upon under local anesthesia, whereas another 26% of the procedures had been started as a local anesthetic and were converted to general anesthesia. Usual reasons for conversion were loss of consciousness during the operation as a result of severe hypovolemic shock or severe discomfort from the rupture and the endovascular instrumentation of the aorta and iliac arteries [8,18,48]. As a result, not all authors share the same enthusiasm about local anesthesia [8,10,48]. Movement artifact due to patient discomfort has been reported to be the reason for inadvertent coverage of the renal arteries or lower placement of the main body of the device resulting in inadequate aneurysm exclusion [8,18,48].

Stent-graft configuration

The choice of endograft type, i.e., bifurcated versus aorto-uni-iliac, in the RAAA setting is a matter for debate. Both approaches have theoretical and real advantages and disadvantages. Because most of the elective cases are performed by using commercially available modular bifurcated endografts, applying this expertise to emergency cases is crucial in achieving rapid and safe deployment of the graft and early hemorrhage control [8,18,48,56]. Several series in which commercially available modular bifurcated systems were largely used, confirm this (Fig. 1) [12,18,23,25,29]. A potential drawback is the time taken to cannulate the contralateral stump of the main device and deploy the contralateral iliac limb. Adjuncts, such as crossover catheter techniques (used by the Ulm group) and occlusion balloons inflated within the stent graft after deployment of the main body (used in the Zurich series), may overcome this. Alternatively, an aorto-uni-iliac stent-graft may be deployed [56]. Although there are advantages, such as the technical simplicity, speed of deployment, and higher eligibility rate, this option also has all the disadvantages of an extra-anatomic approach. Across different series, the decision to use one approach over another depends on several factors, namely as the expertise and preference of the operator, endograft availability at the time of presentation, and anatomic characteristics of the aneurysm. For example, if a bifurcated approach is to be used, patients with small or stenotic iliac arteries are better suited to the lower-profile Excluder graft (Gore, Flagstaff, AZ), whereas a Talent (Medtronic, Santa Rosa, CA) or a Zenith Flex (Cook Medical Inc., Bloomington, IN) graft would have been more appropriate for aneurysms with a short proximal neck that required suprarenal fixation. When an aorto-uni-iliac approach is chosen, an Endofit (LeMaitre Vascular Inc., Burlington, MA), Talent or Zenith graft may offer quick exclusion of the aneurysm and, thus, better hemodynamic conditions (Fig. 2). Details on the type of stent-graft implanted were available in 504 of the 857 patients presented in Table I. A bifurcated stent-graft was employed in 227 (45%) cases and an aorto-uni-iliac stent-graft was used in 260 (52%). Additionally, a straight tube graft was employed in 17 (3%).

Hemodynamic instability

Cardiovascular instability is one of the most important determinants of survival in RAAA patients undergoing open repair. The same applies to pa-

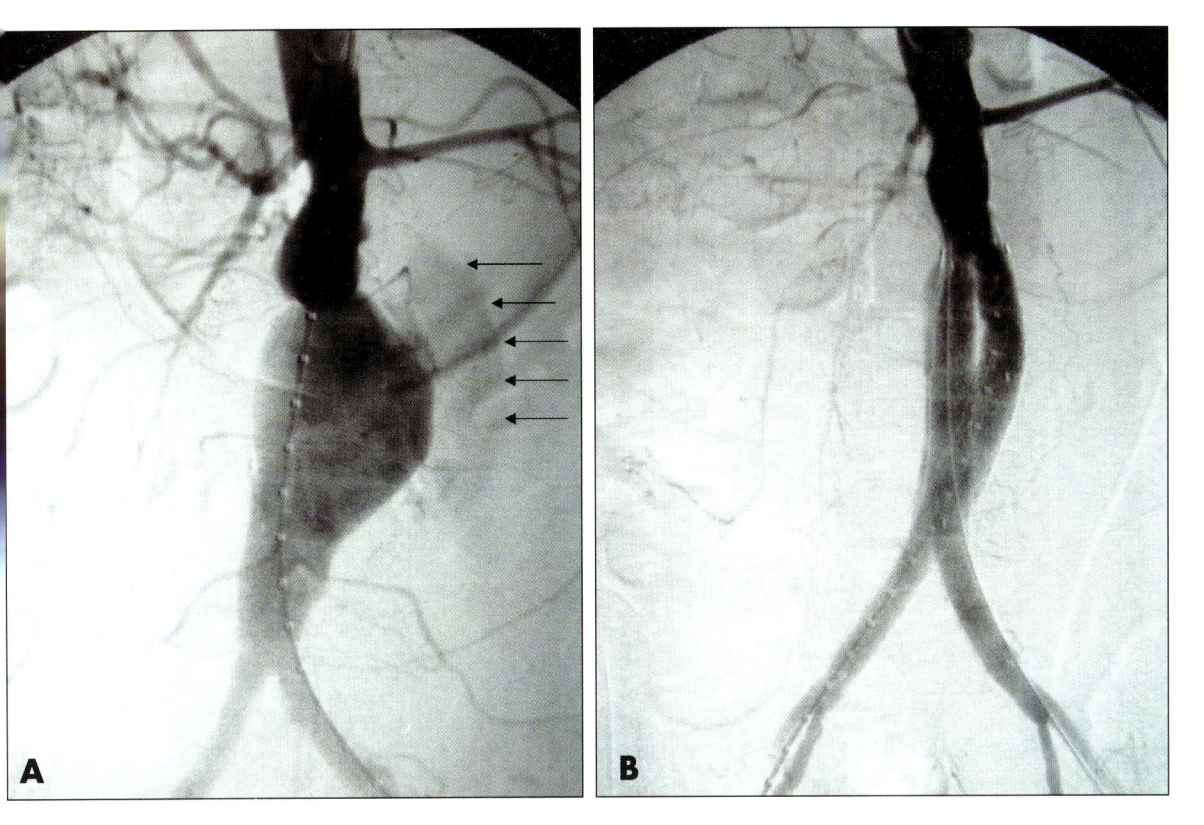

FIG. 1 A - Intra-operative angiogram performed through a pigtail calibrating catheter introduced via the left groin. Contrast extravasation (black arrows) can be seen to the left peri-aortic area suggesting active hemorrhage. B - Completion angiogram after successful aneurysm exclusion with a bifurcated stent-graft.

tients undergoing endovascular aneurysm exclusion. The majority of RAAA patients tend to be relatively stable for a short while at least, but the duration of this window of opportunity is unpredictable [56]. In fact, one study from Colorado suggested that the "stable" RAAA gives a false sense of security [57]. Normal admission blood pressure led to a decreased sense of urgency, creating avoidable delays and missed opportunities for salvage. Another study on the blood pressure of patients who presented with RAAA found 28% to be hypotensive on admission (systolic blood pressure <100 mmHg), which increased to 44% on reaching the operating theatre for open repair [58]. The majority of RAAA treated with endovascular techniques in the literature were hemodynamically stable and, therefore, able to tolerate the inevitable logistical delays. Naturally, this means exclusion of all those patients that are hemodynamically unstable at presentation and who would then need open repair. What constitutes "hemodynamic instability", however, is a matter for debate. Some authors use a cut-off point of <100 mm Hg in the systolic blood pressure, others <90 mm Hg or <80 mm Hg. The Montefiore group prefers even a lower limit at 50 mmHg to keep hemostatic hypotension [9,41,45]. On the other hand, a French group believes that the systemic blood pressure should be kept over 80 mmHg to avoid cardiac, splanchnic, renal and brain ischemia [22,47]. The Thessaloniki group would accept a lower than 80 mmHg pressure as long the patient is conscious and able to protect the airway [18]. This implies a great heterogeneity between studies with regards to case selection, a fact that would certainly have an impact on reported mortality figures.

Hemodynamic instability does not prevent the use of the endovascular technique, however, the outcome would largely depend how quickly aneurysm exclusion can be achieved. In fact, there are centers (Modena, Italy; Thessaloniki, Greece; Calgary, Canada; Albany, New York) which would not exclude hemodynamically unstable patients and in which endovascular repair is offered based mainly on anatomical and not on hemodynamic criteria [18,33,59]. Collective data from the 28 studies pre-

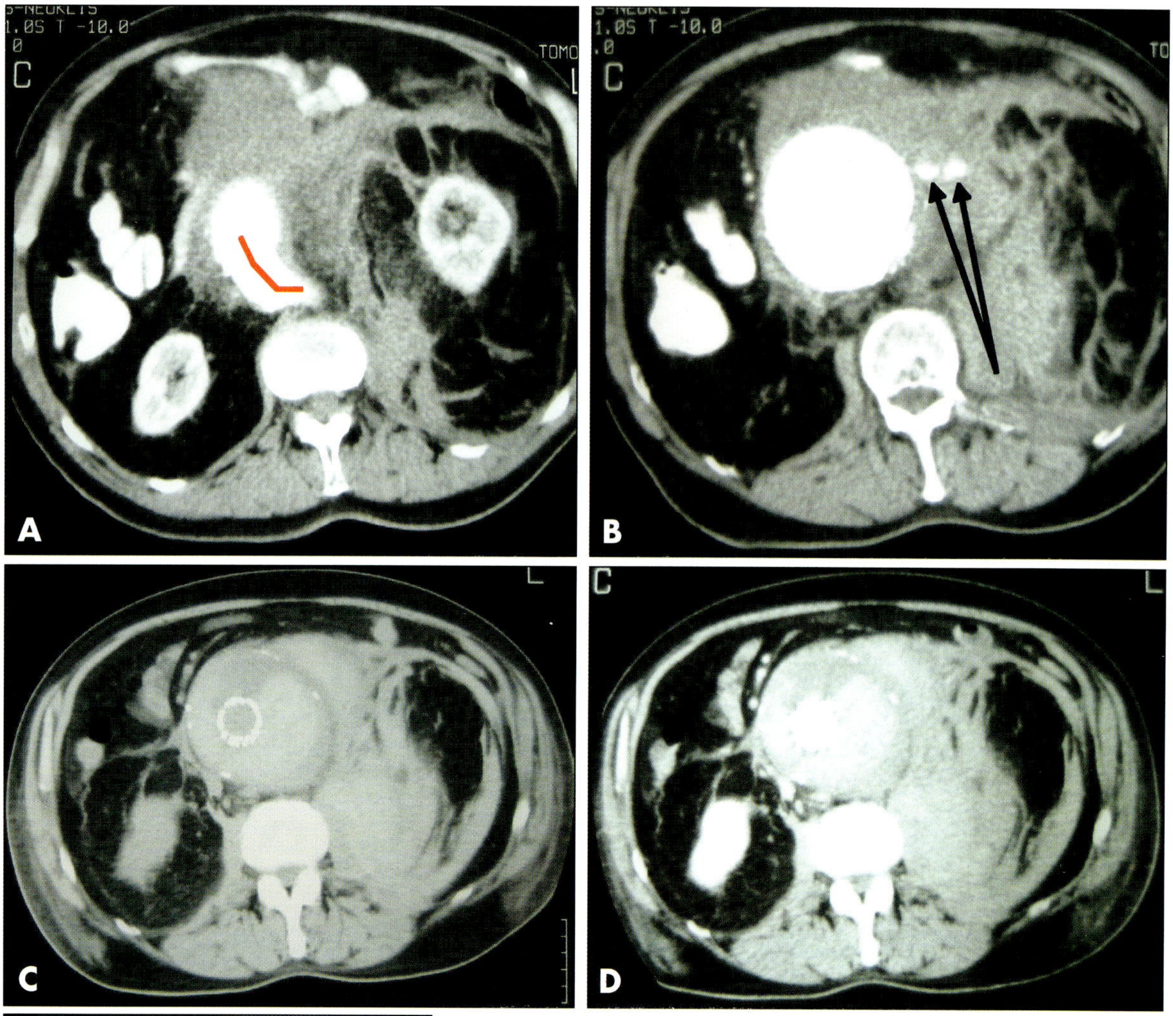

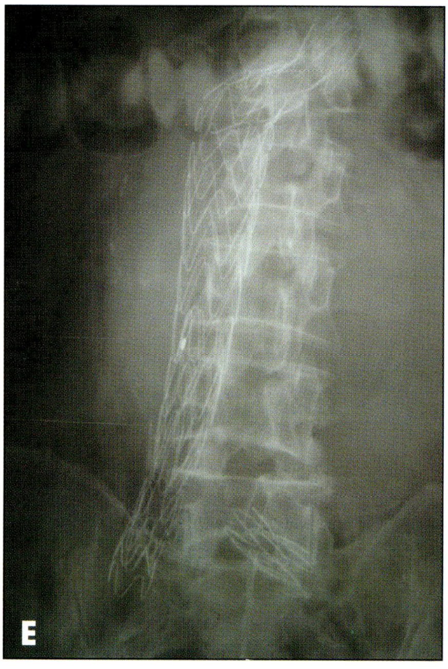

FIG. 2 A - An 80-year-old male patient collapsed whilst inpatient in the medical ward. CT scan shows a RAAA with a large retroperiteoneal hematoma, displacing the left kidney anteriorly. B - Contrast extravasation (black arrows) can be seen filling the peri-aortic hematoma, indicative of active bleeding. The aneurysm was suitable for endovascular repair having a long (>2 cm) but angulated infrarenal neck (red line). He underwent a successful repair under local anesthetic using an aorto-uni-iliac stent-graft (Endofit). CT scan the next day was suspicious of an endoleak, but imaging was suboptimal. Repeat CT 8 days later showed successful aneurysm exclusion. Intra-sac thrombus density was identical prior to (C) and after administration of intravenous contrast (D) with similar appearances to the scan performed the 1st postoperative day. Plain abdominal x-ray illustrating the metal skeleton of the stent-graft and the occluder in the left common iliac artery. E - He had an otherwise uneventful recovery (courtesy of Professor Thomas Gerassimidis, Thessaloniki, Greece).

sented in Table I indicate that hemodynamic instability was present in 221 of the 789 patients (28%) with available information. However, before interpreting these results, one should take into account that the term "hemodynamic instability" was used loosely, accepting the authors' arbitrary definitions even though these were different in different studies. A Canadian study, using predictive models (CUSUM analysis), demonstrated improved RAAA mortality figures following the introduction of an endovascular program, and, in particular, suggested that unstable patients may be particularly benefited by endovascular techniques and should not be excluded from repair [59]. Similar results have been reported by others [33]. In their randomized trial, Hinchcliffe et al. [30] excluded from randomization patients who were so unstable that the surgeon deemed CT scanning unethical. These patients did badly with open repair anyway and, they are, perhaps, those who have most to gain from endovascular repair.

Use of intra-aortic occlusion balloon

The use of intra-aortic occlusion balloons to provide temporary hemostasis before definitive aneurysm exclusion is another controversial issue. Some surgeons use occlusion balloons selectively in hemodynamically unstable patients in whom adequate systolic blood pressure cannot be maintained despite resuscitation measures (Fig. 3). The balloon catheters can be introduced via the brachial artery, as advocated by the Montefiore group [9,41,45], or transfemorally, as described by the Nottingham [30,48], Zurich [23,36], and Malmö [13] groups. The aortic occlusion balloon represents a theoretical advantage because it mimics surgical clamping and immediately slows down the hemorrhage [33]. However, no dedicated occlusion balloons are available on the market, and the use of non-dedicated balloons is problematic, mainly because of balloon instability and diameter, the flexibility of the catheters, and problems linked to executing angiography appropriately [33,60]. Last, and most important, is that insertion of the balloon requires an additional step in the procedure that may consume precious time [61]. As a result, others favor expeditious graft deployment without the use of occlusion balloons. How-

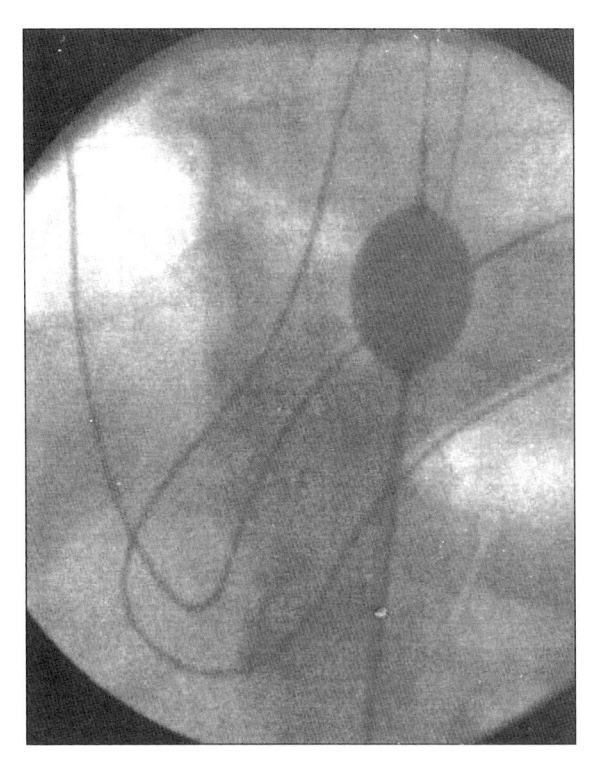

FIG. 3 Intra-aortic balloon occlusion in a hemodynamically unstable patient. This maneuver was used in 17% of patients across the 28 studies. The majority of authors preferred its introduction through the femoral route *(courtesy of Professor Thomas Gerassimidis, Thessaloniki, Greece)*.

ever, there is no doubt that an occlusion balloon may buy time in the very unstable patient, in cases of intra-operative difficulties, or when an immediate conversion to open repair becomes necessary. Nineteen studies in Table I provided information with regards to the use of aortic occlusion balloons. In 13 of these, investigators employed balloon occlusion selectively, whereas 6 centers never used a balloon. The utilization rate ranged from 0%-100%. Across the total population, 17% (62/369) of patients required balloon occlusion.

Conversion to open repair

Immediate conversion to open repair may occasionally be required during endovascular repair because of intra-operative problems and seems to carry a poor prognosis. Primary, i.e. intra-operative, conversion to open repair was necessary in 42 of the 742 patients (6%) with available information across the 28 studies reviewed here. Details regarding the reasons for immediate conversion

Table II. REASONS FOR IMMEDIATE CONVERSION TO OPEN REPAIR IN THE 22 PATIENTS WITH AVAILABLE INFORMATION

Reasons for immediate conversion	N
Access difficulties	5
Type I endoleak and/or stent-graft migration	4
Continued blood loss	4
Inadvertent renal artery overstenting	1
Stent-graft thrombosis	1
Inability to catheterize the contralateral limb	1
Unspecified endoleak	1
Technical error	1
Information not available	4

were only available in 22 cases and these are summarized in Table II. Data on outcome were available in 18 of these. Only 4 patients survived, the overall mortality being 78%. Additionally, there were 6 secondary conversions occurring during hospital stay, 4 because of endoleaks, 1 because of dissection and hemorrhage, and 1 due to inadvertent occlusion of both renal arteries. Conversion to open repair involved 20 out of 290 patients in a large American series [28]. Surprisingly, the mortality among these conversions was only 35%.

Mortality after endovascular repair

The reported mortality rates vary a great deal in the literature. In particular, in-hospital and/or 30-day mortality ranged between 0% and 54% across the 28 different series. These figures cover the whole range "from undeniably superior to frustratingly equivalent" when compared with open repair [56]. The highest mortality was encountered in the context of a randomized trial [30].

This is not surprising since it is well-known that selected case-series invariably produce better results than randomized controlled studies. There may be other contributory factors, including patient selection and the experience of the team available. When all series were combined, the overall mortality was 30% (256/857 patients). In a collective world experience with information from 48 centers on 442 RAAAs, Veith [62] reported a 30-day mortality of 18%. Two meta-analyses have also attempted to calculate the overall mortality after endovascular repair [63,64]. First, Harkin et al. [63] reported an estimated mortality rate of 18% (0%-53%) after analyzing the only one randomized controlled trial available and 33 case-series (24 retrospective and 9 prospective). The second meta-analysis examined 10 studies with 478 procedures (148 endovascular, 330 open) and estimated the pooled 30-day mortality after endovascular repair to be 22% [64]. All these results are much better than those traditionally reported in the literature for open repair. However, it should be stressed that these figures may reflect increasing experience and patient selection. Furthermore, they originate from pioneering centers from around the world with significant experience in elective endovascular aneurysm repair [48].

In particular, there are three groups of patients in which selection may influence the results [18,56]. First, most studies report on hemodynamically stable patients. In fact, only 28% of patients in the 28 series were hemodynamic unstable. Excluding patients with free intraperitoneal rupture, instability, and hypotension, cases that may not be associated with survival at open repair, would certainly improve the results. In the Zurich series, for example, 58% of patients were excluded from endovascular repair because of hemodynamic contraindications [36]. Second, several reports have identified patients who would normally be turned down for open repair because of serious comorbidities but who subsequently undergo successful endovascular surgery and survive [56]. In the series from Nottingham, 8 of 20 cases had been refused open surgery [8]. Also, all 5 patients in the Philadelphia series [16] and another 3 patients described by Greenberg et al. [7] had been previously turned down for open repair. They all underwent successful endovascular aneurysm repair. Finally, some reports also include patients with an acute, symptomatic AAA without documented rupture. The Eindhoven, Rotterdam, and Groningen series contain 24 emergent patients with symptomatic non-ruptured aneurysms; all underwent successful endovascular aneurysm repair with no mortality [10,35,44]. When performing the present literature review, we have set out to exclude all such cases.

Comparison of endovascular to open RAAA repair may be misleading, because endovascular repair cannot be performed in all patients, and selection bias may explain the superior performance of any given strategy [59]. Harkin et al. [63], in their pooled analysis, estimated an overall mortality of 18% and 34% after endovascular and open repair, respectively [63]. The Dutch meta-analysis attempted to compare open and endovascular repair after adjustment for the presence or absence of hemodynamic instability [64]. The pooled 30-day mortality was 22% (95% CI: 16%, 29%) for endovascular repair and 38% (95% CI: 32%, 45%) for open surgery. The crude odds ratio (OR) 30-day mortality for endovascular repair compared with open surgery was 0.45 (95% CI: 0.28, 0.72). After adjustment for patients' hemodynamic condition, the OR was 0.67 (95% CI: 0.31, 1.44), i.e., a benefit in 30-day mortality for endovascular repair was observed, but this was not statistically significant.

Morbidity

Patients undergoing endovascular repair for RAAA are prone to the usual complications of open surgery, as well as to morbidity related to the endovascular technique itself [47]. It is of note that little reference is made with regards to the cardiopulmonary complications, which are very common after open repair [56]. Whether these problems are not seen, which is rather unlikely, or they not as significant an issue after endovascular repair, remains to be clarified. A recent study by Greco et al. examined the discharge data sets from the four states of California, Florida, New Jersey, and New York, for patients undergoing open (n=5 508) or endovascular (n=290) RAAA repair for the period 2000-2003[28]. Cardiac event rates were not different in the two groups (12.7 versus 15.2%, p=0.2), however, there were fewer respiratory complications in the endovascular group (32.4 vs 21.7%, p=0.002).

Renal failure
Renal failure after open RAAA repair has been reported in up to 29% of cases and has been shown to independently predict mortality and prolonged hospital stay [1-3,5]. Deterioration of renal function may also occur after endovascular repair and is associated with a high mortality. This is despite the fact that these patients are spared the ischemic insult of aortic cross-clamping and have less perioperative hemorrhage than open repair [38]. Renal failure was seen in 6, and was fatal in 4 patients in the initial Nottingham experience [8]. In the early Zurich series, Lachat et al. [36] reported renal impairment in 28%, although only 2 out of 6 required renal replacement therapy. Renal failure may be due to several reasons, such as inadvertent coverage of one or both renal arteries by the stent-graft, as seen in the Nottingham and Thessaloniki series; large doses of potentially nephrotoxic intravenous contrast; and endovascular manipulation of the abdominal aorta which carries a risk for kidney embolization. The risk for renal failure is increased in patients with pre-existing renal impairment, hemodynamic compromise and large contrast volumes. Similar to open aortic surgery, this renal deterioration may simply be in the form of worsening renal function or may require temporary or permanent hemodialysis. In the study from Greco et al. [28], the incidence of renal failure after endovascular repair in the 4 states was 14.8%, less common than that encountered after open repair (24.8%, p<0.001). Hichcliffe et al. [48] suggest the use of dilute contrast, carbon dioxide angiography, and IVUS as potential ways to reduce the contrast volume and nephrotoxicity.

Visceral ischemia
Infarction of the sigmoid colon remains one the most frequent fatal complications in published open RAAA series, with an incidence reaching 10% to 20% after endovascular repair [47,48]. Although in the elective setting, the latter is associated with less colonic ischemia than open repair, RAAA patients with preoperative hypotension are more likely to develop colonic ischemia [47,65]. In elective endovascular procedures, occlusion of one or both internal iliac arteries may be achieved safely, albeit observations regarding bilateral internal iliac occlusion are derived from a limited number of patients and the procedure is usually being done in a staged fashion [47,48,50]. On the other hand, all observations of colonic ischemia after endovascular RAAA repair had occurred in patients with occlusion of at least one of the internal iliac arteries. Therefore, it is difficult to predict who will develop splanchnic ischemia postoperatively, but a sensible policy would be the conservation of the hypogastric circulation whenever possible. Of course, in cases of unfavorable iliac anatomy and

need for sacrificing one or two internal iliac arteries, the operator needs to make a prompt and balanced decision between completely excluding the rupture on the one hand, and preventing colonic ischemia on the other. Splanchnic ischemia was no different between open and endovascular RAAA repair groups in the American state-wide experience (5.2 vs 6.9%, p=0.2) [28].

COMPARTMENT SYNDROME

The abdominal compartment syndrome is an important cause of multiple organ failure and is increasingly recognized as a major cause for morbidity and mortality following emergency open repair. The closed nature of endovascular repair has raised concerns that the incidence of abdominal compartment syndrome may be higher using the latter approach. As a result, close monitoring of intra-abdominal pressure may be required in patients with a large intra-abdominal or retroperitoneal hematoma on CT scan. Raised intra-abdominal pressure along with multiple organ dysfunction may well require decompression, either through a laparotomy or a translumbar extraperitoneal approach [11,12]. Nevertheless, many patients may respond well to supportive therapy and not require decompression [47,48]. A novel technique using a percutaneous puncture and installation of tissue plasminogen activator (tPA) in the hematoma has also been described [66].

ENDOLEAKS

Although the significance of endoleaks after elective endovascular repair has been more or less established, their behavior in the presence of a ruptured aneurysm sac is less well documented. Continued perfusion of the aneurysm in the presence of rupture is of major concern, but, fortunately, the reported incidence is low [56]. Proximal type I endoleak is the most serious cause and, apart from immediate conversion, other strategies include laparotomy and banding of the aortic neck [10] or secondary endovascular interventions [36,56]. Continued bleeding due to type II endoleak is a less common occurrence and does not appear to be a significant issue. Rarely, this may lead to persistent blood loss and increase of the retroperitoneal hematoma. Coil embolization has been reported to successfully resolve this problem [61].

The need for prompt interpretation of the CT images in the emergency setting may result in less accurate measurements, which, in turn, may potentially lead to an increase of the incidence of endoleaks above the rate normally expected for elective endovascular repair. In the Zurich series, there was a high overall endoleak rate of 35% which required in-hospital secondary endovascular interventions in 58% of cases [23]. Accurate planning, is therefore crucial to minimize both early and late technical failures. In addition, suprarenal stents, with separate "anchorage" and "seal" zones, and a large Palmaz stent (Cordis Corp., Johnson and Johnson Interventional Systems, Warren, NJ) to improve seal and alignment, all useful adjuncts for difficult necks in elective cases, may prove valuable in the emergency setting as well. This can be difficult to achieve in the "heat of the moment", but may be completed, if necessary, by secondary procedures before discharge [38,47,48].

Successful exclusion of the ruptured sac is associated with resorption of the retroperitoneal hematoma in most cases [18,36,38]. Furthermore, as seen after elective repair, it may be associated with sac shrinkage. Hechelhammer et al. [23] reported that nearly 40% of treated patients had a size reduction of minimum 5 mm at a mean follow-up of 24 months. Lee et al. [14] encountered a higher shrinking rate of 54% in a shorter follow-up of 6.8 months.

Logistical issues

Setting up an emergency endovascular program presents several logistical problems [56]. First of all, there is a need for appropriately trained medical personnel along with the implementation of an out-of-hours emergency endovascular on-call rota. Such a set-up requires a sufficient number of enthusiastic vascular surgeons and interventional radiologists. This is only likely to occur in vascular centers experienced in elective endovascular aneurysm repair with a sufficient workload in high-volume hospitals. Urgent access to CT is also mandatory, along with experienced radiology personnel able to perform an urgent CT scan and then operate the C-arm during the procedure. Operating theatre staff, experienced in both open and endovascular aortic surgery, and anesthetic staff with appropriate training for such challenging cases are both crucial to the success. A further major issue is the availability of a wide range of stent-grafts. Some units have an in-house stock of commercially available endografts, whereas others, such as ours, emergency access to suitable endografts is through the locally based company representatives [18]. Although this policy can potentially lead to inevitable logistical delays, in our experience, frequent communication with the company representatives resulted in timely endograft availability. Naturally, this would largely depend on the local circumstances. One last logistical issue has to do with the centralization of the vascular services. It is likely that offering an emergency RAAA endovascular service will be possible only in major vascular centers. That would mean that patients may have to be transferred to tertiary centers from outlying units. Of course, others may argue that as endovascular technology becomes more and more commonplace, the ease of these procedures might, indeed, make it the preferred option for aneurysm repair: only patients unsuitable for endovascular repair would be selected to go to tertiary centers for complex open surgery [18].

It is now recognized that establishing a standardized protocol is crucial for the successful start of an endovascular RAAA program. The early results show that emergent endovascular treatment of both hemodynamically stable and unstable patients is associated with a reduction in mortality [59,67]. This requires a multidisciplinary approach that includes vascular surgeons, emergency department physicians, anesthesiology and operating room staff, radiology technicians, and availability of a variety of stent-grafts to expedite endovascular repair [59,67].

Conclusion

Emergency endovascular RAAA repair is now technically feasible. To date, several reports from major centers with small numbers, one randomized controlled trial, one collective world experience and two meta-analyses have appeared in the literature suggesting that the results may be the same as or better than seen with open repair. The logistics behind the initiation of an endovascular RAAA service are complex and there are many problems to overcome, such as organization difficulties, availability of a wide range of endografts, appropriate training of medical and paramedical personnel, implementation of an out-of-hours emergency endovascular on-call rota, and centralization of the vascular services. Urgent CT scanning is the imaging of choice in order to determine suitability for endovascular repair. This ranges from 34%-100% in various centers, but could reach an average of around 70%-80% [56,63]. The implanted endograft may be modular bifurcated or aorto-uni-iliac depending on aneurysm morphology, device availability, personal expertise and hemodynamic instability. The majority of units had initially offered endovascular repair to stable patients, but, with increasing experience, this has extended to unstable cases as well, so that some centers would consider endovascular treatment as the procedure of choice for all-comers, irrespective of hemodynamic condition. However, the take home message is that endovascular RAAA repair is associated with a formidable learning curve which is different and, certainly, longer than that of elective cases. That is why such cases should be attempted only by major units that have extensive elective endovascular experience. A large, multicenter, prospective randomized trial would be the ideal way to answer whether endovascular repair is superior to open surgery. However, such a trial is difficult to organize due to logistical issues, recruitment difficulties, and ethical questions. As a result, the alternative would be for major centers to continue to develop their endovascular programs and gain significant experience. The evidence would come from prospective studies and registries, as well as comparisons of the modern results of endovascular treatment - beyond the early learning curve - with historical controls undergoing open repair. The debate for the future would be not which technique is superior, but to define exactly the role of endovascular repair as an additional therapeutic option for RAAAs.

REFERENCES

1 Heller JA, Weinberg A, Arons R et al. Two decades of abdominal aortic aneurysm repair: have we made any progress? *J Vasc Surg* 2000; 32: 1091-1100.

2 Noel AA, Gloviczki P, Cherry KJ Jr et al. Ruptured abdominal aortic aneurysms: the excessive mortality rate of conventional repair. *J Vasc Surg* 2001; 34: 41-46.

3 van Dongen HP, Leusink JA, Moll FL et al. Ruptured abdominal aortic aneurysms: factors influencing postoperative mortality and long-term survival. *Eur J Vasc Endovasc Surg* 1998; 15: 62-66.

4 Ingoldby CJ, Wujanto R, Mitchell JE. Impact of vascular surgery on community mortality from ruptured aortic aneurysms. *Br J Surg* 1986; 73: 551-553.

5 Bown MJ, Sutton AJ, Bell PR et al. A meta-analysis of 50 years of ruptured abdominal aortic aneurysm repair. *Br J Surg* 2002; 89: 714-730.

6. Yusuf SW, Whitaker SC, Chuter TA et al. Emergency endovascular repair of leaking aortic aneurysm. *Lancet* 1994; 344: 1645.

7. Greenberg RK, Ouriel K, Shortell C et al. An endoluminal method of hemorrhage control and repair of ruptured abdominal aortic aneurysms. *J Endovasc Ther* 2000; 7: 1-7.

8. Hinchliffe RJ, Yusuf SW, Macierewicz JA et al. Endovascular repair of ruptured abdominal aortic aneurysm—a challenge to open repair: results of a single centre experience in 20 patients. *Eur J Vasc Endovasc Surg* 2001; 22: 528-534.

9. Veith FJ, Ohki T. Endovascular approaches to ruptured infrarenal aortoiliac aneurysms. *J Cardiovasc Surg* 2002; 43: 369-378.

10. Yilmaz N, Peppelenbosch N, Cuypers PW et al. Emergency treatment of symptomatic or ruptured abdominal aortic aneurysms: the role of endovascular repair. *J Endovasc Ther* 2002; 9: 449-457.

11. Van Herzeele I, Vermassen F, Durieux C et al. Endovascular repair of aortic rupture. *Eur J Vasc Endovasc Surg* 2003; 26: 311-316.

12. Scharrer-Pamler R, Kotsis T, Kapfer X et al. Endovascular stent-graft repair of ruptured aortic aneurysms. *J Endovasc Ther* 2003; 10: 447-452.

13. Resch T, Malina M, Lindbland B et al. Endovascular repair of ruptured abdominal aortic aneurysms: logistics and short-term results. *J Endovasc Ther* 2003; 10: 440-446.

14. Lee WA, Hirneise CM, Tayyarah M et al. Impact of endovascular repair on early outcomes of ruptured abdominal aortic aneurysms. *J Vasc Surg* 2004; 40: 211-215.

15. May J, White GH, Stephen MS et al. Rupture of abdominal aortic aneurysm: concurrent comparison of outcome of those occurring after endovascular repair versus those occurring without previous treatment in an 11-year single-center experience. *J Vasc Surg* 2004; 40: 860-866.

16. Lombardi JV, Fairman RM, Golden MA et al. The utility of commercially available endografts in the treatment of ruptured abdominal aortic aneurysm with hemodynamic stability. *J Vasc Surg* 2004; 40: 154-160.

17. Arya N, Lee B, Loan W et al. Change in aneurysm diameter after stent-graft repair of ruptured abdominal aortic aneurysms. *J Endovasc Ther* 2004; 11: 319-322.

18. Gerassimidis TS, Papazoglou KO, Kamparoudis AG et al. Endovascular management of ruptured abdominal aortic aneurysms: 6-year experience from a Greek center. *J Vasc Surg* 2005; 42: 615-623.

19. Larzon T, Lindgren R, Norgren L. Endovascular treatment of ruptured abdominal aortic aneurysms: a shift of the paradigm? *J Endovasc Ther* 2005; 12: 548-555.

20. Brandt M, Walluscheck KP, Jahnke T et al. Endovascular repair of ruptured abdominal aortic aneurysm: feasibility and impact on early outcome. *J Vasc Interv Radiol* 2005; 16: 1309-1312.

21. Peppelenbosch N, Cuypers PW, Vahl AC et al. Emergency endovascular treatment for ruptured abdominal aortic aneurysm and the risk of spinal cord ischemia. *J Vasc Surg* 2005; 42: 608-614.

22. Alsac JM, Desgranges P, Kobeiter H et al. Emergency endovascular repair for ruptured abdominal aortic aneurysms: feasibility and comparison of early results with conventional open repair. *Eur J Vasc Endovasc Surg* 2005; 30: 632-639.

23. Hechelhammer L, Lachat ML, Wildermuth S et al. Midterm outcome of endovascular repair of ruptured abdominal aortic aneurysms. *J Vasc Surg* 2005; 41: 752-757.

24. Vaddineni SK, Russo GC, Patterson MA et al. Ruptured abdominal aortic aneurysm: a retrospective assessment of open versus endovascular repair. *Ann Vasc Surg* 2005; 19: 782-786.

25. Castelli P, Caronno R, Piffaretti G et al. Ruptured abdominal aortic aneurysm: endovascular treatment. *Abdom Imaging* 2005; 30: 263-69.

26. Dalainas I, Nano G, Bianchi P et al. Endovascular techniques for the treatment of ruptured abdominal aortic aneurysms: 7-year intention-to-treat results. *World J Surg* 2006; 30: 1809-1814.

27. Oranen BI, Bos WT, Verhoeven EL et al. Is emergency endovascular aneurysm repair associated with higher secondary intervention risk at mid-term follow-up? *J Vasc Surg* 2006; 44: 1156-1161.

28. Greco G, Egorova N, Anderson PL et al. Outcomes of endovascular treatment of ruptured abdominal aortic aneurysms. *J Vasc Surg* 2006; 43: 453-459.

29. Visser JJ, Bosch JL, Hunink MG et al. Endovascular repair versus open surgery in patients with ruptured abdominal aortic aneurysms: Clinical outcomes with 1-year follow-up. *J Vasc Surg* 2006; 44: 1148-1155.

30. Hinchliffe RJ, Bruijstens L, MacSweeney ST et al. A randomised trial of endovascular and open surgery for ruptured abdominal aortic aneurysm - Results of a pilot study and lessons learned for future studies. *Eur J Vasc Endovasc Surg* 2006; 32: 506-513.

31. Acosta S, Lindblad B, Zdanowski Z. Predictors for outcome after open and endovascular repair of ruptured abdominal aortic aneurysms. *Eur J Vasc Endovasc Surg* 2007; 33: 277-284.

32. Peppelenbosch N, Geelkerken RH, Soong C et al. Endograft treatment of ruptured abdominal aortic aneurysms using the Talent aortouniiliac system: An international multicenter study. *J Vasc Surg* 2006; 43: 1111-1122.

33. Coppi G, Silingardi R, Gennai S et al. A single-center experience in open and endovascular treatment of hemodynamically unstable and stable patients with ruptured abdominal aortic aneurysms. *J Vasc Surg* 2006; 44: 1140-1147.

34. Franks S, Lloyd G, Fishwick G et al. Endovascular treatment of ruptured and symptomatic abdominal aortic aneurysms. *Eur J Vasc Endovasc Surg* 2006; 31: 345-350.

35. van Sambeek MRHM, van Dijk LC, Hendriks JM et al. Endovascular versus conventional open repair of acute abdominal aortic aneurysm: feasibility and preliminary results. *J Endovasc Ther* 2002; 9: 443-448.

36. Lachat ML, Pfammatter T, Witzke HJ et al. Endovascular repair with bifurcated stent-grafts under local anaesthesia to improve outcome of ruptured aortoiliac aneurysms. *Eur J Vasc Endovasc Surg* 2002; 23: 528-536.

37. Orend KH, Kotsis T, Scharrer-Pamler R et al. Endovascular repair of aortic rupture due to trauma and aneurysm. *Eur J Vasc Endovasc Surg* 2002; 23: 61-67.

38. Piffaretti G, Caronno R, Tozzi M et al. Endovascular versus open repair of ruptured abdominal aortic aneurysm. *Expert Rev Cardiovasc Ther* 2006; 4: 839-852.

39. Badger SA, O'Donnell ME, Makar RR et al. Aortic necks of ruptured abdominal aneurysms dilate more than asymptomatic aneurysms after endovascular repair. *J Vasc Surg* 2006; 44: 244-249.

40. Carpenter JP, Woo EY. Popliteal venous aneurysm. *J Vasc Surg* 2006; 44: 1361-1362.

41. Ohki T, Veith FJ, Sanchez LA et al. Endovascular graft repair of ruptured aortoiliac aneurysms. *J Am Coll Surg* 1999; 189: 102-113.

42. Chiesa R, Setacci C, Tshomba Y et al. Ruptured abdominal aortic aneurysm in the elderly patient. *Acta Chir Belg* 2006; 106: 508-516.

43. Acosta S, Ogren M, Bergqvist D et al. The Hardman Index in

patients operated on for ruptured abdominal aortic aneurysm: a systematic review. *J Vasc Surg* 2006; 44: 949-954.

44 Kapma MR, Verhoeven EL, Tielliu IF et al. Endovascular treatment of acute abdominal aortic aneurysm with a bifurcated stent graft. *Eur J Vasc Endovasc Surg* 2005; 29: 510-515.

45 Ohki T, Veith FJ. Endovascular grafts and other image-guided catheter-based adjuncts to improve the treatment of ruptured aortoiliac aneurysms. *Ann Surg* 2000; 232: 466-479.

46 Teijink JA, Odink HF, Bendermacher B et al. Ruptured AAA in a patient with a horseshoe kidney: emergent treatment using the Talent acute endovascular aneurysm repair kit. *J Endovasc Ther* 2003; 10: 240-243.

47 Alsac JM, Kobeiter H, Becquemin JP et al. Endovascular repair for ruptured abdominal aortic aneurysm: a literature review. *Acta Chir Belg* 2005; 105: 134-139.

48 Hinchliffe RJ, Braithwaite BD, Hopkinson BR. The endovascular management of ruptured abdominal aortic aneurysms. *Eur J Vasc Endovasc Surg* 2003; 25: 191-201.

49 Adam DJ, Bradbury AW, Stuart WP et al. The value of computed tomography in the assessment of suspected ruptured abdominal aortic aneurysm. *J Vasc Surg* 1998; 27: 431-437.

50 Thompson MM, Sayers RD. Arterial aneurysms. In: Beard JD, Gaines PA, eds. *Vascular and Endovascular Surgery*. London: WB Saunders Company Ltd, 1998: pp 253-285.

51 Bradbury AW, Makhdoomi KR, Adam DJ et al. Twelve year experience of the management of abdominal aortic aneurysm. *Br J Surg* 1998: 84: 1705-1707.

52 Walker EM, Hopkinson BR, Makin GS. Unoperated abdominal aortic aneurysm: presentation and natural history. *Ann R Coll Surg Engl* 1983; 65: 311-313.

53 Lloyd GM, Bown MJ, Norwood MG et al. Feasibility of preoperative computer tomography in patients with ruptured abdominal aortic aneurysm: a time-to-death study in patients without operation. *J Vasc Surg* 2004; 39: 788-791.

54 Adam DJ, Mohan IV, Stuart WP et al. Community and hospital outcome from ruptured abdominal aortic aneurysm within the catchment area of a regional vascular surgical service. *J Vasc Surg* 1999; 30: 922-928.

55 Lindbland B. Ruptured abdominal aortic aneurysms: will endovascular repair take over? *International Symposium on Controversies in Vascular Surgery*. August 2002, Copenhagen.

56 Brennan J, McWilliams R. The endovascular treatment of ruptured abdominal aortic aneurysms. In: Wyatt MG, Watkinson AF, eds. *Endovascular intervention: current controversies*. Shrewsbury: tfm Publishing Ltd, 2004: p 19-25.

57 Weinstein ES, Cooper M, Hammond S et al. The "stable" ruptured abdominal aortic aneurysm gives a false sense of security. *Am J Surg* 1999; 178: 133-135.

58 Lawrie GM, Morris GC Jr, Crawford ES et al. Improved results of operation for ruptured abdominal aortic aneurysms. *Surgery* 1979; 85: 483-488.

59 Moore R, Nutley M, Cina CS et al. Improved survival after introduction of an emergency endovascular therapy protocol for ruptured abdominal aortic aneurysms. *J Vasc Surg* 2007; 45: 443-450.

60 Malina M, Veith F, Ivancev K et al. Balloon occlusion of the aorta during endovascular repair of ruptured abdominal aortic aneurysm. *J Endovasc Ther* 2005; 12: 556-559.

61 Hartung O, Vidal V, Marani I et al. Treatment of an early type II endoleak causing hemorrhage after endovascular aneurysm repair for ruptured abdominal aortic aneurysm. *J Vasc Surg* 2007; 45: 1062-1065.

62 Veith F. Update on endovascular repair of ruptured abdominal aortic and thoracic aneurysms: the collected world experience. *The 32nd Annual Veith Symposium*, November 2005, New York.

63 Harkin DW, Dillon M et al. Endovascular ruptured abdominal aortic aneurysm repair (EVRAR): A systematic review. *Eur J Vasc Endovasc Surg* 2007; 34: 673-681.

64 Visser JJ, van Sambeek MR, Hamza TH et al. Ruptured abdominal aortic aneurysms: endovascular repair versus open surgery - systematic review. *Radiology* 2007; 245: 122-129.

65 Elmarasy NM, Soong CV, Walker SR et al. Sigmoid ischaemia and the inflammatory response following endovascular abdominal aortic aneurysm repair. *J Endovasc Ther* 2000; 7: 21-30.

66 Larzon T. Tips and tricks to facilitate endovascular repair of ruptured AAAs, including fascial closure of femoral puncture sites. *The 34th Annual Veith Symposium*, November 2007, New York.

67 Mehta M, Taggert J, Darling RC 3rd et al. Establishing a protocol for endovascular treatment of ruptured abdominal aortic aneurysms: Outcomes of a prospective analysis. *J Vasc Surg* 2006; 44: 1-8.

16

ENDOVASCULAR TREATMENT OF ANASTOMOTIC FALSE ANEURYSMS OF THE ABDOMINAL AORTA

PIERRE-EDOUARD MAGNAN, NABIL SEDKI, MICHEL BARTOLI
ALAIN BRANCHEREAU

Anastomotic false abdominal aortic aneurysms (AFAA) represent a rare but serious complication of abdominal aortic reconstructive surgery. The incidence varies between 1%-8% [1-8], depending on the diagnostic means. Indication for treatment relates to the high mortality rate associated with the complications of AFAA like rupture or development of duodenal fistulae [5,8-11]. Mortality of conventional surgical treatment is elevated, varying between 8% and 28% [9-12]. Endovascular treatment, avoiding repeat abdominal access and aortic cross clamping, represents an attractive, therapeutic alternative, the feasibility of which has been demonstrated [13-20]. The aim of this chapter is to describe short- and mid-term results of endovascular repair based on the literature and personal experience in 22 patients treated for AFAA.

Epidemiology and pathophysiology

The etiology of anastomotic false abdominal aortic aneurysms (AFAA) is most often multifactor: rupture of suture, degeneration of prosthetic material and arterial wall deterioration. Weakness of the arterial wall can be caused by progressive arterial disease, previous interventions, chronic use of tobacco, arterial hypertension and technical factors like small suture bites, prosthetic implantation on a fragile, endarterectomized arterial wall, end-to-side anastomosis and peri-operative complications jeopardizing the organization of peri-anastomotic fibrous tissue like lymph cyst or hematoma [5]. Low grade infections like coagulated negative staphylococcus biofilm infection can also be responsible for false aneurysm formation [4].

The exact incidence of AFAA is difficult to assess since they remain asymptomatic for long times as compared to false aneurysms in the groin. The time to occurrence can vary considerably, varying between months and many years. Early occurrence within 5 years is most often caused by peri-operative local or general (respiratory failure, renal failure, sepsis) complications and if the patient was operated on in emergency setting.

The natural history of false aneurysms is dominated by their rate of growth which can be progressive or develop with serious complications including:
1) compression of surrounding tissue or organs;
2) acute thrombosis;
3) distal embolization;
4) rupture, with or without prosthetic-enteric fistula.

Independent from the technique of discovering an AFAA, a general assessment is mandatory in order to search for associated false aneurysms: 25% of aortic false aneurysms are associated with at least one femoral false anastomotic aneurysm [8].

Surgical treatment

Conventional surgical treatment of AFAA is technically challenging. Repeat access of the aorta is associated with more bleeding and risk of injuring the duodenum, inferior vena cava and renal veins due to sclerosed tissue.

One of the encountered problems during this kind of surgery is the level of aortic clamping. In order to perform the proximal anastomosis it is often required to clamp above the renal arteries or even above the celiac axis, subsequently causing renal or mesenteric ischemia. Therefore, the choice of surgical access is important. By using the transperitoneal approach it might be necessary to detach the posterior mesogastrium by phrenotomy in order to clamp the supravisceral aorta. This extended visceral mobilization augments the risk of injuries, especially the pancreas and spleen. Dividing the left renal vein, sometimes necessary for improved exposure, increases bleeding and the risk of postoperative renal insufficiency. In case sufficient aortic tissue for adequate infrarenal anastomosis is lacking, supravisceral clamping is required to anastomose the graft to the inter-renal level. This maneuver comprises elevated risk of renal embolization and prolonged renal ischemia.

The increased morbidity and mortality rates of these interventions (Table I) are ascribed to cardiac stress related to prolonged surgery and proximal aortic clamping in older patients with extensive general atherosclerotic disease, presenting with severe comorbidities [9-12]. Intestinal ischemia is an additional complication of this kind of surgery. The latter is often due to embolization during dissection and clamping and sometimes caused by torsion of the ostium of the superior mesenteric artery by the suprarenal clamp.

The therapeutic alternative, particularly attractive with regard to this morbidity and mortality, constitutes of implantation of a covered endograft.

Table I	Morbidity and mortality of surgical AFAA repair			
First author [ref.]	*Year*	*Number of cases*	*Morbidity (%)*	*Mortality (%)*
Treiman [9]	1998	18	36	28
Curl [10]	1992	21	-	24
Allen [11]	1993	31	73	21
Mulder [12]	1998	135	-	7.6

Endovascular treatment

Preoperative imaging

Endovascular treatment of AFAA requires exact morphological assessment in order to choose the correct endoprosthesis. The parameters to consider are more numerous and complex when compared to endovascular treatment of native aortic aneurysms. The images should inform on the different diameters and lengths of the AFAA and depict the quality of the aortic wall at the level of the anticipated areas of deployment. The required measurements include: diameter of the interrenal aorta, diameter of the aortic neck, maximal diameter of the aneurysm, diameter of the prosthetic graft and side branches (if any), and diameters of the common and external iliac arteries. Additional assessment includes the length of the proximal neck, the length between the renal arteries and the end or bifurcation of the prosthesis as well as the length of undiseased and/or aneurysmal parts of the iliac arteries. Besides these diameter and length measurements, angulations of the false aneurysm and access arteries are assessed as well as the presence of thrombus or calcifications at the zones of deployment. Severe stenoses and excessive tortuosities of iliac axes or anatomotic anomalies like accessory renal arteries should be identified.

In case the AFAA occurs at a proximal end-to-side anastomosis it is mandatory to visualize patency of the native aorta distal to the false aneurysm as well as the side branches (lumbar arteries, inferior mesenteric artery) and the iliac arteries. In fact, implantation of an endograft abolishes any access to these branches to perform embolization in case of persistent indirect endoleakage. Embolization procedures if considered necessary, should therefore be carried out some days prior to endograft implantation. Basically these morphologic investigations are performed by means of computed tomography (CT)-angiography, however, if not conclusive or in case of interest in flow direction into side branches, catheter angiography could be considered. In the majority of cases, CT-angiography is the only imaging modality which is necessary to perform the previously described measurements and choose the correct endograft. Multislice CT-scanning with millimeter slices are routinely performed, providing high spatial resolution. Only 100 mL of contrast is required and MIP-reconstructions and 3D images are obtained on the working station. Quantification of lengths and diameters are performed by means of 2D centerline reconstructions.

Choice of endograft

Endovascular treatment is only applicable in the presence of an adequate infrarenal aortic neck of at least 15 mm length, without major calcifications or intraluminal thrombus. The proximal diameter of the endograft is 10%-15% larger than the diameter of the aorta at the level of the renal arteries. Bifurcated grafts, either modular or single body, are less applicable in anastomotic false aortic aneurysms. The length between the level of the renal arteries and the bifurcation of the surgically implanted graft is often less than 80 mm, not allowing adequate deployment the contralateral limb of the currently available bifurcated endografts. Furthermore, the lower part of the initial graft is often too straight, including both limbs, to implant the legs of a bifurcated endograft.

In our experience the aorto-uni-iliac endografts are more practical since they avoid these pitfalls. The results of femoro-femoral cross-over bypasses are satisfactory in patients operated on for aneurismal disease and better than in patients with occlusive arterial disease.

Personal experience

Patients and methods

Between 1998 and 2006, 22 patients (all male) were treated for an AFAA by means of endograft implantation. The mean age was 75 years (range 55-86 years). The initial procedure was an aorto-bifemoral graft for occlusive disease in 14 patients with a proximal end-to-end anastomosis in 3 cases and an end-to-side anastomosis in 11 cases. In 8 patients, an inlay technique was used for treatment of an abdominal aortic aneurysm (AAA) (Table II). In 4 of 8 patients initially operated on for AAA, the false aneurysm had developed at the distal anastomosis of the tube graft. The mean time of the interval between the initial intervention and discovery of the AFAA was 14.7 years (range 6-25 years). Sixteen patients were asymptomatic and one patient presented with signs of a ruptured aneurysm. Comorbidities of the patients are summarized in Table III: 6 patients had a left ventrical ejection

Table II — PREOPERATIVE DATA OF OUR PATIENTS

Patient	Years	ASA	Initial pathology	Initial procedure (type aortic anastomosis)	Delay (years)	Localization	Maximum AFAA diameter (mm)	Diameter proximal neck (mm)	Distance renal artery-aortic bifurcation (mm)	Associated lesions	Preoperative embolization
1	55	3	OAIL	ABFB (ES)	18	Proximal	52	18	92	Occlusion SFA	-
2	72	3	OAIL	ABFB (ES)	21	Proximal	76	18	102	-	Aorta + lumbars
3	83	4	OAIL	ABFB (EE)	17	Proximal	60	22	75	Occlusion SFA	-
4	67	2	OAIL	ABFB (EE)	14	Proximal	54	25	99	F An femoral	-
5	74	3	AAA	ABIB (EE)	11	Proximal	48	22	73	-	-
6	86	3	OAIL	ABFB (ES)	11	Proximal	53	20	85	Occlusion left limb	Common iliac
7	82	2	OAIL	ABFB (ES)	10	Proximal	56	22	99	-	-
8	81	3	AAA	ABIB (EE)	8	Proximal				F An iliac	-
9	69	3	AAA	Tube (EE)	19	Distal	63	25	130	-	Lumbars
10	78	3	OAIL	left AFB (ES)	25	Proximal	65	23	50	-	-
11	79	3	OAIL	ABFB (ES)	17	Proximal	45	30	100	F An femoral	-
12	79	3	AAA	ABIB (EE)	13	Proximal	63	18	89	-	-
13	73	3	AAA	Tube (EE)	6	Distal	68	30	115	F An iliac	-
14	81	3	OAIL	ABFB (ES)	18	Proximal	54	25	99	-	-

Table II — PREOPERATIVE DATA OF OUR PATIENTS

Patient	Years	ASA	Initial pathology	Initial procedure (type aortic anas-tomosis)	Delay (years)	Localization	Maximum AFAA diameter (mm)	Diameter proximal neck (mm)	Distance renal artery-aortic bifurcation (mm)	Associated lesions	Preoperative embolization
15	84	3	AAA	Tube (EE)	7	Distal	50	23	124	-	-
16	76	2	OAIL	ABFB (ES)	17	Proximal	52	18	84	F An femoral + Occlusion SFA	-
17	61	3	OAIL	ABFB (ES)	13	Proximal	67	15	96	Occlusion 2 limbs	-
18	76	3	OAIL	ABFB (ES)	14	Proximal	70	24	115	-	-
19	60	3	OAIL	ABFB (ES)	18	Proximal	56	25	90	-	-
20	80	3	OAIL	ABFB (ES)	19	Proximal	77	24	98	Occlusion right limb	Internal iliac
21	80	4	AAA	ABFB (EE)	20	Proximal	36	22	80	F An femoral	-
22	75	3	AAA	Tube (EE)	11	Distal	47	24	100	-	Internal iliac

AAA: abdominal aortic aneurysm
SFA: superficial femoral artery
AFAA: anastomotic false abdominal aortic aneurysm
F An: false aneurysm
AOIL: occlusive aorto-iliac lesions
EE: end-to-end
ES: end-to-side
ABIB: aorto-bi-iliac bypass
ABFB: aortobifemoral bypass
AFB: aortofemoral bypass

Table III	Comorbidities of our patients
	Number
Hypertension	14
Respiratory failure	2
Renal insufficiency	5
Coronary artery disease	9
Heart failure	6
Paraplegia	1

fraction of less than 40%; 2 patients suffered from severe respiratory insufficiency and 5 patients had renal failure with blood creatinine levels above 120 micromol/L. One patient was paraplegic following thoracoabdominal aortic repair 20 years after AAA surgery. According to the American Society of Anesthesiology (ASA) classification, 17 patients corresponded to class 3 and 2 patients to class 4 (Table II). All patients had pre-operative contrast enhanced CT-angiography. Mean diameter of the false aneurysm was 55.3 mm (range 36-76 mm). Mean diameter and length of the proximal neck were 23 mm (range 15-30 mm) and 33 mm (range 18-85 mm), respectively. Mean length between the lowest renal artery and the aortic bifurcation or the aortabifemoral graft was 95.4 mm (range 50-130 mm). Mean diameter of the iliac arteries or prosthetic branches serving as access site for endograft implantation was 12.3 mm (range 10-15 mm). In the 11 patients in whom the initial procedure was an aortobifemoral graft with proximal end-to-side anastomosis, the aorta was patent distal to the false aneurysm in 7 cases. Associated arterial lesions existed in 11 patients (Table II): iliac aneurysm in 2 cases, degradation of the entire graft with femoral anastomotic aneurysm in one patient (Fig. 1), occluded aortobifemoral graft in one, occlusion of one of the aortobifemoral branches in 2, false femoral anastomotic aneurysms in 4 and symptomatic superficial femoral artery occlusion in 3 cases. Five patients underwent percutaneously performed embolization pre-operatively with a mean of 10 days prior to the intervention: 2 for occlusion of the aorta distal to the false aneurysm (Fig. 2), one for closure of two large lumbar arteries communicating with the aneurysm sac and 2 for excluding the internal iliac artery prior to endovascular treatment of an associated iliac aneurysm. All patients were informed about the advantages and complications of the endovascular technique and signed a consent. All procedures were performed in the operating room using fluoroscopy and automatic contrast injection; 19 patients had general anesthesia and 3 had local anesthesia. All patients received heparin 100 units/kg and antibiotic prophylaxis. The following endografts were

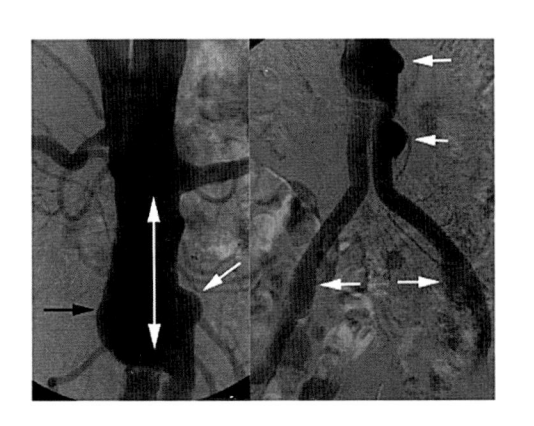

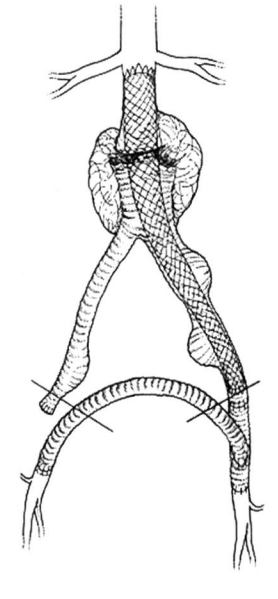

FIG. 1 Generalized degradation of aortic prosthesis. A - Angiography demonstrates several false aneurysms at the aortic anastomosis (black arrow) and in the graft itself (white arrows). The distance between the level of the renal arteries and the bifurcation of the graft was 50 mm. B - The implanted aorto-uni-iliac endograft covers the degenerated prosthesis and the procedure is completed with a femoro-femoral cross-over bypass.

implanted: 20 aorto-uni-iliac: 11 Zenith (Cook®), 3 AneuRx (Medtronic®), 2 Powerlink (Endologix®), 3 Talent (Medtronic®), 1 handmade and 2 aortic tube prostheses (1 Talent, 1 handmade). In 20 patients an associated surgical procedure was performed (Table IV). Two patients underwent a retroperitoneal approach to the common iliac artery: in 1 to exclude an aneurysm with preservation of the internal iliac artery and in 1 to perform an ileofemoral graft allowing introduction of the endoprosthesis and to revascularize the legs in a patient who presented with occlusion of both external iliac arteries (Fig. 3). Graft resection of a femoral false aneurysm was performed in 4 patients. A femoro-femoral cross-over bypass was implanted in 18 of 20 patients treated with an aorto-uni-iliac system; in 2 patients a cross-over graft was already carried out because of an occluded aorto-bifemoral limb. Three patients received a femoropopliteal bypass. Before discharge or within the 8 postoperative day all patients had plain abdominal X-ray (anterior, lateral and three-quarter left-

FIG. 2 False aneurysm at the proximal end-to-side anastomosis of an aortobifemoral graft. Angiography (A) and CT (B) demonstrate the false aneurysm and patency of the distal abdominal aorta (white arrow) as well as a large lumbar artery (black arrow). The latter and the internal iliac artery were embolized (C) prior to the final repair (D).

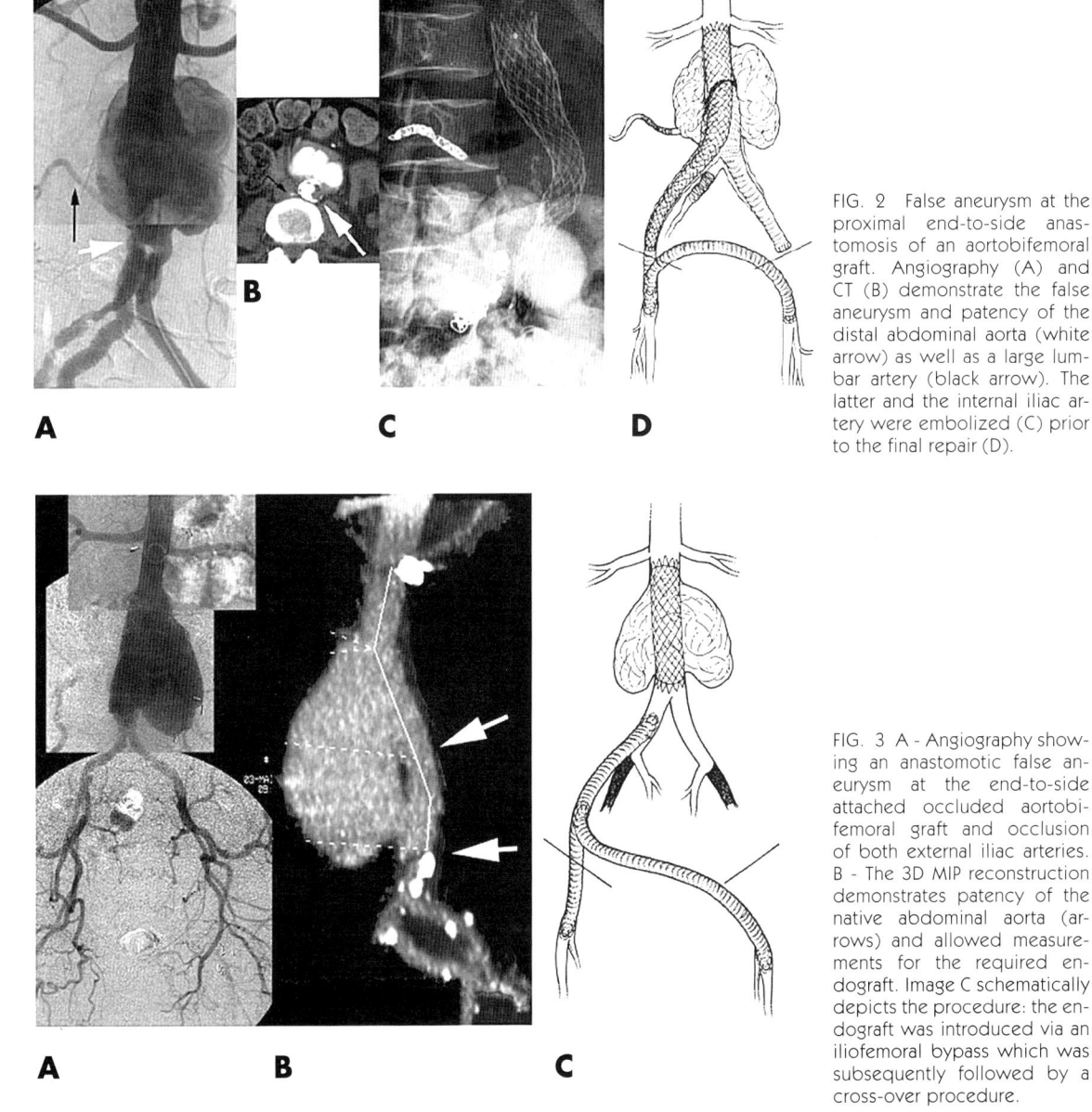

FIG. 3 A - Angiography showing an anastomotic false aneurysm at the end-to-side attached occluded aortobifemoral graft and occlusion of both external iliac arteries. B - The 3D MIP reconstruction demonstrates patency of the native abdominal aorta (arrows) and allowed measurements for the required endograft. Image C schematically depicts the procedure: the endograft was introduced via an iliofemoral bypass which was subsequently followed by a cross-over procedure.

Table IV — PERI-OPERATIVE AND POSTOPERATIVE DATA OF OUR PATIENTS

Patient	Endoprothesis	Associated procedures	Fluoroscopy time min	Intervention time min	Postoperative complications	Hospital stay	Follow-up months	Outcome	Aneurysm sac
1	Aorto-iliac	Cross-over + FPB	19	240	-	8	2	Death	
2	Aorto-iliac	Cross-over	24	180	-	12	12	Death	
3	Aorto-iliac	Cross-over	17	130	-	9	24	-	Stable
4	Tube	F An femoral	12	150	-	7	108	-	Complete regression
5	Aorto-iliac	Cross-over	-	190	Digestive bleeding + ARF	30	6	Dialysis	Stable
6	Aorto-iliac	Previous cross-over	10	60	-	5	48	-	Complete regression
7	Aorto-iliac	Cross-over	12	120	Prostatitis	28	5	Death	
8	Aorto-iliac	Cross-over	45	205	-	10	40	-	Complete regression
9	Aorto-iliac	Cross-over	14	165	-	9	76	Occlusion of endograft	-23 mm
10	Aorto-iliac	Previous cross-over	17	110	-	3	27	-	Complete regression
11	Aorto-iliac	F An femoral + cross-over	-	240	-	7	24	-	-15 mm

Table IV — PERI-OPERATIVE AND POSTOPERATIVE DATA OF OUR PATIENTS

Patient	Endoprosthesis	Associated procedures	Fluoroscopy time min	Intervention time min	Postoperative complications	Hospital stay	Follow-up months	Outcome	Aneurysm sac
12	Aorto-Iliac	Cross-over	11	150	ARF	17	6	-	-14 mm
13	Aorto-Iliac	Iliac angioplasty + cross-over	7	175	-	5	6	-	Stable
14	Aorto-Iliac	Cross-over	16	120	-	10	42	-	Stable
15	Aorto-Iliac	Cross-over	12	120	-	6	10	Death	
16	Aorto-Iliac	F An femoral + cross-over + FPB	10	300	Ileofemoral infection	20	36	-	-10 mm
17	Tube	IFB + cross-over	19	300	-	15	73	-	-36 mm
18	Aorto-Iliac	Cross-over	17	190	-	18	27	-	-23 mm
19	Aorto-Iliac	Cross-over	10	190	ARF	9	3	Death	
20	Aorto-Iliac	Cross-over	14	110	-	5	13	-	-27 mm
21	Aorto-Iliac	F An femoral + cross-over + FPB	19	255	-	6	74	Thrombosis cross-over	Complete regression
22	Aorto-Iliac	Cross-over	14	120	-	19	1	-	Stable

ARF: acute renal failure
IFB: iliofemoral bypass
FPB: femoropopliteal bypass
F An: false aneurysm

right) and a contrast enhanced CT-angiography. At one month the plain abdominal X-ray and contrast enhanced Duplex were performed. Plain X-ray, Duplex and CT-angiography were realized at 3, 6, 12, 18 and 24 months and repeated annually in case no complications were encountered.

Results

Mean intervention time was 173 minutes (range 60-300 minutes) and mean fluoroscopy time was 16 minutes (range 7-45 minutes) with a mean volume of contrast of 155 mL (range 100-260 mL). All implantations were technically successful. During the first 30 postoperative days mortality did not occur and we have observed complications in 5 patients (three acute renal insufficiency, one iliofemoral infection, one prostatitis). Two patients, one with respiratory failure and one with cardiac insufficiency, required intensive care treatment during 24 and 48 hours, respectively. Five patients received a mean of 2.6 units of blood transfusion. CT-angiography demonstrated complete exclusion of the AFAA in all cases. Mean hospitalization stay was 12 days (range 3-30 days) and mean follow-up was 30.3 months (range 1-108 months): 5 patients died during this period at 3, 4, 6, 10 and 13 months, respectively due to cancer (n=4) and cardiac failure (n=1). In all patients the AFAA remained excluded without detectable endoleak. We have not observed any migration or deformation of the endograft. In total, 15 living patients have had a follow-up of 6 months or longer (5 deaths, one refusing control CT, one with shorter follow-up): in all patients a significant diameter reduction of the AFAA sac larger than 10 mm (mean 23 mm, range 10-36 mm) was observed. In 5 patients the aneurysm sac disappeared completely and in 4 the diameter remained unchanged. The paraplegic patient presented with an occlusion of the aorto-uni-iliac endograft 7 months after the procedure and was treated with an axillobifemoral bypass. In one patient a severe stenosis at the distal end of the aorto-uni-iliac endograft was detected by Duplex scanning at the 6th month follow-up and successfully treated by percutaneous balloon dilatation. In one patient thrombectomy of the cross-over bypass and femoral artery plasty was necessary at 36 months follow-up. Finally, one patient suffered from a transient ischemic attack due to a carotid artery stenosis, which was successfully operated (Table IV).

Discussion

To our knowledge this report on 22 patients represents the largest published series today after the publications of Morrissey et al. [19] on 11 cases and van Herwaarden et al. [21] on 6 cases. Our experience confirms the feasibility of the endovascular treatment of AFAA with acceptable postoperative morbidity, as published in a previous report [22]. Series on this subject are rare and the number of

Table V	Endovascular treatment of AFAA: outcome in literature and personal experience						
First author [ref]	Year	Number of cases	AUIE	Tube	Bifurcated	Postoperative mortality	Follow-up (months)
Morrissey [19]	2001	11	7	2	2	0	21
van Herwaarden [21]	2004	6	0	3	3	0	12
Zhou [24]	2006	5	-	5	0	0	10
El Sakka [25]	2007	3	2	1	-	0	28
Pers. exp.	2007	22	20	2	-	0	30

AUIE: aorto-uni-iliac endograft

cases limited (Table V). The interest of our series, besides shown efficacy, is based on the homogenecity of cases and the regular CT-angiography follow-up, allowing accurate assessment of the results at mid-term. Morrissey et al. [19] described an inhomogeneous series of 36 para-anastomotic aneurysm cases of which 11 were a mixture of AFAA or real para-anastomotic aneurysms of the infrarenal aorta; in the other cases the aneurysms were located in the thoracic aorta or iliac arteries. This experience has recently been updated in a publication reporting on 53 patients in which it is not possible to identify the number of AFAA treated by means of endovascular technology [23]. Zhou et al. [24] described 5 patients treated with an endovascular tube graft. In the 8 patients of El Sakka et al. [25] only 3 had AFAA.

The mechanically induced AFAA most often occur more than 10 years after the initial procedure (Table II), in older patients in whom the atherosclerotic disease progressed, and severe comorbidities are present. These risk factors explain the elevated postoperative morbidity and mortality rates after open surgical repair [9-12] (Table I). In the present series of endovascular treatment postoperative morbidity was limited and mortality did not occur in unselected patients suffering from serious comorbidities. This improved morbidity-mortality is confirmed in other previously published experiences [13-20] (Table IV).

The feasibility of the endovascular treatment and the choice of the correct endograft are basically determined by high quality pre-operative imaging. Among all vascular imaging techniques, CT-angiography is certainly the most appropriate to assess the extent of the AFAA and the morphological characteristics (Fig. 3). We believe that aorto-uni-iliac endografts are technically the most suitable since they allow to avoid the pitfalls described above. In contrast, the use of a tube endograft requires an usable length for distal implantation at the level of the graft body already in place of at least 15 mm, and identical diameters of the proximal and distal necks. Therefore, in the present series, we have only been able to implant a tube endograft in two patients: in one the distance between the lowest renal artery and the bifurcation of the graft was largely enough (Table II,IV, case 4) and the aortic prosthetic body long enough (20 mm) to implant the device safely; the second patient (Table II, IV, case 17) presented with a false aneurysm at the end-to-side proximal anastomosis of an occluded aortobifemoral graft associated with occlusion of both external iliac arteries. The endograft was implanted through the native aorta in order to maintain its patency and preserve pelvic circulation. An iliofemoral graft was implanted first to accommodate the implantation (Fig. 3).

The use of non-modular endografts comprises the advantage of simplifying implantation of the endograft which is certainly of benefit in these prolonged procedures requiring additional surgical strategies to treat associated vascular lesions. In some cases (four times in this series) it is necessary to perform a custom-made endograft in order to cope with specific morphologic characteristics. Also, it is desirable, if possible, to cover the old graft as much as possible and minimize the contact of circulating blood with the old polyester prosthesis, preventing further degradation (Fig. 1).

The durability of endovascular AFAA repair is still uncertain, especially when the late complications of endovascular AAA are considered. In the experience of van Herwaarden [21], 2 of 6 patients required conversion to open surgery because of extending aneurysm diameter; one patient suffered from rupture and did not survive the procedure. The authors report difficulties with sealing of the endograft in the prosthetic polyester graft and they implanted an additional tube endograft in two patients. In our experience, the false aneurysms behaved differently after endovascular treatment since we observed significant diameter regression of the aneurysm sac in all patients and disappearance of the AFAA in five patients. Application of single body aorto-uni-iliac endografts might explain these results.

Conclusion

Endovascular treatment of AFAA seems to provide adequate outcome and might be favorable to conventional surgical repair. Therefore, this approach might be considered the first option in these patients at high surgical risks.

Endovascular treatment of AFAA, however, appears to be more complex than endovascular AAA repair since it frequently requires pre-operative embolization and associated surgical reconstructions. Long-term follow-up is necessary in order to confirm the observed excellent short- end mid-term results in this series.

REFERENCES

1 Kalman PG, Johnston KW. Regarding "The value of late computed tomographic scanning in identification of vascular abnormalities after abdominal aortic aneurysm repair". *J Vasc Surg* 1999; 30: 961-962.

2 Hallett JW Jr, Marshall DM, Petterson TM et al. Graft-related complications after abdominal aortic aneurysm repair: reassurance from a 36-year population-based experience. *J Vasc Surg* 1997; 25: 277-284.

3 Hagino RT, Taylor SM, Fujitani RM Mills JL. Proximal anastomotic failure following infrarenal aortic reconstruction: late development of true aneurysms, pseudoaneurysms, and occlusive disease. *Ann Vasc Surg* 1993; 7: 8-13.

4 Sciannameo F, Ronca P, Caselli M et al. The anastomotic aneurysms. *J Cardiovasc Surg* 1993; 34: 145-151.

5 Edwards JM, Teefey SA, Zierler RE et al. Intraabdominal paraanastomotic aneurysms after aortic bypass grafting. *J Vasc Surg* 1992; 15: 344-350.

6 van den Akker PJ, Brand R, van Schilfgaarde R et al. False aneurysms after prosthetic reconstructions for aortoiliac obstructive disease. *Ann Surg* 1989; 210: 658-666.

7 Sieswerda C, Skotnicki SH, Barentsz JO et al. Anastomotic aneurysms underdiagnosed complication after aorto-iliac reconstructions. *Eur J Vasc Surg* 1989; 3: 233-238.

8 Dennis JW, Littooy FN, Greisler HP et al. Anastomotic pseudoaneurysms. A continuing late complication of vascular reconstructive procedures. *Arch Surg* 1986; 121: 314-317.

9 Treiman GS, Weaver FA, Cossman DV et al. Anastomotic false aneurysms of the abdominal aorta and the iliac arteries. *J Vasc Surg* 1988; 8: 268-273.

10 Curl GR, Faggioli GL, Stella A et al. Aneurysmal change at or above the proximal anastomosis after infrarenal aortic grafting. *J Vasc Surg* 1992; 16: 855-859.

11 Allen RC, Schneider J, Longenecker L et al. Paraanastomotic aneurysms of the abdominal aorta. *J Vasc Surg* 1993; 18: 424-431.

12 Mulder EJ, van Bockel JH, Maas J et al. Morbidity and mortality of reconstructive surgery of noninfected false aneurysms detected long after aortic prosthetic reconstruction. *Arch Surg* 1998; 133: 45-49.

13 White RA, Donayre CE, Walot I et al. Endoluminal graft exclusion of a proximal para-anastomotic pseudoaneurysm following aortobifemoral bypass. *J Endovasc Surg* 1997; 4: 88-94.

14 Schonolz C, Donnini F, Naselli G et al. Acute rupture of an aortic false aneurysm treated with a stent graft. *J Endovasc Surg* 1999; 6: 293-296.

15 Grabs AJ, Irvine CD, Lusby RJ. Stent-graft treatment for bleeding from a presumed aortoenteric fistula. *J Endovasc Ther* 2000; 7: 236-239.

16 Chuter TA, Lukaszewicz GC, Reilly LM et al. Endovascular repair of a presumed aortoenteric fistula: late failure due to recurrent infection. *J Endovasc Ther* 2000; 7: 240-244.

17 Brittenden J, Gillespie I, McBride K et al. Endovascular repair of aortic pseudoaneurysms. *Eur J Vasc Endovasc Surg* 2000; 19: 82-84.

18 Tiesenhausen K, Hausegger KA, Tauss J et al. Endovascular treatment of proximal anastomotic aneurysms after aortic prosthetic reconstruction. *Cardiovasc Intervent Radiol* 2001; 24: 49-52.

19 Morrissey NJ, Yano OJ, Soundararajan K et al. Endovascular repair of para-anastomotic aneurysms of the aorta and iliac arteries: Preferred treatment for a complex problem. *J Vasc Surg* 2001; 33: 503-512.

20 Matsumoto T, Komori K, Furuyama T et al. Alternative approach to endoluminal treatment of an anastomotic aneurysm. *J Cardiovasc Surg* 2002; 43: 403-406.

21 van Herwaarden JA, Waasdorp EJ, Bendermacher BL et al. Endovascular repair of paraanastomotic aneurysms after previous open aortic prosthetic reconstruction. *Ann Vasc Surg* 2004; 18: 280-286.

22 Magnan PE, Albertini JN, Bartoli JM et al. Endovascular treatment of anastomotic false aneurysms of the abdominal aorta. *Ann Vasc Surg* 2003; 17: 365-374.

23 Sachdev U, Baril DT, Morrissey NJ et al. Endovascular repair of para-anastomotic aortic aneurysms. *J Vasc Surg* 2007; 46: 636-641.

24 Zhou W, Bush RL, Bhama JK et al. Repair of anastomotic abdominal aortic pseudoaneurysm utilizing sequential AneuRx aortic cuffs in an overlapping configuration. *Ann Vasc Surg* 2006; 20: 17-22.

25 El Sakka K, Halawa M, Cotze C et al. Complications of open abdominal aortic surgery: the endovascular solution. *Interact Cardiovasc Thorac Surg* 2007 6. [Epub ahead of print].

17

ENDOVASCULAR TREATMENT OF INFECTED AORTIC ANEURYSMS

MERYL DAVIS, PETER TAYLOR

Infected aortic aneurysms are rare and occur in 0.65% to 1.3% of all aortic aneurysms [1-3]. The more common secondary aorto-enteric fistulae occur in 0.4%-4% of cases after aortic prosthetic graft placement after an average interval of approximately six years although it has been described as early as two weeks after aortic surgery [4,5].

The natural history of infected aortic aneurysms is associated with a significant mortality and morbidity. Conventional treatment has included ligation or excision of the aneurysm with debridement and in-situ or extra-anatomical surgical revascularization with the use of appropriate antibiotics. The role of endoluminal treatment is controversial and there is no level one evidence to support it. The advent of branched and fenestrated stent grafts has allowed infected aneurysms close to important side branches such as the origins of the visceral vessels to be treated by endoluminal techniques. However, endovascular treatment may only be a temporizing measure used to control hemorrhage in the emergency situation before definitive repair is undertaken at a later date.

This chapter reviews the literature and suggests reasons why the endovascular treatment of infected aortic aneurysms may have advantages over open surgery in certain situations. A randomized controlled trial or at least an international registry is required to determine the optimal treatment for this difficult problem.

History and background

In the last fifteen years endovascular aortic repair (EVAR) for degenerative aneurysms of the thoracic and abdominal aorta has become established as a realistic alternative to open surgery with lower mortality and morbidity [6]. There has been an increasing number of reports published on the subject of infected aortic aneurysms showing successful outcomes with EVAR; however, most papers have small numbers of patients and the majority comprise just single case reports. The use of EVAR in infected aortic aneurysms offers a less invasive approach and appears to have an improved mortality rate as compared with open surgery. Caution, however, does need to be observed as there are several important questions as yet unanswered which include:
1) what is the rate of infection of endografts when they are placed in potentially infected tissue or in a septic patient?
2) Can the residual infection be overcome with antibiotics?
3) Should an endovascular device be regarded only as a temporizing measure until open definitive surgery can be carried out?

Diagnosis and presentation

Early diagnosis and intervention is paramount for survival as over 50% of mycotic aneurysms present with rupture [7]. In a series of 13 patients presenting with infected aortic or iliac artery aneurysms the following findings were noted: abdominal pain, fever, leucocytosis, positive blood cultures, palpable mass and rupture (Table I [2]).

The symptoms may be non specific, however, a high index of suspicion is needed in any patient with a history of fever, and raised inflammatory markers with positive blood cultures. The first presentation of an uncalcified aneurysm after bacterial sepsis with erosion of a vertebra should also raise the possibility of the diagnosis of infected aortic aneurysm.

The distribution of mycotic aneurysms is different from that seen in degenerative aneurysms. The thoracic, supra or juxta renal aorta is the site of almost 70% of mycotic aneurysms with the infra renal aorta being involved in 32% [8]. It should also be noted that mycotic aneurysms are often multiple in nature, thus compounding the complexity of the surgery with the possible need for the patient to require both a thoracotomy and laparotomy. In the presence of serious comorbidities this could offer significant challenges both to the patient and surgeon.

Table II indicates the cultured organisms from infected aneurysms. Table III summarizes the cultured organisms in patients with infected aortic aneurysms treated with endoluminal grafts, as reviewed by Kan et al. [10].

Table I — FINDINGS IN PATIENTS PRESENTING WITH INFECTED AORTIC OR ILIAC ARTERY ANEURYSMS

Marker	Number of patients (%)	N
Abdominal pain	92	12
Fever	77	10
Leucocytosis	69	9
Positive blood cultures	69	9
Palpable abdominal mass	46	6
Rupture	31	4

Conventional open surgery

The determinants of outcome following open surgery are the location of the aneurysm, the presence or absence of rupture, the presence of established infection and the virulence of the organism and the presence of significant comorbidities. In the clinical situation where there is prosthetic graft in-situ (secondary infected aneurysms) there is also the dilemma of whether the graft should be removed.

Open surgery for infected aortic aneurysms consists of debridement or excision of infected tissue and in-situ homograft or extra-anatomical reconstruction with aortic ligation or oversew. In addition the graft needs to be removed if there is a second-

Table II Organisms cultured from infected aneurysms [9]

Organisms	Before 1965 N (%)	1965-1984 N (%)	Total N (%)
Salmonella spp	14 (38%)	15 (10%)	29 (15%)
Staphylococcus aureus	7 (19%)	47 (30%)	54 (28%)
Streptococcus spp	5 (14%)	15 (10%)	20 (10%)
Pseudomonas spp	1	6	7
Staphylococcus epidermidis	1	5	6
Escherichia coli		4	4
Proteus spp	2	1	3
Serratia spp		3	3
Enterobacter spp		3	3
Neisseria spp		3	3
Clostridium spp		2	2
Enterococcus group		2	2
Bacteroides spp		2	2
Candida spp		2	2
Klebsiella spp		2	2
Culture negative	7 (19%)	41 (25%)	48 (25%)

ary aorto-enteric fistula [31]. This surgery carries a high peri-operative mortality ranging from 25%-90% with an average mortality rate in the region of 27%-36% [2,3,32]. These operations also carry a high risk of both amputation (5%-25%) and aortic stump rupture (10%-50%) [33,34].

Vascular reconstruction can be performed in many ways with oversewing of the proximal and distal aorta followed by extra-anatomical reconstruction. Alternatively, in-situ replacement can be performed using various conduits including prosthetic grafts, arterial and venous homografts and allografts. In-situ replacement is associated with an early mortality of 27% and up to 20% of these patients require further surgery due to infection of the in-situ graft [32,35]. The use of antibiotic impregnated or antibiotic coated grafts would be a logical step in such an environment [36]. Unfortunately, the results of randomized trials of such grafts (in non infected tissue) have failed to show a benefit [37,38]. Similarly silver coated or Triclosan bonded grafts have not been shown to be of benefit in the treatment of vascular graft infection [39,40].

Cryopreserved arterial allografts

The use of cryopreserved arterial allografts for infected aortic grafts or mycotic aneurysms ob-

Table III Infected aortic aneurysms treated with endoluminal grafts. Summary of published data [23]

First author/Year [ref.]	Age/Sex	Site	Rupture/Fistula	Organism	Follow-up	Persistent infection	Mortality
Jones/2005 [11]	58/F	Th	A-enteric fistula	Not proven	62	?yes	62 months (hematemesis)
	64/F	Th & AAA	No	Not proven	56		
	62/M	Th x 2	No	Not proven	0		<30 days
	76/M	Th	No	MRSA	43	Yes	-
	60/F	Th	No	Salmonella	36		
	69/F	Th	A-cut fistula	Not proven	5	Rebleeding	5 months
	72/F	Th	A-bronchial fistula	Not proven	28		
	80/M	Th & AAA	No	Salmonella	27	Rebleeding	
	40/M	AAA	No	Pneumococcus	16		
Ting/2006 [12]	87/M	Th	A-enteric fistula	Staph aureus	3	Sepsis	
	37/M	Th	No	Staph aureus	38		
	59/M	Th	No	Salmonella	35		
	68/M	Th	A-enteric fistula	Candida albicans	34		
	77/M	Th	No	Salmonella	7		
	59/M	Th	A-enteric fistula	Not proven	3	Stentgraft	
	90/M	Th	No	Not proven	4		
Lee/2006 [13]	65/F	AAA	No	Staph aureus	36		

Table III INFECTED AORTIC ANEURYSMS TREATED WITH ENDOLUMINAL GRAFTS. SUMMARY OF PUBLISHED DATA [23]

First author/Year [ref.]	Age/Sex	Site	Rupture/Fistula	Organism	Follow-up	Persistent infection	Mortality
	58/M	AAA	No	G neg bacteria	48		
	56/M	AAA	No	TB	96		
	30/F	Th	No	Enterococcus	0	A-enteric fistula/sepsis	<30 days
	85/M	AAA	A-enteric fistula	Staph aureus	0	Rebleeding/sepsis	<30 days
Stanley/2003 [14]	64/M	Th	No	Strep	12		
	62/M	Th	No	Staph aureus	15		
	77/M	Th	Rupture	Enterococcus	10		
	79/F	AAA	No	Streptococcus	2		
Sayed/2005 [15]	46/F	Th	No	Not proven	12		
	77/F	Th	A-bronchial fistula	Not proven	26		
	50/F	Th	A-bronchial fistula	Not proven	12		
Semba/1998 [16]	64/M	Th	A-bronchial fistula	Proteus mirabilis	25		25 months (cardiac arrest)
	70/M	Th	No	Not proven	24		
	69/F	Th	Rupture	Clostridium septicum	4		
Forbes/2006 [17]	73/M	AAA	No	Salmonella	48		
	83/F	AAA	No	Salmonella	5	Sepsis/bacteremia	
Gonzalez-Fajardo/2005 [18]	75/M	AAA	A-enteric fistula	Not proven	2	Sepsis	2 months

Table III Infected aortic aneurysms treated with endoluminal grafts. Summary of published data [23]

First author/Year [ref.]	Age/Sex	Site	Rupture/Fistula	Organism	Follow-up	Persistent infection	Mortality
Liu/2000[19]	68/M	Th	A-enteric fistula	Salmonella	0	Sepsis/bleeding	<30 days
	42/F	AAA	No	TB	24		
	41/M	AAA	Rupture	TB	18		
Alpagut/2006[20]	38/M	Th	No	Not proven	7		
Jorna/2006[21]	79/F	Th	Rupture-contained	Streptococcus	6		
Corso/2005[22]	62/M	AAA	Rupture-contained	Staph aureus	12		
Koeppel/2004[23]	47/M	AAA	No	Salmonella	12		
Kotzampassakis/2004[24]	84/F	Th	A-bronchial fistula	Salmonella	6		
Rayan/2004[25]	51/M	Th	Rupture-contained	Staph aureus	7		
Van Doorn/2002[26]	66/F	Th	A-enteric fistula	Clostridium septicum	24		
Ishida/2002[27]	81/F	Th	Rupture	Staph aureus	0	Rupture/sepsis	<30 days
Berchtold/2002[28]	60/M	AAA	No	Salmonella	48		
Madhaven/2000[29]	50/M	AAA	No	Staph aureus	12		
Kinney/2000[30]	55/F	AAA	No	Escherichia coli	10		10 months (MI)

AAA: abdominal aortic aneurysm
Th: thoracic aortic aneurysm
A-bronchial fistula: aorto-bronchial fistula
A-enteric fistula: aorto-enteric fistula
A-cut fistula: aorto-cutaneous fistula

viates the need for extra-anatomical reconstruction. In the published series the mortality rate is low and the mid-term results are good with no recurrence of infection, no suture line problems and no homograft stenoses or aneurysms seen. A retrospective study [41] compared in-situ repair and extra-anatomical reconstruction (n=38) with cryopreserved arterial allografts (n=34). Patients who received allografts had a better survival and lower re-operation rate with less days in hospital, less complications and better rates of infection elimination. In another publication from the same group 49 patients with mycotic aneurysms or infected prosthetic aortic grafts had a 30 day mortality rate of 6% for the whole series. In this paper [42] the mortality decreased to 2.6% for the last 39 patients with no recurrence of infection or allograft-related late death. This improvement was due to the use of higher quality allografts, allograft strips supporting large anastomoses, antibiotic impregnated fibrin glue for better hemostasis and the use of sutures rather than clips for occluding side branches. Cryopreserved arterial allografts are not widely available in the United Kingdom and their use is currently limited in Europe.

Antibiotic irrigation and conservative surgery

A novel method of treating prosthetic graft infection has been described in ten patients with infected aortic grafts. All grafts were found to be either bathed in frank pus or gastro-intestinal effluent at the time of operation. Patients underwent exposure of the infected graft via an extra-peritoneal approach, the sac opened and infected tissue removed. Silicone drains were then brought out via the skin and irrigation using antibiotics was performed until sterile effluent cultures were achieved (with a recommendation that this should be performed for at least 14 days). Patients were subsequently maintained on oral antibiotics for several weeks. The 30 day mortality was 10% with a one year survival of 80%; and at five years the surviving patients remained free from infection [43]. In certain cases this may be an appropriate treatment modality and offers a good outcome both in terms of infection free survival and in limb preservation.

Advantages of endovascular repair

The endoluminal treatment of mycotic aneurysms offers several advantages, however, it also raises various dilemmas. The practice of endovascular repair of infected aortic aneurysms is contrary to the surgical principles of debridement and revascularization in non-infected planes. The potential benefits of EVAR include no aortic cross clamp with consequent decrease in end organ ischemia, general anesthesia may not be required, smaller incisions, a decrease in blood loss, subsequent reduction in the length of stay in intensive care or high dependency units and in hospital stay. A faster return to daily activities and normal life is anticipated.

The low peri-operative mortality of endovascular repair both in the thoracic and abdominal aorta compared with open surgery has led to the use of stent grafts in the treatment of infected aortic aneurysms. Table III summarizes the reported cases of EVAR used in the treatment of mycotic aortic aneurysms. EVAR may help in temporarily controlling blood loss in a patient with a ruptured infected aortic aneurysm who can then be optimized with regard to their comorbidities and subsequently have definitive surgery.

EVAR for infected aortic aneurysms

Table III is a summary of the English literature which revealed 22 reports with a total of 48 patients [10]. The study group included 29 men and 19 women with a median age of 64 (range 30-90) years. The median follow-up was 12 (range 0-96) months. Infected aortic aneurysms were located in two thirds of cases in the thoracic aorta with the remainder in the abdominal aorta. A significant proportion 37.5% (n=18) required an emergency EVAR due to symptoms of rupture reflecting the urgent nature of this disease. Table IV below summarizes the organisms found and it is noteworthy that an infecting organism was not found in 27% (n=13) of patients.

Most patients received broad spectrum antibiotics and 46% (n=22) had received antibiotics for more than 7 days before EVAR was performed. At the time of deployment, 44% (n=21) had a fever

Table IV	Organisms identified in patients with infected aortic aneurysms and treated with EVAR [10]		
	Organism	%	N
	Salmonella species	21	10
	Staphylococci	21	10
	Streptococci	6	3
	Mycobacteria	6	3
	Other species	19	9
	Not isolated	27	13

Table V	Treatments received by patients (N=15) with secondary aorto-enteric fistulae [44]	
	Number of patients (%)	Device
	9 (60%)	Aorto-uni-iliac and femoro-femoral cross over graft
	4 (27%)	Aorto-bi-iliac
	1 (7%)	Open division of fistula; 4 days later endovascular tube stent graft
	1 (7%)	Proximal and distal occluders and gentamicin sponge; right axillofemoral bypass graft

with a raised temperature. Persistent infections manifesting with prolonged fever, sepsis and rupture or bleeding occurred in 23% (n=11) patients. The 30 day mortality of EVAR in infected aortic aneurysms was 10.4% (n=5). Late mortalities occurred in a further 10.4% (n=5). Subdividing the group reveals an one year survival rate of 94% (+/-4%) for the non-infected and 39% (+/-17%) for the infected patients (p<0.05). There is no published data as to the outcome of patients who presented with an infected aortic aneurysm and were treated conservatively. One assumes that the mortality rate in this group would be high, as rupture would almost inevitably lead to death.

Endovascular repair in secondary infected aortic aneurysms

A multicenter study aimed to evaluate the use of endoprostheses in patients with secondary aorto-enteric fistulae was recently reported from Belgium and The Netherlands [44]. In six years, fifteen patients with an aorto-enteric fistula were treated endovascularly of whom thirteen (87%) had previously undergone aortic or iliac surgery. The outcome in terms of morbidity, mortality, re-infection or fistula recurrence was analyzed. All patients showed signs of bleeding (either clinically or biochemically), eight patients (53%) were in shock and required treatment on an emergency basis and five (33%) had systemic signs of infection. Table V outlines the treatment received.

Success in sealing the fistula was achieved in all cases. The 30 day mortality was 0% with an in-hospital mortality of 7%. The overall survival at six months was 92% falling to 79% and 66% at one and two years respectively. The mean hospital stay was 20 (8-21) days. All fifteen patients received antibiotics postoperatively for at least 14 days. Twelve patients (67%) were prescribed life long antibiotic treatment although half the group voluntary stopped their antibiotics after a time. The freedom from recurrence of an aorto-enteric fistula was 65% (confidence interval 40-90%) at 6 months 71% of all patients had a recurrent infection or new aorto-enteric fistula within one year despite antibiotic treatment. The authors concluded that endovascular repair can control the rupture from an aorto-enteric fistula and this allows time to treat shock, local and systemic infection and optimize comorbidites. Subsequently these patients can then have definitive open surgery with better outcome.

A more optimistic outcome was found in a small series of seven patients presenting with aorto-enteric fistulae (two primary and five secondary) treated with endovascular repair [45]. One patient was treated with coil embolization while six patients received stent grafts (3 aorto-uni-liac, 2 tube and 1 bifurcated). One patient died and there were three late deaths not related to the procedure or fistula formation. Three patients were alive and well an average of 36 months after the procedure with no evidence of infection.

The management of infected endovascular grafts

The risk of endografts becoming infected is low with an incidence of 0.4% compared with 1.3% for open vascular surgery [46]. This is likely to be an underestimation and partly reflects the short time that endovascular procedures have been performed. There is a paucity of data published on this topic. It does seem that endovascular grafts are protected from infection once they are incorporated at approximately three months post implantation [47]. A theory has been suggested that once an infection is established endovascular devices are at a disadvantage as their position within the artery acts as a protective layer against host organ defences and may reduce the treatment potential of antibiotics. Conversely endoprostheses are in close proximity to blood and therefore adjacent to the highest concentration of antibiotics administered intravenously.

A review of 62 cases of infected endovascular grafts found that the majority were treated surgically by graft explantation and extra-anatomic bypass or in-situ graft replacement (79%; n=49) which resulted in a mortality rate of 16%. Conservative therapy included antibiotics with or without drainage of collections was given to 18% (n=11) of patients with a higher mortality rate of 36% at a mean of 11.5 weeks [46].

Disadvantages of endovascular treatment

There is a risk of ongoing sepsis and subsequent rupture of the aorta or the development of pseudoaneurysms at the site of the device due to the lack of debridement and the placement of stent grafts in infected tissues. This problem is almost certain to occur when the mycotic aneurysm contents are not sterile and continuing virulent infection spreads to contaminate the endoprosthesis. Figs. 1 and 2 demonstrate the initial success of endovascular techniques with subsequent serious complications.

Successful EVAR treatment can be achieved and results in a better clinical outcome than conventional open surgery, with a 94% one year survival rate.

Persistent infection in the presence of a stent graft offers only a 39% one year survival rate. Multivariate analysis of Table III reveals that the significant independent predictors of poor outcome are aneurysm rupture (including the presence of fistulae) and fever at the time of device deployment. A more favourable outcome is associated with antibiotics for greater than one week prior to procedure, and the use of additional procedures combined with EVAR. These include drainage, bowel diversion in patients with sepsis due to colonic fistulae, debridement and irrigation.

Reservations/unanswered questions with endovascular treatment of infected aneurysms

The lack of debridement of infected tissue together with the ongoing presence of the infected source would seem to be risks associated with endoluminal repair. One explanation for the apparent success of EVAR in such an environment is that most patients receive broad spectrum antibiotics as soon as the diagnosis is made and so the infection that caused the aneurysm may have been treated and eliminated with antibiotics. Therefore the risk of endograft infection is low as the patient no longer carries active microbes at the time of implantation.

The duration of antibiotics post procedure is also not clear. Some would advocate antibiotics 'for life'; while others would suggest a length of time (possibly six weeks) on initially intravenous and then oral antibiotics. These should ideally be continued until there is no abnormality in the white cell count, C reactive protein or the erythrocyte sedimentation rate. Pragmatically, most patients stop their antibiotics of their own volition in due course. Irrespective of the antibiotic regimen it is paramount that these patients are monitored for life with laboratory and radiological monitoring.

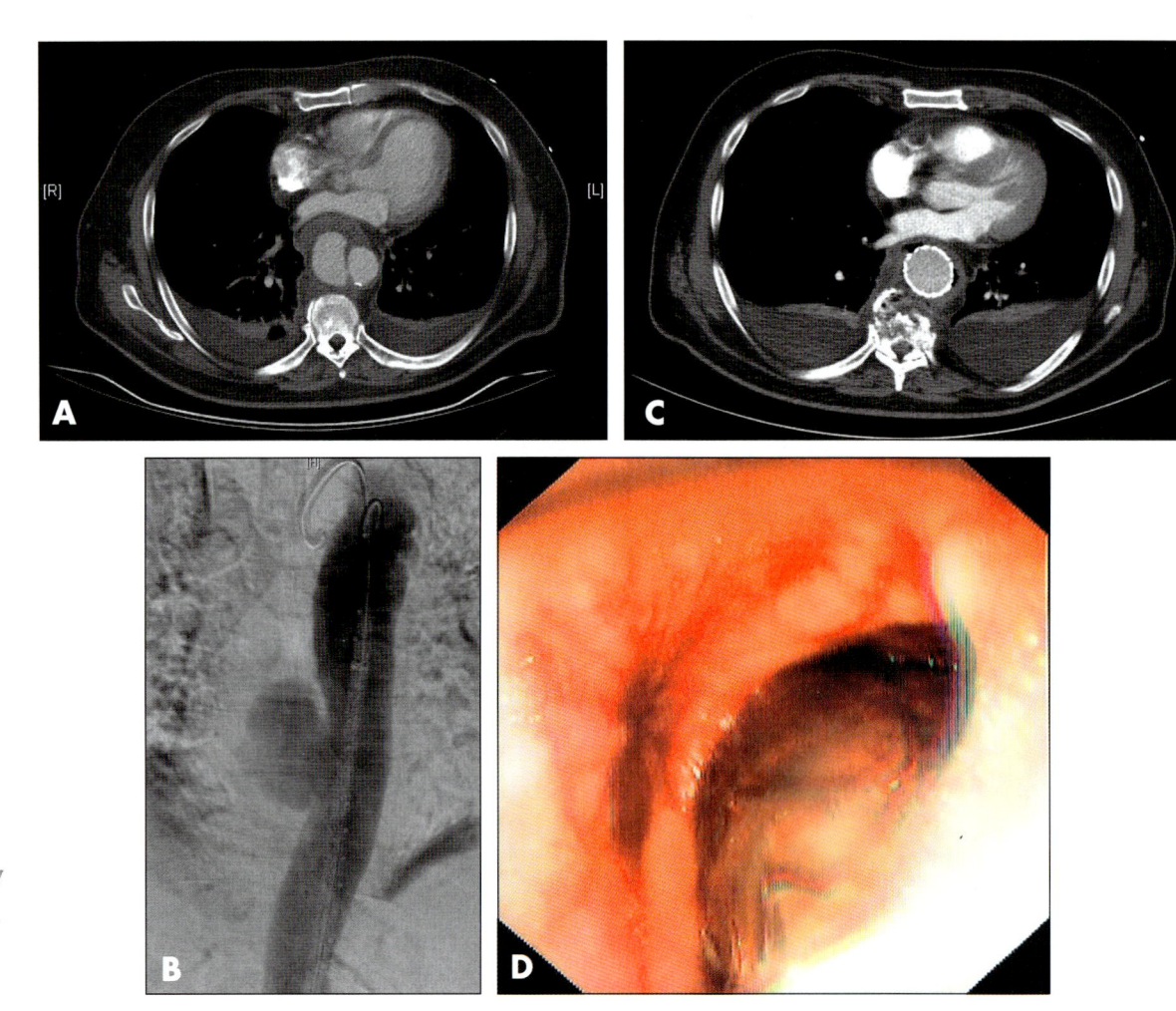

FIG. 1 A - Eighty-two year old man was admitted to his local hospital with diarrhea, Salmonella spp was isolated from the stool, appropriate antibiotics were given and the patient was discharged home. He represented four weeks later with shortness of breath and chest pain; he had hematemesis and required a blood transfusion. Endoscopy revealed only mild erosions of the esophagus. He had no fever, a moderate leucocytosis and a raised CRP; blood cultures were negative. He was referred to the Vascular Unit where CT scan was performed. B - Angiogram, showing the saccular aneurysm. C - Post stent graft the patient recovered slowly and was discharged home. He represented approximately six weeks later with weight loss, fever and indigestion. CT findings revealed bilateral pleural effusions, gas around the stent graft with significant destruction of the thoracic vertebra, endoscopy revealed an aorto-esophageal fistula. A decision was taken that no further active management was appropriate and he died following a large hematemesis. D - Endoscopic findings of an aorto-esophageal fistula with stent graft seen via the esophagus.

Conclusion

There are no level one data to determine the use of stent grafts for infected aortic aneurysms. There is no definitive answer as to the duration of antibiotics and as to the format and length of surveillance.

Certain variables predict the presence of persistent infection and this is associated with a less favourable outcome: rupture, presence of a fistula and fever at the time of operation. EVAR can be used as a means of achieving hemodynamic stability when patients present with rupture or fever. However, if there is evidence of ongoing infection, then a definitive open surgical option needs to be considered before rupture occurs.

Endovascular aortic stent graft placement in the presence of aorto-enteric fistulae is a safe and effective method of controlling hemorrhage. Endovascular therapy must be regarded as either palliative, in patients who are too sick to undergo open surgery, or a temporizing measure until definitive

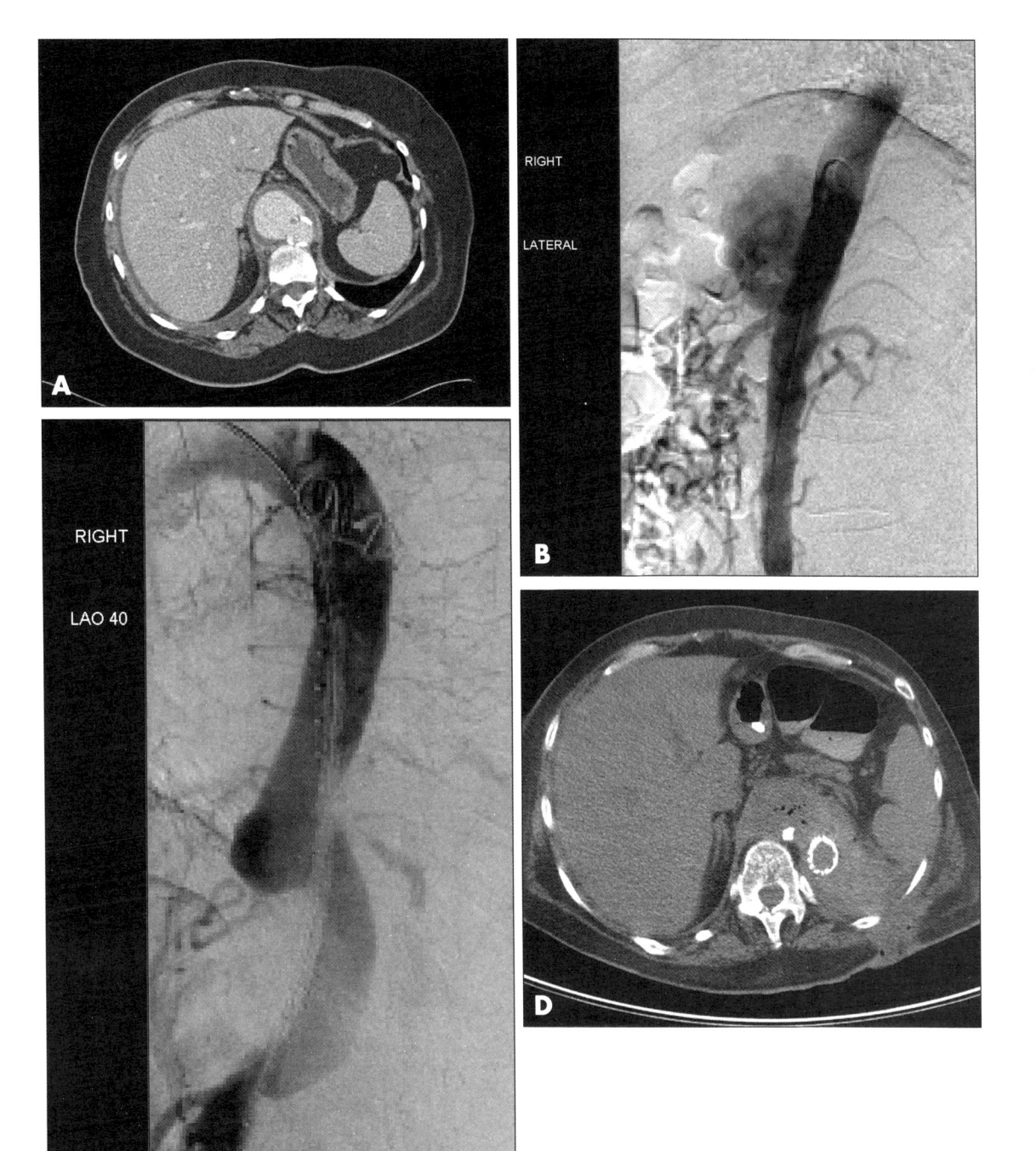

FIG. 2 A - A woman aged 78 years was referred to the Vascular Unit with a six months history of epigastric pain; there was no history or clinical investigations to suggest infection. She had been extensively investigated and found to have a saccular aneurysm, as shown on CT. B - Angiography to ascertain the proximity of the visceral vessels. C - The celiac and superior mesenteric vessels were considered to be too close to a possible landing zone for a stent graft and therefore she underwent open surgery. A thoracotomy was performed and a prosthetic graft was sutured end-side proximally and end-end to the aorta just above the visceral vessels with oversewing of the aorta. The patient recovered well although developed a superficial wound dehiscence which required debridement and resuturing on day 12, and she was discharged home on the fouteenth day postoperatively. She represented four weeks later with sepsis and pus extruding from her thoracotomy wound. She also required a 4 unit blood transfusion. CT findings revealed a collection around the graft which communicated with the thoracotomy wound. An angiogram revealed a proximal leak and this was treated with a stent graft. D - Post procedure she subsequently developed widespread infection and died of sepsis and multiorgan failure. CT scan two days post stent graft.

surgery can be conducted. It cannot be regarded as definitive treatment without debridement of contaminated tissue or removal of prosthetic graft material. Complete eradication of infection may not be possible, however, life long antibiotics may suppress sepsis.

In the future stent grafts may be available with antimicrobial surfaces specifically designed for this scenario, or alternatively devices may be produced that are resistant to infection; at present these are not economically viable. In certain low grade infections EVAR may be the answer for some patients but life long follow-up for these patients is essential.

It would be very difficult to perform a randomized controlled trial to determine the best treatment for infected aortic aneurysms due to the low incidence of cases. Therefore the only practical way of improving our knowledge and treatment will be an international registry.

REFERENCES

1. Chan FY, Crawford ES, Coselli JS et al. In situ prosthetic graft replacement for mycotic aneurysm of the aorta. *Ann Thorac Surg* 1989; 47:193-203.
2. Reddy DJ, Shepard AD, Evans JR et al. Management of infected aortoiliac aneurysms. *Arch Surg* 1991; 126:873-878.
3. Muller BT, Wegener OR, Grabitz K et al. Mycotic aneurysms of the thoracic and abdominal aorta and iliac arteries: experience with anatomic and extra-anatomic repair in 33 cases. *J Vasc Surg* 2001; 33:106-113.
4. Barry PA, Molland JG, Falk GL. Primary aortoduodenal fistula. *Aust N Z J Surg* 1998; 68:243-244.
5. Busuttil SJ, Goldstone J. Diagnosis and management of aortoenteric fistulas. *Semin Vasc Surg* 2001; 14:302-311.
6. Anonymous. Endovascular aneurysm repair versus open repair in patients with abdominal aortic aneurysm (EVAR trial 1): randomised controlled trial. *Lancet* 2005; 365:2179-2186.
7. Oderich GS, Panneton JM, Bower TC et al. Infected aortic aneurysms: aggressive presentation, complicated early outcome, but durable results. *J Vasc Surg* 2001; 34:900-908.
8. Macedo TA, Stanson AW, Oderich GS et al. Infected aortic aneurysms: imaging findings. *Radiology* 2004; 231:250-257.
9. Brown SL, Busuttil RW, Baker JD et al. Bacteriologic and surgical determinants of survival in patients with mycotic aneurysms. *J Vasc Surg* 1984; 1:541-547.
10. Kan CD, Lee HL, Yang YJ. Outcome after endovascular stent graft treatment for mycotic aortic aneurysm: A systematic review. *J Vasc Surg* 2007; 46:906-912.
11. Jones KG, Bell RE, Sabharwal T et al. Treatment of mycotic aortic aneurysms with endoluminal grafts. *Eur J Vasc Endovasc Surg* 2005; 29:139-144.
12. Ting AC, Cheng SW, Ho P et al. Endovascular stent graft repair for infected thoracic aortic pseudoaneurysms–a durable option? *J Vasc Surg* 2006; 44:701-705.
13. Lee KH, Won JY, Lee DY et al. Stent-graft treatment of infected aortic and arterial aneurysms. *J Endovasc Ther* 2006; 13:338-345.
14. Stanley BM, Semmens JB, Lawrence-Brown MM et al. Endoluminal repair of mycotic thoracic aneurysms. *J Endovasc Ther* 2003; 10:511-515.
15. Sayed S, Choke E, Helme S et al. Endovascular stent graft repair of mycotic aneurysms of the thoracic aorta. *J Cardiovasc Surg* (Torino) 2005; 46:155-161.
16. Semba CP, Sakai T, Slonim SM et al. Mycotic aneurysms of the thoracic aorta: repair with use of endovascular stent-grafts. *J Vasc Interv Radiol* 1998; 9:33-40.
17. Forbes TL, Harding GE. Endovascular repair of Salmonella-infected abdominal aortic aneurysms: a word of caution. *J Vasc Surg* 2006; 44:198-200.
18. Gonzalez-Fajardo JA, Gutierrez V, Martin-Pedrosa M et al. Endovascular repair in the presence of aortic infection. *Ann Vasc Surg* 2005; 19:94-98.
19. Liu WC, Kwak BK, Kim KN et al. Tuberculous aneurysm of the abdominal aorta: endovascular repair using stent grafts in two cases. *Korean J Radiol* 2000; 1:215-218.
20. Alpagut U, Ugurlucan M, Kafali E et al. Endoluminal stenting of mycotic saccular aneurysm at the aortic arch. *Tex Heart Inst J* 2006; 33:371-375.
21. Jorna FH, Verhoeven EL, Bos WT et al. Treatment of a ruptured thoracoabdominal aneurysm with a stent-graft covering the celiac axis. *J Endovasc Ther* 2006; 13:770-774.
22. Corso JE, Kasirajan K, Milner R. Endovascular management of ruptured, mycotic abdominal aortic aneurysm. *Am Surg* 2005; 71:515-517.
23. Koeppel TA, Gahlen J, Diehl S et al. Mycotic aneurysm of the abdominal aorta with retroperitoneal abscess: successful endovascular repair. *J Vasc Surg* 2004; 40:164-166.
24. Kotzampassakis N, Delanaye P, Masy F et al. Endovascular stent-graft for thoracic aorta aneurysm caused by Salmonella. *Eur J Cardiothorac Surg* 2004; 26:225-227.
25. Rayan SS, Vega JD, Shanewise JS et al. Repair of mycotic aortic pseudoaneurysm with a stent graft using transesophageal echocardiography. *J Vasc Surg* 2004; 40:567-570.
26. Van Doorn RC, Reekers J, de Mol BA et al. Aortoesophageal fistula secondary to mycotic thoracic aortic aneurysm: endovascular repair and transhiatal esophagectomy. *J Endovasc Ther* 2002; 9:212-217.
27. Ishida M, Kato N, Hirano T et al. Limitations of endovascular treatment with stent-grafts for active mycotic thoracic aortic aneurysm. *Cardiovasc Intervent Radiol* 2002; 25:216-218.
28. Berchtold C, Eibl C, Seelig MH et al. Endovascular treatment and complete regression of an infected abdominal aortic aneurysm. *J Endovasc Ther* 2002; 9:543-548.
29. Madhavan P, McDonnell CO, Dowd MO et al. Suprarenal mycotic aneurysm exclusion using a stent with a partial autologous covering. *J Endovasc Ther* 2000; 7:404-409.
30. Kinney EV, Kaebnick HW, Mitchell RA et al. Repair of mycotic

paraviscceral aneurysm with a fenestrated stent-graft. *J Endovasc Ther* 2000; 7:192-197.

31. Hsu RB, Chen RJ, Wang SS et al. Infected aortic aneurysms: clinical outcome and risk factor analysis. *J Vasc Surg* 2004; 40:30-35.

32. Kyriakides C, Kan Y, Kerle M et al. 11-year experience with anatomical and extra-anatomical repair of mycotic aortic aneurysms. *Eur J Vasc Endovasc Surg* 2004; 27:585-589.

33. Kuestner LM, Reilly LM, Jicha DL et al. Secondary aortoenteric fistula: contemporary outcome with use of extraanatomic bypass and infected graft excision. *J Vasc Surg* 1995; 21:184-195.

34. Yeager RA, McConnell DB, Sasaki TM et al. Aortic and peripheral prosthetic graft infection: differential management and causes of mortality. *Am J Surg* 1985; 150:36-43.

35. Smith JJ, Taylor PR. Endovascular treatment of mycotic aneurysms of the thoracic and abdominal aorta: the need for level I evidence. *Eur J Vasc Endovasc Surg* 2004; 27:569-570.

36. Gupta AK, Bandyk DF, Johnson BL. In situ repair of mycotic abdominal aortic aneurysms with rifampin-bonded gelatin-impregnated Dacron grafts: a preliminary case report. *J Vasc Surg* 1996; 24:472-476.

37. Earnshaw JJ, Whitman B, Heather BP. Two-year results of a randomized controlled trial of rifampicin-bonded extra-anatomic dacron grafts. *Br J Surg* 2000; 87:758-759.

38. Braithwaite BD, Davies B, Heather BP et al. Early results of a randomized trial of rifampicin-bonded Dacron grafts for extra-anatomic vascular reconstruction. Joint Vascular Research Group. *Br J Surg* 1998; 85:1378-1381.

39. Hernandez-Richter T, Schardey HM, Lohlein F et al. The prevention and treatment of vascular graft infection with a Triclosan (Irgasan)-bonded Dacron graft: an experimental study in the pig. *Eur J Vasc Endovasc Surg* 2000; 20:413-418.

40. Illingworth BL, Tweden K, Schroeder RF et al. In vivo efficacy of silver-coated (Silzone) infection-resistant polyester fabric against a biofilm-producing bacteria, Staphylococcus epidermidis. *J Heart Valve Dis* 1998; 7:524-530.

41. Vogt PR, Brunner-La Rocca HP, Carrel T et al. Cryopreserved arterial allografts in the treatment of major vascular infection: a comparison with conventional surgical techniques. *J Thorac Cardiovasc Surg* 1998; 116:965-972.

42. Vogt PR, Brunner-LaRocca HP, Lachat M et al. Technical details with the use of cryopreserved arterial allografts for aortic infection: influence on early and midterm mortality. *J Vasc Surg* 2002; 35:80-86.

43. Morris GE, Friend PJ, Vassallo DJ et al. Antibiotic irrigation and conservative surgery for major aortic graft infection. *J Vasc Surg* 1994; 20:88-95.

44. Danneels MI, Verhagen HJ, Teijink JA et al. Endovascular repair for aorto-enteric fistula: a bridge too far or a bridge to surgery? *Eur J Vasc Endovasc Surg* 2006; 32:27-33.

45. Burks JA, Jr., Faries PL, Gravereaux EC et al. Endovascular repair of bleeding aortoenteric fistulas: a 5-year experience. *J Vasc Surg* 2001; 34:1055-1059.

46. Fiorani P, Speziale F, Calisti A et al. Endovascular graft infection: preliminary results of an international enquiry. *J Endovasc Ther* 2003; 10:919-927.

47. Parsons RE, Sanchez LA, Marin ML et al. Comparison of endovascular and conventional vascular prostheses in an experimental infection model. *J Vasc Surg* 1996; 24:920-925.

18

ENDOVASCULAR TREATMENT OF TRAUMATIC AORTIC RUPTURES

GEERT WILLEM SCHURINK, TANJA LETTINGA VAN DE POLL
THOMAS KOEPPEL, STEPHAN LANGER, GOTTFRIED MOMMERTZ
MICHIEL DE HAAN, MICHAEL JACOBS

Traumatic rupture of the thoracic aorta is a surgical emergency usually related to blunt thoracic trauma. It results from a sudden deceleration tearing the fixed thoracic arch from the mobile aorta mostly at the level of the isthmus. Trauma mechanism includes frontal or side collisions, falls from height and explosions. Blunt traumatic aortic rupture (BTAR) is the direct cause of death in 18% of all road accident fatalities [1]. In 80% of the cases the victim dies at the scene of the accident. Of the patients reaching the hospital alive, 30% will die within 6 hours and 40%-50% will not survive the first 24 hours if left untreated [2,3]. In patients who initially survive, the rupture is contained by the integrity of the adventitia and surrounding mediastinal structures. The natural course of this contained rupture is unfavorable, since a third of those patients eventually dies from subsequent complications [4].

Change of strategy

Until several years ago, treatment of choice was immediate surgical intervention with direct suture or interposition of a prosthetic graft [5]. However, surgical mortality rate ranges from 9% to 15% [6] and is about 10% in stabilized patients [7-9]. Surgical intervention can lead to severe morbidity such as paraplegia and cerebrovascular accidents. Paraplegia incidence varies from 2.3% [6] using active distal aortic perfusion to 19.2% with "clamp and sew"-technique [10].

More recently, endovascular treatment of traumatic thoracic aortic ruptures has been introduced

[11]. Although initial results seem promising, the true benefit and long-term results of endovascular treatment of BTAR remains to be established. In 2003 in the EVC book on Vascular Emergencies, Roberto Chiesa et al. wrote a chapter on "Traumatic rupture of the thoracic aorta" [12]. Since this time endovascular treatment has been treatment of first choice. In this chapter, diagnostic and technical aspects of the endovascular treatment of BTAR will be discussed.

Trauma mechanism

BTAR typically involves a transverse tear in the wall of the aorta. The aortic injury can be mild and only involve the intimal layer, or may extent into the medial layer of the aortic wall [13]. In these state of situations, the intact advential layer may be strong enough to prohibit a prompt free rupture and the victim can reach the hospital alive. The damage of the arterial wall will cause a false aneurysm or, when blood is forced between the layers of the aortic wall, an aortic dissection. In more severe cases, the aortic transaction will involve all three layers and the victim will usually die shortly after the accident due to massive hemorrhage. Richens et al. [14] reported a 90% prehospital mortality of the BTAR victims in the United Kingdom between 1992 and 1999.

Almost 90% of the BTAR injuries are located at the aortic isthmus. Hunt et al. [15] reported BTAR in the ascending aorta and the aortic arch in 3.2% and 1.6%, respectively. Rupture of the ascending aorta was more common in unbelted victims compared with belted victims. Rupture at the isthmus was equally common in the two groups [16].

Involvement of the distal descending thoracic aorta was even more infrequent (0.8%) [15] and was often associated with fracture of the thoracic vertebra. Rupture of the distal descending aorta was more common in belted persons than unbelted persons [16].

The most common theory on the mechanism of BTAR is the massive deceleration during trauma causing rupture of the aorta at the level of the aortic isthmus a few centimeters distal to the left subclavian artery (ligamentum arteriosum). The heart and aortic arch can displace during deceleration, while the descending thoracic aorta being fixed to the spine via the segmental arteries remains fixed. Other theories on the trauma mechanism of BTAR suggest that it is a complex multivariate process secondary to a combination of stresses [17]:
1) stretching of the aorta;
2) intravascular pressure;
3) water-hammer effect;
4) osseous pinch of the aorta between the osseous body of the chest.

Several cadaveric studies and finite element models investigating the trauma mechanism of BTAR are performed. Finite element analysis demonstrated that the simulated impact studies induce the maximal peak stress at the aortic isthmus [18]. The cadaveric study of Baqué et al. [19] support the theory of aortic stretching, but found no evidence of the osseous pinch being an important factor.

A simple analytic model by Kivity et al. [20] confirms that a sudden occlusion of the blood flow in the aorta, e.g. by extreme abdominal compression, would lead to a significant pressure pulse in the aorta, possibly able to create an aortic rupture.

Diagnosis

The treatment of the seriously injured patients requires rapid assessment of the injuries and institution of life-preserving therapy according to the Advanced Trauma Life Support principles. Persistent and recurrent hypotension is usually due to an unidentified bleeding site, like an aortic rupture. Specific sign and symptoms are frequently absent. A high index of suspicion triggered by a history of deceleration force and characteristic radiological findings are the elements to make the diagnosis. Radiological sign on the chest X-ray which can indicate major thoracic vascular injury include:
1) widened mediastinum. The positive predictive value (PPV) of a widened mediastinum for BTAR is about 15% [21].
2) Fractures of the first and second ribs. This sign has a very low PPV [22].
3) Obliteration of the aortic knob.
4) Opacification of the aorto-pulmonary window.
5) Deviation of the trachea and/or the esophagus to the right site.
6) Presence of a pleural cap.
7) Elevation of the right and/or deviation of the left mainstem bronchus.

Sensitivity and specificity of chest X-ray in diagnosis of BTAR in patients with blunt thoracic trauma is 56% and 64%, respectively [23].

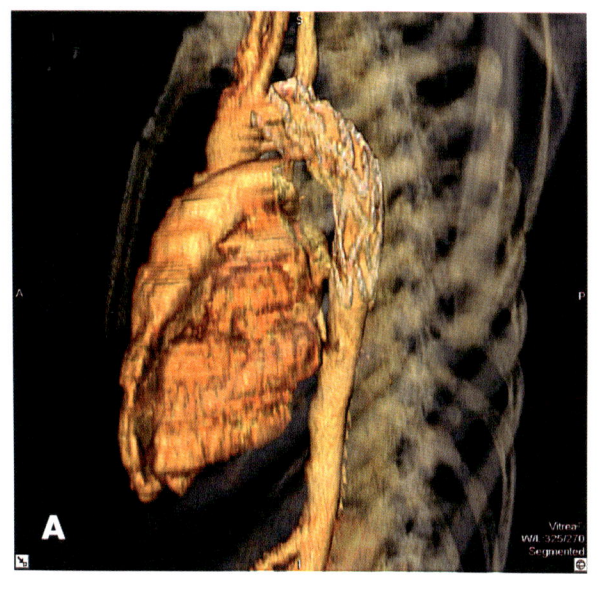

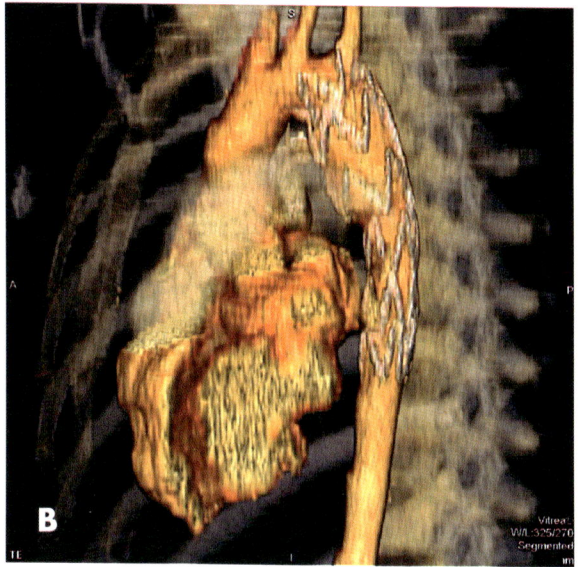

FIG. 1 In patient A, the stent-graft in the BTAR aortic segment has a normal diameter, suggesting partial aortic wall rupture. In patient B, the stent-graft has reached its maximal diameter, suggesting complete aortic wall rupture.

Although arteriography has long been considered the gold standard for the diagnosis of BTAR [24], multiplane transesophageal echocardiography (TEE) [25,26] and contrast-enhanced spiral computed tomography (CT) of the chest are accurate alternative imaging modalities [27,28].

Helical CT scanner has been reported to diagnose BTAR with a sensitivity of 100% [23,29]. However, specificity is about 83%-95%, leaving some indication for conventional angiography. CT scanning is also valuable in the evaluation of the other injuries, which are common in these mostly multitrauma patients.

The reliability of TEE in the diagnosis of BTAR involving the aortic isthmus depends upon the performance of a meticulous examination by an experienced echocardiographer. Due to the diagnostic accuracy and availability of both TEE and helical CT, indications of aortography are now principally restricted to the suspicion of injuries to the aortic arch or the brachiocephalic arteries, and when TEE or CT findings are not characteristic of BTAR. In addition, TEE is highly sensitive for the diagnosis of limited aortic injuries, and allows a gradation of severity of aortic trauma [30]:
- Grade 1 BTAR corresponds to superficial lesions that can safely and efficiently be managed conservatively.
- Grade 2 aortic injuries represent subadventitial BTAR that require surgical repair.
- Grade 3 BTAR corresponds to aortic transsection with blood extravasation or aortic obstruction with ischemia and must be operated on promptly.

Preoperative CT angiography does not enable this kind of gradation. However, postoperative stent-graft behavior can possibly suggest the presence or absence of aortic wall at the BTAR location (Fig. 1).

Timing of treatment

The management of traumatic rupture of the thoracic aorta has evolved significantly over the past decades. The early pharmalogical reduction of the blood pressure can markedly reduce the risk of free rupture [31]. In the era of open surgical repair of BTAR, it has been demonstrated that in high risk patients, due to other traumatic injuries, delayed repair of the BTAR is safe under appropriate treatment. Symbas et al. [32] reported that in a group of 14 patients who had associated injuries that were likely to increase the risk of surgical death, operation was postponed for more than 48 hours. Keeping their mean arterial pressure at less than 70 mmHg with medication, none of these patients had a rupture of their BTAR. After the introduction of the endovascular treatment of BTAR, many contraindications for immediate

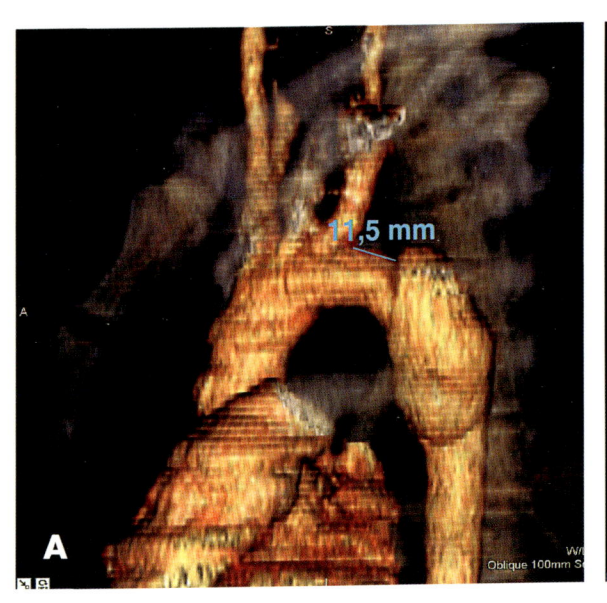

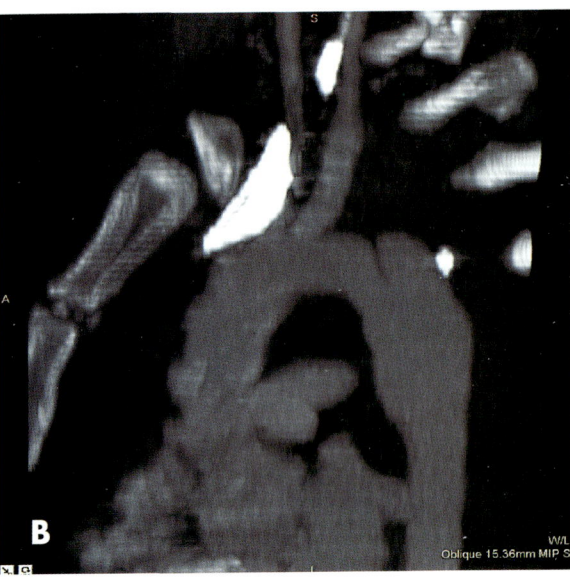

FIG. 2   Patient with BTAR at the level of the aortic isthmus. SSD-CT reconstruction (A) suggests only a short proximal neck (11.5 mm). MPR-CT reconstruction (B) shows a more proximal extent of the false aneurysm, leaving a longer proximal neck.

open repair expire. Because of a shorter operation time of the endovascular treatment, chances of developing complications due to other, unrecognized injuries will be reduced. The avoidance of the extra-corporeal circulation used in open procedures with distal aortic perfusion, eliminates the need to use heparin. This means that (intra-abdominal) hemorrhage, head injuries and multiple fractures, no longer (relatively) contraindicate direct treatment for BTAR. In case of combined injury of the thoracic aorta and the spleen and/or liver a combined procedure of endovascular treatment for BTAR and embolizing bleeding of the intra-abdominal parenchymatous organs is possible. Because endovascular treatment avoids the necessity of thoracotomy patients with lung contusion or other pulmonary injuries benefit from this minimal invasive procedure. The loss of these contraindications eliminates the necessity to postpone acute treatment of this potentially life-threatening situation.

The ideal timing of the procedure remains a point of debate. Patients with TRA will have other organ injuries in 90% of the cases [31,32], which may at times make it difficult to decide which injury to treat first. The estimated mortality of stable patients with rupture of the aorta (TRA) is 25% and is more often due to these other injuries [33]. Although in trauma surgery the adage "treat first what kills first" still stands, this may not always be as obvious as it sounds. In polytraumatized patients with TRA the surgeon has to weigh the chances of rupture against the lethality of the remaining injuries. Adequate blood pressure control minimizes the risk of free rupture [31,32], but the risk of free rupture still remains and is up to 4% during delay of treatment [2,31,34,35]. The question is whether the introduction of the endovascular approach changes the timing of BTAR treatment.

In a recent review [36] concerning endovascular treatment of BTAR, a large number of delayed treatments (88 of 284 cases) was encountered, suggesting that still many authors consider the risk of rupture smaller then the advantages of stabilizing multiple injured patients. The major advantage of endovascular repair of BTAR is that it enables immediate stabilization of a potentially lethal injury making treatment of other acutely threatening but less potentially dangerous injuries possible, while at the same time avoiding comorbidity of open surgery.

Immediate endovascular treatment of BTAR is recommended, not only in patients with a high risk of free rupture (such as an increasing hemothorax or increasing rupture size), but also in patients that are clinically stable. Endovascular stent grafting should be done as soon as primary survey is completed and the patient is stabilized. This is generally within 4 to 6 hours after the trauma. At the present time there are no means of predicting which will remain stable and which will eventually progress to uncontrolled hemorrhage [35]. Delaying the procedure should only be considered when the patient is respiratory or hemodynamically instable (from other causes than BTAR). When delaying treatment, blood pressure should be kept below 140 mmHg [31].

Technical considerations and technique

Thoracic endovascular aortic repair (TEVAR) of various thoracic aortic pathology is being performed for many years with satisfactory results. The first report on TEVAR already included "post-traumatic true and false aneurysms" [11]. In case of a BTAR at the level of the aortic isthmus, endovascular treatment looks quite easy and harmless, because of the short pathologic aortic segment in a mostly undiseased thoracic aorta in a often young patient. However, several issues can complicate this procedure.

Standard access for a thoracic stent-graft is performed by common femoral artery cut down. Most thoracic devices are loaded in (or need for introduction) a 22 French sheath (or more), requiring a common femoral and external iliac artery of 8 mm in diameter. BTAR patients often are younger than patients with thoracic aneurysms or dissections. Although the access vessels are usually healthy, free of calcifications and will stretch easily, their diameter can be to small, needing introduction of the stent-graft system through the common iliac artery. In a review of the literature, 79% of the BTAR patients had access through the common femoral artery [36]. In 15% the common iliac artery was used and in 3% direct aortic access was performed. The direct aortic access was combined with laparotomy for different traumatic reasons.

The left subclavian artery (LSA) is usually just proximal to the BTAR. In literature, partial or complete coverage of the orifice of the LSA was reported in 26% of the cases [36]. The necessity of covering the LSA is not very clear. In the endovascular treatment of thoracic aortic aneurysms in the distal aortic arch, a proximal neck of two centimeters is required to obtain a secure seal. In the distal arch, the length of the proximal neck measured on the inner and outer curve of the arch can differ significantly. Borsa et al. [37] descibe the anatomical characteristics of the thoracic aorta in 50 BTAR patients. The mean distance from the LSA to the superior aspect of the injury measured 5.8 mm along the lesser curve and 14.9 mm along the outer curve. Neschis et al. [38] reported a mean distance between the LSA and the proximal end of the tear of 19.9 mm, whereas in 70% of the cases the distance was over 20 mm. It can be difficult to interpret the images from computer tomography or angiography with regard to exact location of the aortic tear. Often a false aneurysm extends more proximal than the level of the tear, concealing the exact length of the proximal neck (Fig. 2). Looking at the results of Borsa et al. [37] LSA overstenting will be necessary in the majority of the cases, whether according to the measurements of Neschis et al. [38] a sufficient proximal neck distal to the LSA is mostly present. It has become fairly well accepted that covering the LSA is safe. However, this young and active patient group will probably complain more frequently about arm ischemia and will need secondary subclavian revascularization. Ischemia of the left arm in BTAR patients after TEVAR has been reported five times in literature [36].

At the moment, small thoracic aorta diameter and steep curvature of the aortic arch are the biggest problem. Current commercially available devices were designed for aneurysmal disease in older patients with usually wider and elongated thoracic aortas. Borsa et al. reported a mean diameter of the thoracic aorta in BTAR patients of 19.3 mm. (range 14.1 to 40.6 mm) The use of commercially available stent-grafts in these patients often leads to a degree of oversizing which is more than advised in the instructions for use. Several industries have introduced smaller diameter thoracic grafts. At the moment a 22 mm thoracic graft is the smallest available (Zenith TX2, William Cook Europe, Denmark). The Gore TAG (W.L. Gore, Flagstaff, AZ, USA) has a minimal diameter of 26 mm and requires a smaller degree of oversizing compared to the other stent-grafts. For this reason the use of abdominal extension cuffs has been recommended by some authors [38], however their short length, requiring the use of multiple devices, creates a potential risk for device separation and endoleak. Also the length of the abdominal introduction devices can be insufficient for thoracic use. The radius of the aortic arch in younger patients is much tighter than in older patients. Introduction of a very stiff guide wire (e.g. Lunderquist or Backup Meier) can be difficult, resulting in permanent bending of the

Table I PERSONAL EXPERIENCE WITH ENDOVASCULAR TREATMENT OF BTAR

Case	1	2	3	4	5
Age (yrs)/(sex)	20/m	24/m	65/m	31/m	19/m
Trauma	Car vs tree	Motor vs car	Fall from tree	Suicide jump	Motor vs car
Location BTAR	Aortic isthmus	Aortic isthmus	Aortic isthmus	Aortic isthmus	Aortic isthmus
Concomitant injuries	Lung contusion, splenic rupture, femoral fracture, vertebral fractures	Lung contusion, minor hepatic and pancreatic rupture.	Lung contusion, multiple rib fractures, spleen rupture	Hemothorax, Lungcontusion	Hemothorax, Lung contusion
Delay of operation (hr:min)	5:03	4:58	0:55	1:25	2:40
Introduction stent graft	Left femoral artery	Left femoral artery	Left femoral artery	Left femoral artery	Right femoral artery
Graft/diameter (mm)	Talent/32	Talent/28	Talent/42	Talent/28	Talent/30
Stent-graft oversizing (%)	14	17	17	17	67
Subclavian artery	Overstented	Overstented	Overstented	Overstented	Overstented
Complications during procedure	None	None	None	None	Endoleak
Operation time (hr:min)	0:52	0:47	0:51	0:45	1:35
Post operative complications	-	-	-	Died due to lungcontusion and psychiatric prognosis	Type 1a endoleak (sealed spontaneously)
Hospital stay (days)	14	10	16	5	27
Follow-up (months)	49	36	33	0	27

Table I PERSONAL EXPERIENCE WITH ENDOVASCULAR TREATMENT OF BTAR

Case	6	7	8	9	10
Age (yrs)/(sex)	57/m	39/m	70/m	57/m	42/m
Trauma	Car vs car	Motorbike	Motorbike	Motorbike	Motorbike
Location BTAR	Desc. thor. aorta	Aortic isthmus	Aortic isthmus	Aortic isthmus	Aortic isthmus
Concomitant injuries	Lung contusion, multiple rib fractures, bilateral femoral fracture	Lung contusion, fractured pelvis, multiple fractures	Subdural hematoma	Multiple fractures	Lung contusion, abdominal bleeding, lumbar fractures
Delay of operation (hr:min)	8:20	2:25	5:07	10:17	3:17
Introduction stent graft	Left femoral artery	Left femoral artery	Left femoral artery	Right femoral artery	Left femoral artery
Graft/diameter (mm)	Zenith / 30	Zenith/22	Valiant/38	Zenith/26	Zenith/26
Stent-graft oversizing (%)	11	10	6	8	12
Subclavian artery	Open	Open	Overstented	Overstented	Open
Complications during procedure	None	None	None	None	None
Operation time (hr:min)	0:41	1:20	2:15	1:35	2:00
Post operative complications	Minor stroke	Infection osteosynthesis	None	Pulmonary embolus	None
Hospital stay (days)	>30	>30	17	21	8
Follow-up (months)	1	9	5	3	Lost to follow-up

wire [38]. In this setting, prebending the wire or the use of an Amplatz wire is advocated. The very steep aortic arch will often create a mal-alignment of the stent-graft at the inner curve, creating a possible endoleak. The use of a proximal bare stent will reduce this problem, however, it can impose the patient with a life long bare stent position over the orifice of the left carotid artery, possibly inducing embolic complications. The combination of ample oversizing and the a steep aortic arch is probably responsible for the Gore TAG stent-graft collapses reported in literature [38-40]. Collapsed devices were either repaired by another stent-graft or balloon-expandable stent, or removed during open repair. Muhs et al. [40] analyzed collapsed versus non-collapsed Gore TAG devices in BTAR. They concluded that stent-graft collapse occurred in patients who were treated outside the manufacturer's instructions for use for minimum required aortic diameter. The small distal aortic diameter and minimum intragraft aortic diameter predicted collapse. Caution should be exercised when treating BTAR in patients with small (<23 mm) aortic diameters.

Procedure-related complications in BTAR patients were reported in 14% of the cases [36]. No paraplegia after TEVAR for BTAR has been reported. Type 1 endoleaks were noted in 1.4% during the procedure and were resolved by additional stent-graft placement or ballooning. Postoperative endoleaks (type 1 and 3) were found in 5.3% of the cases. Again, the amount of oversizing of the stent-graft and the steep angle of the aortic arch will be partly responsible for the presence of the proximal type 1 endoleak. Mortality in this patient group after endovascular treatment of the BTAR is mainly related to the remaining injuries in the multitrauma patients. Lettinga et al. reported a 5.6% mortality after TEVAR for BTAR, 1.4% being procedure related [36].

Postoperative follow-up

Normal postoperative follow-up schemes will include plain chest X-ray and computed tomography angiography (CTA). In TEVAR for thoracic aneurysms CTA will be performed lifelong. For the younger BTAR patient lifelong can easily be sixty years. Everyone will agree that annual CTA in this group is not advisable, however, there is no consensus about a suitable follow-up scheme. Lifelong yearly CTA has a small, but significant risk of radiation-induced cancer in this group [41]. In literature there is no report on device failure or migration 12 months after initial treatment. Many aortic ruptures will be incomplete and will be less than semi-circular. These lesions will probably heal and the stent-graft is only needed temporary. In case of a complete, circular rupture, the aortic wall retracts and will be repaired with the interposition of connective tissue. Without the support of the stent-graft these lesions will develop into chronic false aneurysms. The position of the stent-graft in the ruptured aorta is thought to be very stable, because of the healthy aorta proximal and distal to the rupture site. Once the rupture has been excluded from the circulation, chances of migration are small. In theory, any change in aortic diameter and stent-graft position can be seen on plain chest X-ray. For this reason, our follow-up policy after two years (in the absence of complications) will be yearly plain chest X-ray in four directions (AP, transverse and oblique (2x)).

Personal experience

From 2002 until now, 10 patients with BTAR have been treated endovascularly. Five of these patients were included in the Dutch experience on endovascular treatment of blunt traumatic aortic rupture [42]. In the same period, no patients died before operation while diagnosed with BTAR. In one patient the BTAR seemed to be located proximal of the left subclavian artery. This patient died during open repair. Characteristics of the endovascular treated patients are given in the Table. One patient died, not directly related to the BTAR. One patient had a minor stroke after treatment, which could be related to the endovascular treatment. These results indicate a 10% mortality rate, which in fact was not related to the aortic trauma.

Conclusion

Traumatic rupture of the thoracic aorta is almost always associated with severe concomitant injuries. The introduction of endovascular aortic repair has significantly contributed to improved outcome of these multitrauma patients when compared to open repair comprising thoracotomy, aortic cross-clamping and heparinization. There is general consensus that endovascular repair is the therapy of choice for traumatic aortic ruptures.

REFERENCES

1. Greendyke RM. Traumatic rupture of aorta; special reference to automobile accidents. *JAMA* 1966; 195: 527-530.
2. Fabian TC, Richardson JD, Croce MA et al. Prospective study of blunt aortic injury: Multicenter Trial of the American Association for the Surgery of Trauma. *J Trauma* 1997; 42: 374-380.
3. Parmley LF, Mattingly TW, Manion WC et al. Nonpenetrating traumatic injury of the aorta. *Circulation* 1958; 17: 1086-1101.
4. Finkelmeier BA, Mentzer RM Jr, Kaiser DL et al. Chronic traumatic thoracic aneurysm. Influence of operative treatment on natural history: an analysis of reported cases, 1950-1980. *J Thorac Cardiovasc Surg* 1982; 84: 257-266.
5. Nagy K, Fabian T, Rodman G et al. Guidelines for the diagnosis and management of blunt aortic injury: an EAST Practice Management Guidelines Work Group. *J Trauma* 2000; 48: 1128-43.
6. Jahromi AS, Kazemi K, Safar HA et al. Traumatic rupture of the thoracic aorta: cohort study and systematic review. *J Vasc Surg* 2001; 34: 1029-1034.
7. Wahl WL, Michaels AJ, Wang SC et al. Blunt thoracic aortic injury: delayed or early repair? *J Trauma* 1999; 47: 254-259.
8. Gammie JS, Shah AS, Hattler BG et al. Traumatic aortic rupture: diagnosis and management. *Ann Thorac Surg* 1998; 66: 1295-1300.
9. Maggisano R, Nathens A, Alexandrova NA et al. Traumatic rupture of the thoracic aorta: should one always operate immediately? *Ann Vasc Surg* 1995; 9: 44-52.
10. von Oppell UO, Dunne TT, De Groot MK et al. Traumatic aortic rupture: twenty-year metaanalysis of mortality and risk of paraplegia. *Ann Thorac Surg* 1994; 58: 585-593.
11. Dake MD, Miller DC, Semba CP et al. Transluminal placement of endovascular stent-grafts for the treatment of descending thoracic aortic aneurysms. *N Engl J Med* 1994; 331: 1729-734.
12. Chiesa R, Castellano R, Lucci C et al. Traumatic rupture of the thoracic aorta. In: Branchereau A, Jacobs M, eds. *Vascular emergencies*. New York: Futura Publishing Co, 2003: pp 107-123.
13. Sevitt S. The mechanisms of traumatic rupture of the thoracic aorta. *Br J Surg* 1977; 64: 166-173.
14. Richens D, Kotidis K, Neale M et al. Rupture of the aorta following road traffic accidents in the United Kingdom 1992-1999. The results of the co-operative crash injury study. *Eur J Cardiothorac Surg* 2003; 23: 143-148.
15. Hunt JP, Baker CC, Lentz CW et al. Thoracic aorta injuries: management and outcome of 144 patients. *J Trauma* 1996; 40: 547-555.
16. Arajarvi E, Santavirta S, Tolonen J. Aortic ruptures in seat belt wearers. *J Thorac Cardiovasc Surg* 1989; 98: 355-361.
17. Richens D, Field M, Neale M et al. The mechanism of injury in blunt traumatic rupture of the aorta. *Eur J Cardiothorac Surg* 2002; 21: 288-293.
18. Richens D, Field M, Hashim S et al. A finite element model of blunt traumatic aortic rupture. *Eur J Cardiothorac Surg* 2004; 25: 1039-1047.
19. Baque P, Serre T, Cheynel N et al. An experimental cadaveric study for a better understanding of blunt traumatic aortic rupture. *J Trauma* 2006; 61: 586-591.
20. Kivity Y, Collins R. Nonlinear wave propagation in viscoelastic tubes: application to aortic rupture. *J Biomech* 1974; 7: 67-76.
21. Barcia TC, Livoni JP. Indications for angiography in blunt thoracic trauma. *Radiology* 1983; 147: 15-19.
22. Livoni JP, Barcia TC. Fracture of the first and second rib: incidence of vascular injury relative to type of fracture. *Radiology* 1982; 145: 31-33.
23. Demetriades D, Gomez H, Velmahos GC et al. Routine helical computed tomographic evaluation of the mediastinum in high-risk blunt trauma patients. *Arch Surg* 1998; 133: 1084-1088.
24. Ben-Menachem Y. Assessment of blunt aortic-brachiocephalic trauma: should angiography be supplanted by transesophageal echocardiography? *J Trauma* 1997; 42: 969-972.
25. Cinnella G, Dambrosio M, Brienza N et al. Transesophageal echocardiography for diagnosis of traumatic aortic injury: an appraisal of the evidence. *J Trauma* 2004; 57: 1246-1255.
26. Vignon P, Lang RM. Use of Transesophageal Echocardiography for the Assessment of Traumatic Aortic Injuries. *Echocardiography* 1999; 16: 207-219.
27. Collier B, Hughes KM, Mishok K et al. Is helical computed tomography effective for diagnosis of blunt aortic injury? *Am J Emerg Med* 2002; 20: 558-561.
28. Patel NH, Stephens KE Jr, Mirvis SE et al. Imaging of acute thoracic aortic injury due to blunt trauma: a review. *Radiology* 1998; 209: 335-348.
29. Fabian TC, Davis KA, Gavant ML et al. Prospective study of blunt aortic injury: helical CT is diagnostic and antihypertensive therapy reduces rupture. *Ann Surg* 1998; 227: 666-676.
30. Goarin JP, Cluzel P, Gosgnach M et al. Evaluation of transesophageal echocardiography for diagnosis of traumatic aortic injury. *Anesthesiology* 2000; 93: 1373-1377.
31. Pate JW, Fabian TC, Walker W. Traumatic rupture of the aortic isthmus: an emergency? *World J Surg* 1995; 19: 119-125.
32. Symbas PN, Sherman AJ, Silver JM et al. Traumatic rupture of the aorta: immediate or delayed repair? *Ann Surg* 2002; 235: 796-802.
33. Mattox KL. Traumatic rupture of the thoracic aorta. *Adv Card Surg* 1998; 10: 271-283.
34. Heijmen RH, Dossche KM, van den Berg JC et al. Two-stage, delayed endovascular treatment of traumatic rupture of the thoracic aorta. *Eur J Vasc Endovasc Surg* 2001; 22: 271-274.
35. Holmes JH 4th, Bloch RD, Hall RA et al. Natural history of traumatic rupture of the thoracic aorta managed nonoperatively: a longitudinal analysis. *Ann Thorac Surg* 2002; 73: 1149-1154.
36. Lettinga-van de Poll T, Schurink GW, De Haan MW, et al. Endovascular treatment of traumatic rupture of the thoracic aorta. *Br J Surg* 2007; 94: 525-533.
37. Borsa JJ, Hoffer EK, Karmy-Jones R, et al. Angiographic description of blunt traumatic injuries to the thoracic aorta with specific relevance to endograft repair. *J Endovasc Ther* 2002;9 Suppl 2: II84-91.
38. Neschis DG, Moaine S, Gutta R et al. Twenty consecutive cases of endograft repair of traumatic aortic disruption: lessons learned. *J Vasc Surg* 2007; 45: 487-492.
39. Idu MM, Reekers JA, Balm R et al. Collapse of a stent-graft following treatment of a traumatic thoracic aortic rupture. *J Endovasc Ther* 2005; 12: 503-507.
40. Muhs BE, Balm R, White GH et al. Anatomic factors associated with acute endograft collapse after Gore TAG treatment of thoracic aortic dissection or traumatic rupture. *J Vasc Surg* 2007; 45: 655-661.
41. de Gonzalez AB, Kim KP, Samet JM. Radiation-induced cancer risk from annual computed tomography for patients with cystic fibrosis. *Am J Respir Crit Care Med* 2007; 176: 970-973.
42. Hoornweg LL, Dinkelman MK, Goslings JC et al. Endovascular management of traumatic ruptures of the thoracic aorta: a retrospective multicenter analysis of 28 cases in The Netherlands. *J Vasc Surg* 2006; 43: 1096-1102.

ENDOVASCULAR TREATMENT OF ACUTE THORACIC AORTIC DISSECTION

JAN BRUNKWALL, VLADIMIR MATOUSSEVITCH, MICHAEL GAWENDA

The acute dissection, with its 1%-2% mortality per hour during the first 24 hours, is a serious disorder with separation in the "media" plane of the aortic wall. Nicholls (1699-1778) in 1760 described acute dissection of the thoracic aorta referring to the autopsy finding of King George II [1]. Among the two classification systems, the later simplified Stanford classification distinguishing between involvement of the ascending aorta (Stanford A) or only of the descending aorta (Stanford B) is less useful than the primary classification by DeBakey, which is more detailed and divides into DeBakey I (both the ascending and descending aorta), DeBakey II (only the ascending aorta) and DeBakey IIIa (only the descending aorta) and DeBakey IIIb (also involving the abdominal aorta). The acute dissection of the descending thoracic aorta particularly starts just below the origin of the left subclavian artery. This chapter will only deal with the acute dissection of the descending aorta, and not the dissection of the ascending aorta or the aortic arch.

Diagnosis

Three different tools are available at the moment including transesophageal echography (TEE), Computer tomography (CT) scanning and magnetic resonance angiography (MRA). These modalities are described in detail in this textbook and will only be depicted briefly. In a meta-analysis by Shiga et al. [2] comparing these modalities, the sensitivity and specificity were approaching 93%-96%, when clinically a high likelihood for aortic dissection was present. On the contrary, for ruling out a dissection, this could be done in 99% of the cases when there was a low clinical suspicion. Due to anatomical reasons, TEE has difficulties in defining the extent of the dissection far distal in the descending aorta, and CT seems to be better for examination of the arch vessels. The advantage of a 64-slice CT in patients with suspicion of an ischemic complication is the speed, high resolution and high accuracy. For planning a surgical or endovascular intervention, the CT and MRA are of more use for the vascular surgeon as the information can be easily transmitted and crosschecked. In a practical routine the patients often have undergone two or more investigations using the three mentioned modalities.

Medical treatment

The primary aim of the medical treatment is to reduce the blood pressure to a level of around 120 mmHg systolic and 80 mmHg diastolic, while maintaining urinary output. The preferred medication is based on beta-blockers, which may have, in addition to its blood pressure lowering effect, an effect per se on the mortality [3]. Best medical therapy (BMT) also includes diuretics, which will initially be used in all subjects, supplemented with ACE-inhibitors and followed by calcium blockers and alpha blockers. The 30-day mortality of 40% in the 1960s decreased to less than 10% at present with monitoring and effective medication. In house mortality from type B dissection is in the range of 10%-17% within the first 30 days [4-6], but with a significant morbidity [6].

In order to detect those patients who will develop an aneurysm rapidly, we perform CT-scan after one week, and when no change has appeared with stable clinical condition and blood pressure control, we make the next CT-scan after another 2 weeks. In case of stable conditions, the interval increases to 3-6 months for the following 2-3 years. If on the other hand morphological alterations of the dissection occur, the interval shortens.

Surgical therapy

The open surgical therapy started more widely after the reports by DeBakey in the years 1955 and 1965, where initially open fenestration was performed [7,8]. The results using this method, however, were not encouraging and closing the false lumen at the proximal tear with its improved outcome became more popular. Since the efficacy of antihypertensive treatment has been shown to be equal to open surgery with respect to mortality, but with less morbidity, there is now no role for open surgery anymore for uncomplicated aortic dissection DeBakey type III.

In the acute setting, surgical therapy may be indicated in patients with overt or pending rupture of the thoracic aorta and this includes closing of the proximal tear, fenestration and aortic resection. Open fenestration eventually in combination with a bypass may be necessary. In patients with ischemic complications like visceral ischemia, renal ischemia or paraplegia, the mortality of open surgery, mainly as the result of multi organ failure reaches 21%-50% and is therefore discouraging [4]. The use of endovascular techniques performing a fenestration and stenting of the orifices may produce good reperfusion results. Slonim et al. [9] showed that balloon fenestration and stenting for life-threatening ischemic complications was feasible: they recanalized 37 of 40 malperfused vessels. However, 30-day mortality was high (25%), reflecting the severity of the disease. In general, emergency surgery or endovascular intervention is indicated in patients with rupture, shock, and hemodynamic instability. Malperfusion of visceral organs and kidneys, as well as spinal cord and lower limbs, requires immediate treatment. An uncomplicated type B dissection which extends retrogradely into the aortic arch necessitates emergency surgery via sternotomy. Urgent repair is indicated in case of unremitting pain, uncontrollable hypertension and rapid aortic expansion.

Endovascular therapy

The first report on endografting in DeBakey type III aortic dissections was reported by Dake et al. 1994 [10], indicating that the stent-grafts could be used also in patients with dissection. The aim is to obliterate the false lumen and restore the normal anatomy, as false lumen obliteration is associated with better long-term outcomes [11,12]. Stent graft therapy will promote false lumen thrombosis and thereby resulting in less aneurysm formation. The main primary goal is to seal the proximal tear thereby compressing the false lumen, which is successful in up to 90%-98% of the cases [13,14]. The anatomical conditions, however, are not always so that the false channel distal to the stent-graft will be obliterated or thrombosed by the stent-graft [13]. The reason for this is the reentry/entries feeding the false channel with pressure from below. The rate of complete apposition of the inner membrane towards the outer wall after closing the proximal tear is not known at the moment and there is no indication in the literature as to how often this appears even though it is clear that it happens.

Several reports on the outcome have been published and a research with retrieval of the data from Pubmed from 1990 and onwards, revealed 50 publications with altogether 3 990 patients dealing with dissection of the thoracic descending aorta. Of these patients, 39 died immediately after admittance. Of the reported patients, 3 502 were acute (within 2 weeks), and 488 had a chronic dissection. Of the 3 990 patients, 2 419 were treated with best medical treatment, 928 were surgically and 604 endovascularly treated. The mortality in the acute group being subjected to best medical treatment was 9.1%. In the open surgery group mortality was 23.4% and 5.7% in the endovascular group. One of the feared complications of open surgery is paraplegia, which in the presented series was 6.6% in the open group and 2.4% in the endovascular group. A risk factor for paraplegia after stent-grafting of the thoracic aorta is the length of the stent-graft; the longer the segment of the thoracic aorta to be covered by the stentgraft, the higher the risk for paraplegia [15]. A recent EUROSTAR analysis [16] assessed the neurologic complications associated with endovascular repair of thoracic aortic pathology. At multivariate regression analysis, independent correlation with spinal cord ischemia was observed for four factors: left subclavian artery covering without revascularization (odds ratio [OR], 3.9), renal failure (OR, 3.6), concomitant open abdominal aorta surgery (OR, 5.5) and three or more stent grafts used (OR, 3.5).

As can be expected, surgically and endovascularly treated patients suffered from the classical symptoms associated with a complicated dissection, whereas the medically treated patients had non-complicated dissection [15]. The endovascular treatment of complicated type B dissection is in several reports conjuncted with a mortality of around 3%-10%, which favors well with the historical mortality rates after open repair [13,14]. Few reports, though, report on solely acute type B dissections and most of the reports are a mixture of acute cases including traumatic transection, ruptured aneurysms and complicated acute type B dissections.

The role of endovascular treatment of uncomplicated acute aortic dissection DeBakey type III (Stanford B) is not clear at the moment. Several authors report that the modulation of the dissected membrane is easier to achieve in the acute phase than in the chronic one, as the membrane in the chronic phase retracts and becomes less elastic. It is thus possible to get a complete dissolution of the false channel, when treating acute dissections, whereas the remodeling takes much longer, if at all, in patients with chronic dissections. Two thirds of the patients occlude their false channel, whereas in chronic dissections, it cannot be expected that the false channel outside the stent-graft will thrombose, but only the portion inside the stentgraft will. This is supported by the findings reported after treatment of acute dissections with a stentgraft [13]. If there is a large false channel one must also suspect a transmission of the blood pressure into the false channel, therefore not excluding the risk for rupture.

As the mortality in the best medical treatment group is still high, when the acute cases are included, the question arises if acute dissection without complication should be treated more invasively than just with best medical treatment. There are no randomized studies on this subject but the case reports speak in favor of such treatment even in the acute cases. The first randomized trials in this patient population will be conducted and the Acute Dissection Stentgrafting OR Best medical treatment (ADSORB) trial is currently being started comparing the best medical treatment with stentgraft plus best medical treatment. This European multicenter trial will include 250 patients and the endpoints include occlusion of the false channel and death, both dissection related and overall mortality after one and three years.

REFERENCES

1 Nicholls F. Observations on the body of his late Majesty. *Philos Trans Lond* 1761; 52: 265-274.

2 Shiga T, Wajima Z, Apfel CC et al. Diagnostic accuracy of transesophageal echocardiography, helical computed tomography, and magnetic resonance imaging for suspected thoracic aortic dissection: systematic review and meta-analysis. *Arch Intern Med* 2006; 166: 1350-1356.

3 Henke PK, Williams DM, Upchurch GR, Jr., et al. Acute limb ischemia associated with type B aortic dissection: clinical relevance and therapy. *Surgery* 2006; 140: 532-540;

4 Carrel T, Nguyen T, Gysi J et al. Acute type B aortic dissection: prognosis after initial conservative treatment and predictive factors for a complicated course. *Schweiz Med Wochenschr* 1997; 127: 1467-1473.

5. Tsai TT, Fattori R, Trimarchi S et al. Long-term survival in patients presenting with type B acute aortic dissection: insights from the International Registry of Acute Aortic Dissection. *Circulation* 2006; 114: 2226-2231.

6. Roseborough G, Burke J, Sperry J et al. Twenty-year experience with acute distal thoracic aortic dissections. *J Vasc Surg* 2004; 40: 235-246.

7. DeBakey ME, Cooley DA, Creech O Jr et al. Surgical considerations of dissecting aneurysm of aorta. *Ann Surg* 1955; 142: 586-612.

8. DeBakey ME, Henly WS, Cooley DA et al. Surgical management of dissecting aneurysms of the aorta. *J Thorac Cardiovasc Surg* 1965;49:130-149.

9. Slonim SM, Miller DC, Mitchell RS et al. Percutaneous balloon fenestration and stenting for life-threatening ischemic complications in patients with acute aortic dissection. *J Thorac Cardiovasc Surg* 1999; 117: 1118-1126.

10. Dake MD, Miller DC, Semba CP et al. Transluminal placement of endovascular stent-grafts for the treatment of descending thoracic aortic aneurysms. *N Engl J Med* 1994; 331: 1729-1734.

11. Marui A, Mochizuki T, Mitsui N et al. Toward the best treatment for uncomplicated patients with type B acute aortic dissection: A consideration for sound surgical indication. *Circulation* 1999; 100(19 Suppl): II275-280.

12. Akutsu K, Nejima J, Kiuchi K et al. Effects of the patent false lumen on the long-term outcome of type B acute aortic dissection. *Eur J Cardiothorac Surg* 2004; 26: 359-366.

13. Schoder M, Czerny M, Cejna M et al. Endovascular repair of acute type B aortic dissection: long-term follow-up of true and false lumen diameter changes. *Ann Thorac Surg* 2007; 83: 1059-1066.

14. Xu SD, Huang FJ, Yang JF et al. Endovascular repair of acute type B aortic dissection: early and mid-term results. *J Vasc Surg* 2006; 43: 1090-1095.

15. Amabile P, Grisoli D, Giorgi R et al. Incidence and Determinants of Spinal Cord Ischaemia in Stent-graft Repair of the Thoracic Aorta. *Eur J Vasc Endovasc Surg* 2008; [Epub ahead of print].

16. Buth J, Harris PL, Hobo R et al. Neurologic complications associated with endovascular repair of thoracic aortic pathology: incidence and risk factors. A study from the European Collaborators on Stent/Graft Techniques for Aortic Aneurysm Repair (EUROSTAR) Registry. *J Vasc Surg* 2007; 46: 1103-1111.

20

ENDOVASCULAR TREATMENT OF CHRONIC DISSECTING ANEURYSMS

MATT THOMPSON, DAVID SAYER, IAN LOFTUS, ROB MORGAN

Type B aortic dissections are classified according to their temporal relationship to the initial onset of symptoms. Acute dissections are defined by an elapsed time period of 2 weeks from the onset of symptoms. Dissections 2 weeks or more after the onset of symptoms are termed chronic. In recent years, several authors have suggested that the definition be refined to include a "sub-acute" category, which would include those dissections between 2 and 6 weeks following symptoms. The reasons for the confusion in classification may be referenced to the surgical modalities available for the treatment of type B dissections [1]. When the only option was open surgery, the operative mortality in treating acute dissections was at its highest within 2 weeks of presentation as the tissue was friable and surgery technically demanding. Nowadays a broader classification may be appropriate to reflect the indications for endovascular repair.

Natural history of chronic type B dissections

The principle complications attributed to chronic type B aortic dissections are those that cause aortic related death, namely chronic aneurysmal degeneration, rupture of the false lumen, repeated acute dissection with complications of rupture or end organ ischemia; and retrograde type A dissection.

The natural history of chronic dissections is not well defined, but in many series, patients appear to have a high long-term mortality. Suzuki et al. [2], reported a 25% mortality rate at 4 years follow up with many of the deaths aortic related; whilst Tsai et al. [3] revealed a 78% 3 year survival in patients treated medically. In contrast to this dire prognosis, Winnerkvist et al. [4] reported the long-term outcome of 66 patients with type B dissection who did not require surgical treatment at the acute stage. Of this cohort, 82% remained free of dissection related death at 10 years. However, 15% of patients had a chronic aneurysm that exceeded 6 cm in diameter, 14% had died of aortic related disease and 7.5% had a diagnosis of a type A dissection.

Onitsuka et al. [5] reported only 4 dissection related deaths in 66 patients treated medically for chronic type B dissections at 52 months. Similarly, Estera et al. [6] demonstrated that 7.6% of patients with chronic dissections required aortic intervention within 6 months of the acute episode.

One interpretation of these series is that a substantial proportion of patients with a stable, asymptomatic type B dissection progress to lesions that cause aortic related death. It seems reasonable that chronic dissections with aneurysmal degeneration should have the same indications for repair as thoracic aneurysms, namely consideration for repair when the diameter of the aorta exceeds 5.5-6.0 cm or acute complications intervene.

Prevention of chronic dissecting aneurysms: repair of uncompleted acute type B dissection

In recent years, endovascular techniques have been successfully applied to the treatment of complicated acute type B aortic dissections. With increasing experience in this field, several authors have suggested that endovascular repair might be considered for uncomplicated lesions, in an attempt to stop these lesions from progressing to chronic aneurysmal dissections [7]. This premise was based on the assumption that a high number of patients with uncomplicated acute type B dissections would progress to chronic aneurysmal degeneration, and that endovascular repair in the acute phase could be performed with adequate safety margins.

Recent evidence has suggested that repair of all uncomplicated type B dissections may be inappropriate. In the acute phase, uncomplicated type B dissections appear to have a relatively low mortality. Estera et al. reported a series of 159 patients presenting with acute type B dissections. Forty-seven percent of patients had complicated dissections and had an overall, in-hospital mortality of 18%. In contrast, the 53% of patients with uncomplicated dissection had medical management with mortality of just 1.2%. Repair of uncomplicated dissections in the acute phase seems unjustified on the basis of these data.

The data from Winnerkvist et al. [4] reported above suggest that the incidence of progression to chronic aneurysmal degeneration is not sufficient to justify the repair of all uncomplicated acute type B dissections to prevent future aneurysm formation. However, the natural history of uncomplicated acute type B dissections is not well defined and further data will be welcome. The INSTEAD study provided some insight into repair of uncomplicated dissections. In this investigation, patients with asymptomatic dissections, 2 weeks or more after the initial event, were randomized to best medical management or endovascular repair. The initial results have suggested no significant differences between the groups in terms of mortality, with the endovascular cohort having a slightly higher mortality rate. Longer follow-up will be invaluable in defining the natural history of the condition. A multicenter trial is currently underway. The Adsorb study is a randomized trial of patients with acute uncomplicated type B dissection. The study will recruit 270 patients from 30 European sites and randomize to endovascular repair or best medical therapy. Primary end points are focused on aortic morphology after treatment and secondary end points include dissection and all cause mortality.

At the present time, endovascular repair cannot be recommended for all patients with acute uncomplicated type B dissection. Clearly, it would be beneficial to identify a sub-group of patients who have a significant chance of rapid progression to chronic aneurysmal degeneration, and several studies have addressed this issue. Identification of patients with an increased risk of aneurysm formation would allow these patients to be treated in the acute phase. Sueyoshi et al. [8] demonstrated that patients with a perfused false lumen demonstrated continued aortic expansion. In a more recent investigation, Song et al. [9] revealed that the best predictor of subsequent event free survival was the maximum diameter of the false lumen in the thorax. Patients with an initial false lumen that exceeded 22 mm in the thorax had significantly reduced event free survival. With further studies, it may well become possible to accurately define a sub-group of patients with uncomplicated dissection that have significantly increased rates of aortic progression to aneurysm formation. This group can then be targeted for early endovascular repair, in the acute phase, when the potential for complete aortic remodelling is at its highest.

Surgical or endovascular repair

Surgical treatment of thoracic and thoracoabdominal dissections often involves a thoraco-laparotomy, left heart bypass and cerebrospinal fluid drainage. The results of these surgical procedures are difficult to define. Certain highly specialized centers report excellent results [10], but a realistic figure for 30-day mortality in a community setting may be 20%. Endovascular techniques have been enthusiastically applied to thoracic dissections due to the encouraging initial results reported for many thoracic aortic pathologies [11]. The treatment of chronic dissections by endovascular techniques has been attempted with mixed results. A summary of current results is given in the Table, although it must be noted that many series are very small.

The data suggest that endovascular treatment of chronic dissections appears to be a well-tolerated procedure with acceptable mortality rates and reasonable paraplegia and stroke rates [51,52]. The major problem associated with this technique appears to be the high rate of intervention required after the primary procedure, and equivocal false lumen thrombosis rates. Unfortunately, at present the data set regarding the outcomes of treatment for chronic dissections is poor with small series, mixing acute and chronic cases. Several registries are now investigating the outcome of endovascular repair of chronic dissections. The Virtue study is a prospective single arm clinical registry designed to evaluate the Valiant endograft [53] in the treatment of acute, sub-acute and chronic type B dissections. The study plans to recruit 100 patients with type B dissection from 18 European centers. The primary end point is procedure, device or disease related mortality at 12 months but, more importantly, patients will be evaluated by serial imaging up to 36 months post-procedure, and a core lab will evaluate the results of computed tomography (CT) imaging. This study will provide reliable data regarding the morphology of the aorta following endovascular treatment, and in particular may help to define the results of endovascular therapy in sub-acute and chronic cases. Both Boston Medical and LeMaitre are acquiring similar registry data.

Endovascular treatment of chronic aortic dissections – St George's Vascular Institute

INDICATIONS FOR TREATMENT, RESULTS AND PROCEDURAL DETAILS

In our center the indications for the endovascular treatment of chronic dissections are an aortic diameter exceeding 5.5 cm (female) or 6.0 cm (male), rapid expansion, or the onset of complications (rupture, visceral ischemia, renal compromise or lower limb ischemia). We accept both chronic type B dissections and chronic type A dissections that have expanded following root replacement for acute type A aortic dissection.

Ideally, the proximal lading zone for endograft placement should measure at least 2 cm on the lesser curvature of the arch. This is often problematic and requires bypass of the great vessels, with carotid-carotid-left subclavian bypass, to ensure a sufficient proximal attachment site (Fig. 1). In cases of chronic type A dissection, bypass from the pre-existing ascending aortic graft to the innominate and left common carotid arteries facilitates endovascular repair (Fig. 2). The left subclavian artery is routinely revascularized with a left carotid-subclavian bypass in all patients requiring left subclavian artery coverage. The origin of the left subclavian artery is occluded with an Amplatzer plug [54].

During endovascular repair, attention is given to covering the primary entry site. The graft is then placed distally to level of the diaphragm, in an attempt to maximize false lumen thrombosis. Early experience with coverage of the primary entry tear and minimal distal extension of the endograft was associated with a high rate of re-intervention. Cross sectional imaging is performed immediately post procedure, at 1 month, 3 months and then 6 monthly to 18 months and annually thereafter.

In total we have treated 40 patients with chronic aortic dissection. Seven of these patients (17.5%) had Marfan syndrome, and 10% presented with rupture. Great vessel bypass was required in 25% of cases. There were no cases of stroke or paraplegia. Three patients died within 30 days of the procedure (7.5%). Two deaths occurred from rupture

Table — COMPARISON OF STUDIES REPORTS OF ENDOVASCULAR TREATMENT OF CHRONIC TYPE B DISSECTION

First author [ref.]	Device	No. of chronic	Total patients	Procedural success	Secondary procedures	Stroke	Paraplegia	Other Morbidity	30 day mortality	Total mortality	Thrombosis	FU
Tespili [12]		27	43	100%	0%	0%	0%	2	NA	9.3%	NA	29 m
Attia [13]	Talent	7	40	86%	0%	0%	14.20%	14.20%	0%	0%	NA	15 m
Livi [14]	Talent, Excluder, Tag, Zenith	2	51	100%	0%	0%	0%	0%	0%	0%	50%	16 m
Chu [15]		3	53	89%	NA	NA	NA	NA	0%	NA	NA	22 m
Czerny [16]	Excluder, Talent, Relay	6	6	100%	0%	0%	0%	16.70%	0	0%	83%	16 m
Yang [17]	Talent, Aegis	40	76	100%	0%	0%	0%	15.80%	NA	1.3%	NA	15 m
Kiyotaka [18]	Gianturco	35	37	100%	5%	0%	0%	72%	0%	3%	81%	44 m
Piffaretti [19]	Excluder, Gore, Talent	6	52	100%	NA	16.70%	0%	NA	3.10%	NA	NA	18 m
Kaya [20]	Talent, Excluder	12	28	100%	14%	0%	14%	3%	3.6%	21.4%	NA	11 m
Chen [21]	Angiolet, Angcover	19	62	100%	0%	0	0%	0	4.8%	5.5%	95.7%	27.7 m
Bockler [22]	Talent, Excluder, endofit	14	37	97%	7%	0%	0%	22%	0%	28%	44%	24 m
Gaxotte [23]	Talent, Excluder	21	50	100%	NA	0%	0%	NA	NA	NA	63%	15 m
Suzuki [24]	Dacron, Z stent	31	45	100%	NA	0%	0%	NA	0%	9.7%	81%	15 m
Dong [25]	Talent, Endofit, Aegis	23	30	83%	3.3%	0%	0%	26.60%	9.00%	9%	86.7%	1-32 m
Guo [26]		102	178	NA	NA	0%	NA	NA	NA	NA	NA	NA
Kusagawa [27]		17	49	100%	0%	0%	NA	NA	0%	0%	36%	42 m
Kato [28]		12	21	90.4%	NA	0%	NA	NA	NA	NA	77%	NA

Table — COMPARISON OF STUDIES REPORTS OF ENDOVASCULAR TREATMENT OF CHRONIC TYPE B DISSECTION

First author [ref.]	Device	No. of chronic	Total patients	Procedural success	Secondary procedures	Stroke	Paraplegia	Other Morbidity	30 day mortality	Total mortality	Thrombosis	FU
Shimono [29]		10	28	NA	NA	NA	NA	NA	NA	NA	NA	NA
Fattori [30]		4	18	NA	NA	NA	NA	NA	NA	NA	NA	NA
Fattori [31]	Talent, Excluder	12	70	100%	0%	0%	0%	4.54%	4.55%	4.55%	90.9%	14 m
Czermak [32]	Vanguard, Talent	2	7	86%	0%	0%	0%	NA	0%	14.2%	55%	25.1 m
Won [33]	Homemade	12	23	91%	0%	0%	0%	NA	0%	NA	83%	
Kato [34]	Homemade	14	15	100%	0%	0%	0%	0%	0%	0%		24 m
Kato [35]	Homemade	14	38	100%	0%	0%	0%	14%	0%	0%	NA	
Duda [36]	Talent, Gore TAG	5	16	NA	NA	NA	NA	NA	NA	NA	NA	NA
Nienaber [37]	Talent	12	12	100%	0%	0%	0%	0%	0%	0%	NA	27 m
Bortone [38]	Talent, Excluder	14	31	61.5%	0%	0%	0%	NA	8.3%	8.3%	NA	NA
Shim [39]	Homemade	15	15	93%	14%	0%	0%	7%	7%	14%	66.6%	31.5 m
Pamler [40]	Talent	13	14	100%	28.6%	0%	7.20%	0%	0%	0%	NA	14 m
Lopera [41]	Homemade	6	10	90%	0%	0%	0%	20%	0%	10%	90%	20 m
Lambrechts [42]	AneuRx, Talent, Excluder	6	26	100%	0%	0%	0%	NA	0%	0%	90.9%	8 m
Lonn [43]	Excluder, Talent	4	20	100%	0%	0%	NA	NA	NA	NA	90%	13 m
Bortone [44]	Talent, Excluder, Zenith, endofit	19	129	95.3%	0%	0%	0%	10.50%	NA	NA	NA	20 m
Destrieux [45]		17	32	100%	NA	0%	0%	NA	NA	NA	NA	13.5 m

Table COMPARISON OF STUDIES REPORTS OF ENDOVASCULAR TREATMENT OF CHRONIC TYPE B DISSECTION

First author [ref.]	Device	No. of chronic	Total patients	Procedural success	Secondary procedures	Stroke	Paraplegia	Other Morbidity	30 day mortality	Total mortality	Thrombosis	FU
Li [46]		8	9	87.5%	12.5%	0%	0%	12%	12.5%	24%	88.9%	7 m
Hansen [47]	AneuRx, Talent, Excluder	8	60	100%	12.5%	0%	0%	50%	13%	13%	100%	24 m
Lee [48]	Homemade	37	46	96%	0%	0%	0%	NA	0%	NA	74%	34 m
Nathanson [49]	Gore TAG	17	40	95%	0%	0%	NA	NA	0%	NA	NA	15 m
Eggebrecht [50]	Talent	28	38	100%	24%	0%	0%	14.2%	0%	40.9%	72%	46 m

*Excluded non-English language
NA: not available

Methods used to compile the table:

- A search of Pub Med was used with the search criteria "endovascular treatment aortic dissections" to identify potential papers. These were then examined to determine those that reported series of patients who were endovascularly treated for chronic type B dissections.
- The column "total patients" reports the total number of patients in a study and "no. of chronic" reports how many of these had chronic type B dissections.
- "Procedural success" is defined as primary sealing of the entry site of the false lumen.
- "Secondary procedures" shows the amount of procedures that were needed subsequently due to failure of treatment, or further complications.
- "Stroke" and "paraplegia" reflects the rate of stroke/TIA and paraplegia following the endovascular intervention.
- "Other morbidity" expresses all other complications other than neurological events and death. It is not explored in further detail as studies vary widely in how morbidity is reported. In some, only serious complications are reported, whereas others report every single adverse event no matter how small.
- "30 day mortality" is the amount of patients who passed away within 30 days of the procedure.
- "Total mortality" is the percentage of patients who died during the entire study length. This is related to the amount of follow up, as the longer studies will naturally have a greater mortality. The literature does not distinguish between death related to the dissection and death from other causes consistently enough to separate it out in this table.
- "Thrombosis" refers to the percentage of patients who have complete thrombosis of the false lumen, at the level of the stent, by the end of the study.
- "Follow up" (FU) is the mean length of follow up for patients in the studies.

Throughout the table 0% represents a rate of zero for the respective data, whereas "n/a" reflects the data is not available. The reason that there are many "n/a s" is that where a study did not distinguish the data for chronic dissections separately from the other pathologies it was not included.

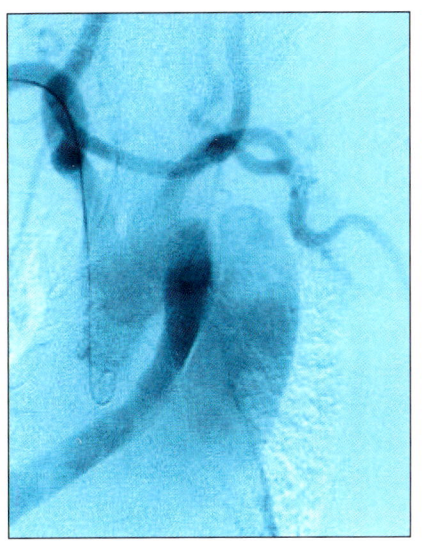

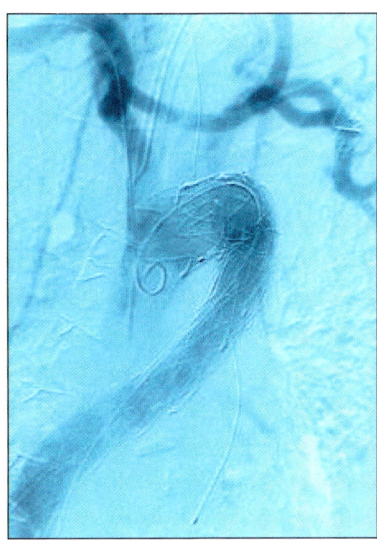

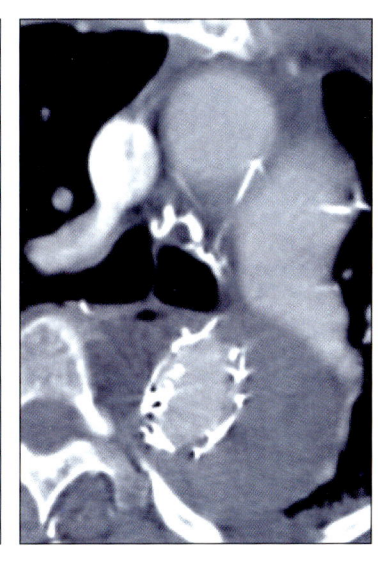

FIG. 1 Patient with Marfan syndrome and a chronic type B dissection. A short proximal landing zone has been modified by a carotid-carotid-left subclavian bypass. The endograft has been positioned satisfactorily.

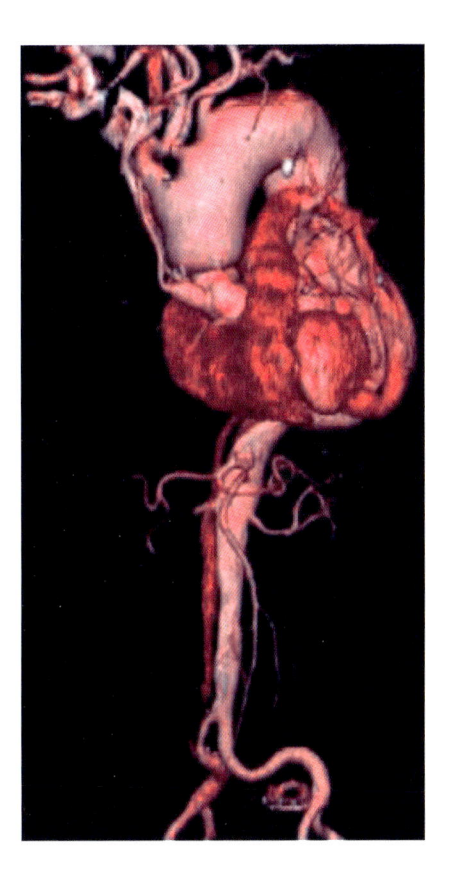

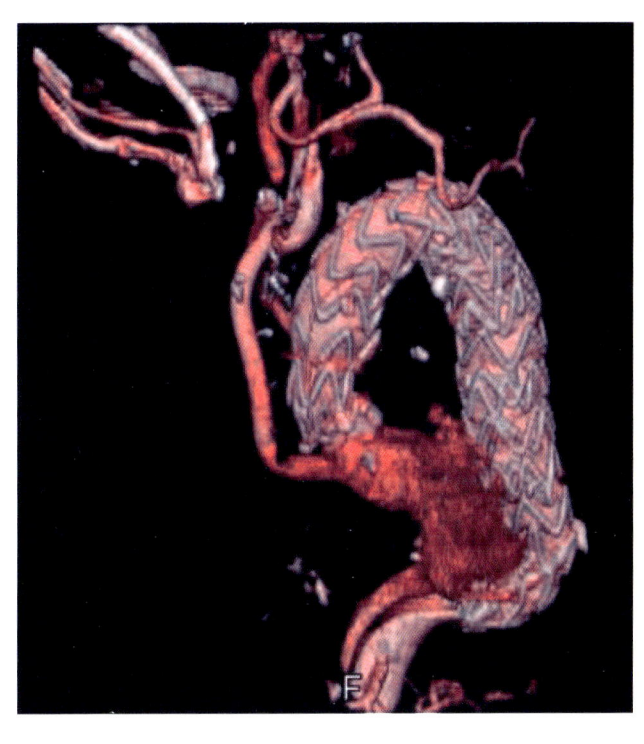

FIG. 2 Patient with a chronic type A dissection and previous ascending aortic replacement. A graft has been performed from the ascending aortic reconstruction to the innominate artery. A carotid-carotid-subclavian bypass completes the revascularization of the great vessels. A stent has then been placed from the ascending aortic graft to the thoracic aorta at the level of the diaphragm.

of the false lumen in the abdomen following patient discharge. The remaining death was due to a retrograde type A dissection. In view of the deaths from false lumen rupture, the follow-up regimen was altered to more frequent cross sectional imaging in the months after the procedure to identify patients with persistent false lumen filling and aneurysm expansion.

AORTIC REMODELLING AFTER ENDOVASCULAR REPAIR AND REINTERVENTIONS

The false lumen thrombosis rates for 40 chronic dissections (CAD), compared to 38 acute dissections (AAD) treated at the St George's Vascular Institute are illustrated in Fig. 3 for the false lumen at the level of the stent, and Fig. 4 for the false

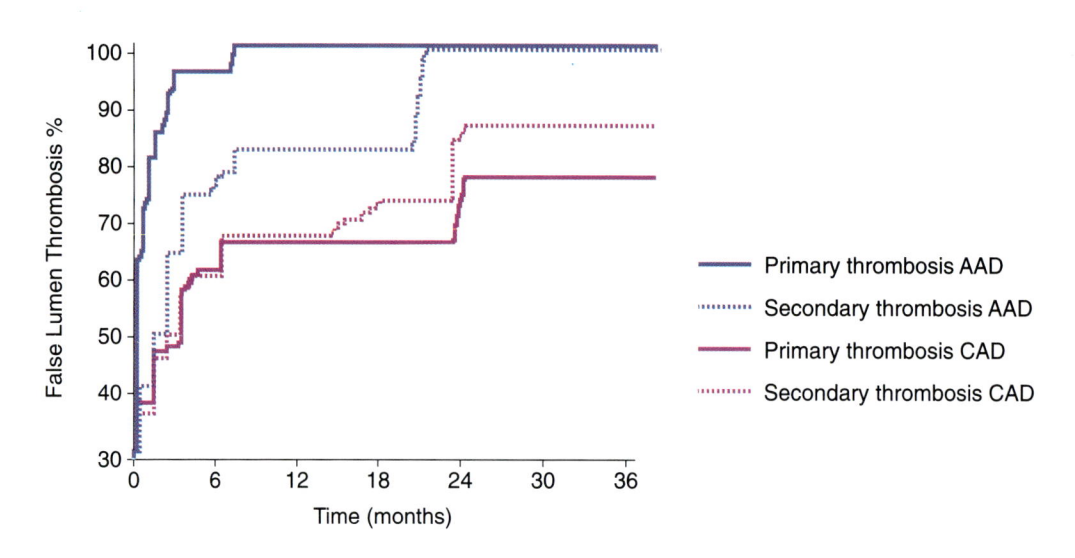

FIG. 3 Graph plotting rates of false lumen thrombosis at the level of the endograft in the thoracic aorta. Data are given as primary and secondary (after re-intervention) thrombosis rates for acute type B dissections (AAD) and chronic type B dissection (CAD).

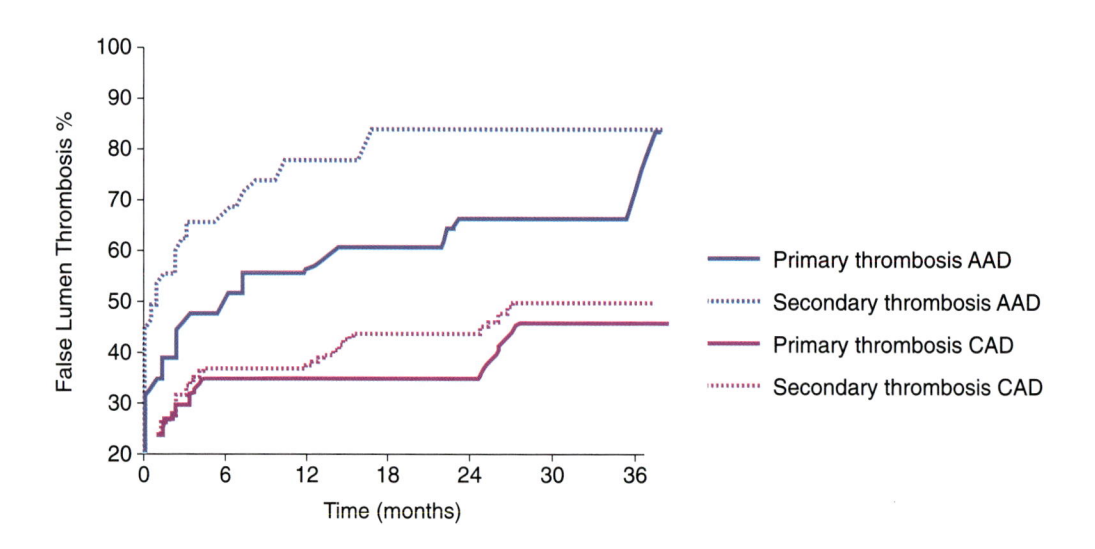

FIG. 4 Graph plotting rates of false lumen thrombosis below the level of the endograft in the thoracic aorta. Data are given as primary and secondary (after re-intervention) thrombosis rates for acute type B dissections (AAD) and chronic type B dissection (CAD).

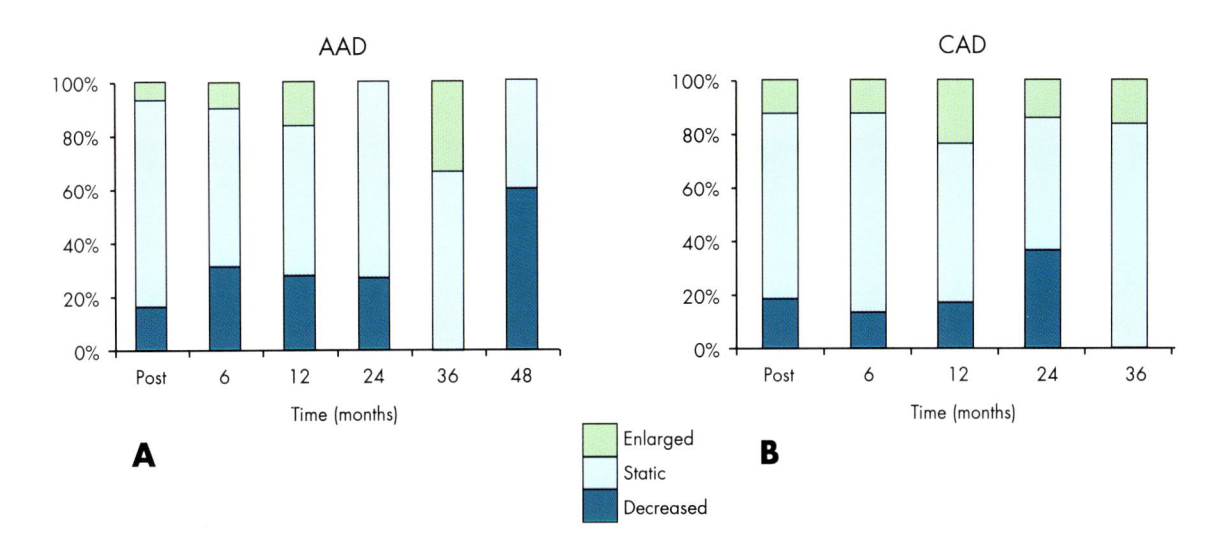

FIG. 5 Graph plotting the change in the maximum short axis diameter of the thoracic aorta following treatment for acute type B dissections (AAD) (A) and chronic type B dissection (CAD) (B). Significant rates of enlargement and regression are defined by a change of 5mm or more from the pre-intervention CT.

lumen of the thoracic aorta below the endograft. The figure illustrates that complete false lumen thrombosis is more easily achieved in acute than chronic cases, and that false lumen thrombosis is more complete at the level of the endograft than below this level. In CAD, the false lumen thrombosis rate exceeds 80% after secondary procedures have been considered. Noticeably, the incidence of false lumen thrombosis is worse below the level of the endograft in both AAD and CAD. There are a significant proportion of patients in whom the maximum thoracic diameter increases after treatment of either AAD or CAD (Fig. 5).

Managing a persistently perfused false lumen at or below the level of the endograft is a particular challenge in patients with chronic dissections as the rate of incomplete thrombosis is high. Assuming that there is no proximal endoleak, we consider re-intervention in patients with persistently perfused false lumens if there is evidence of disease progression or significant aneurysmal degeneration. In these cases, detailed imaging is required to determine whether the perfused false lumen is filling from above, below and where the major re-entry points are situated. In cases where the false lumen is filling form a re-entry point in thoracic aorta, then the endograft may be extended down as far as needed to the level of the celiac axis.

In cases where filling is from a natural fenestration at one of the visceral vessels, three options are available. If there is one major point of re-entry, then consideration may be given to closing this with a covered stent. This would be a relatively unusual appearance in our experience, but presents a less morbid option than closure of multiple fenestrations with either a branched endograft or a visceral hybrid procedure (Fig. 6).

In cases where multiple fenestrations and re-entry sites exist, the endovascular options are more difficult. Two approaches used in our center are either to debranch the visceral and renal arteries from retrograde grafts and then perform total thoracoabdominal stenting into the iliac system (Figs 7,8); alternatively, the thoraco-abdominal aorta may be excluded by the use of a totally fenestrated or branched graft.

Maintaining closure of the false lumen in CAD is difficult and requires constant surveillance and frequent reintervention. In our series, the cumulative re-intervention rate was 35% at 2 years. The most significant re-interventions included 2 distal endograft extensions; 3 visceral hybrid procedures; 2 isolated endovascular abdominal aortic aneurysm repairs and 2 repairs of type A dissections.

Conclusion

Endovascular treatment of chronic dissections is perhaps the least well documented of the endovascular procedures in the thoracic aorta, and has a

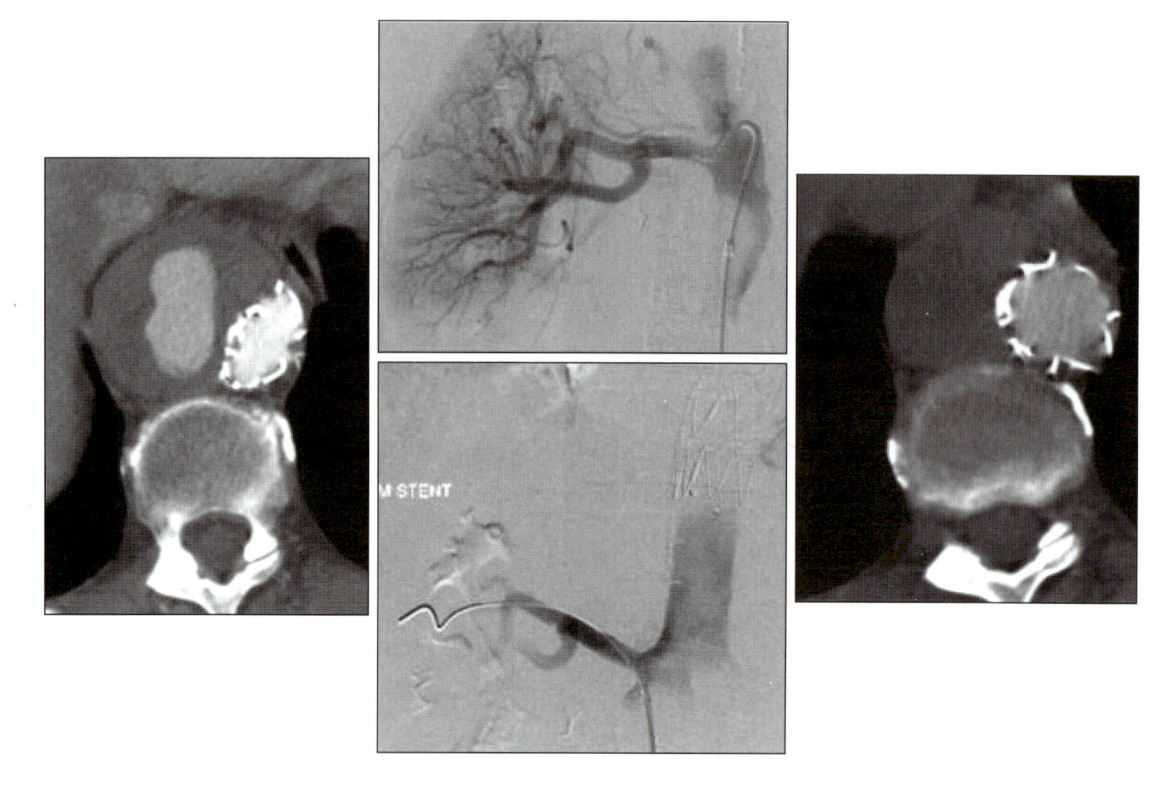

FIG. 6 Patient who developed a persistently perfused false lumen and increasing aortic diameter following treatment of an acute ruptured aortic dissection. Angiography demonstrated that the principle re-entry point involved the origin of the right renal artery. Following stenting of the renal artery, the false lumen thrombosed and the aortic diameter decreased in diameter.

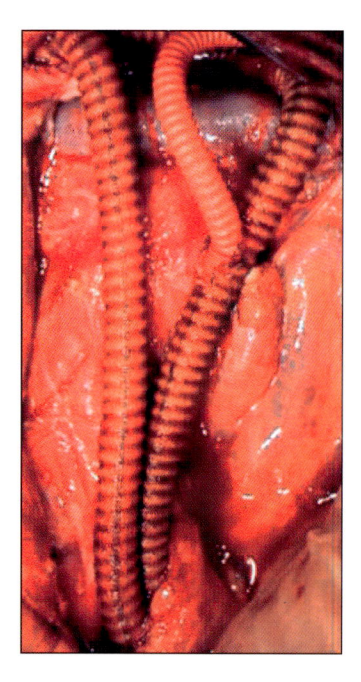

FIG. 7 Preoperative picture of a visceral revascularization that preceded total thoracoabdominal stenting. Grafts are passing from the left iliac artery to superior mesenteric artery, celiac axis and left renal artery.

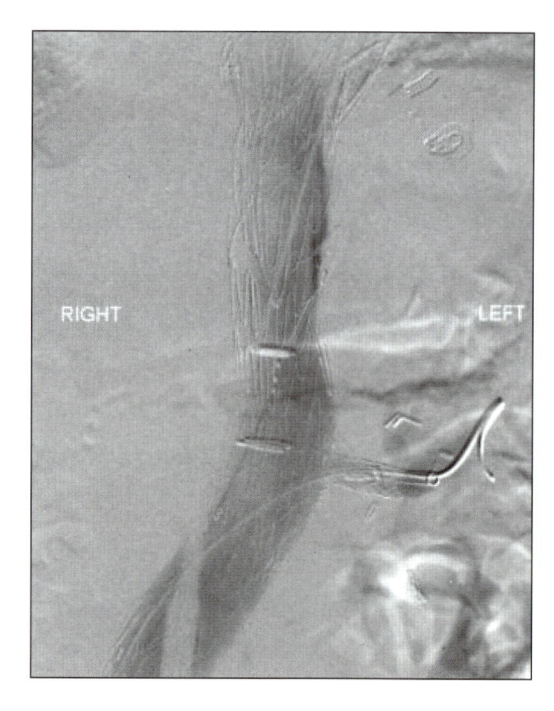

FIG. 8 Repair of a chronic aortic dissecting aneurysm with total thoracoabdominal stenting and a branched graft to the left renal artery.

poor evidence base. The indications for treatment require further definition from sub-group analyzes, especially in the sub-acute stage. The strategy for endovascular repair requires further attention with detail as to the necessity for closure of both primary entry tear and subsequent re-entry sites.

REFERENCES

1 Nienaber CA, Rehders TC, Ince H. Interventional strategies for treatment of aortic dissection. *J Cardiovasc Surg (Torino)* 2006; 47: 487-496.
2 Suzuki T, Mehta RH, Ince H et al. Clinical profiles and outcomes of acute type B aortic dissection in the current era: lessons from the International Registry of Aortic Dissection. *Circulation* 2003; 108 Suppl 1: II312-317.
3 Tsai TT, Fattori R, Trimarchi S et al. Long-term survival in patients presenting with type B acute aortic dissection: insights from the International Registry of Acute Aortic Dissection. *Circulation* 2006; 114: 2226-2231.
4 Winnerkvist A, Lockowandt U, Rasmussen E et al., Radegran K. A prospective study of medically treated acute type B aortic dissection. *Eur J Vasc Endovasc Surg* 2006;32:349-355.
5 Onitsuka S, Akashi H, Tayama K et al. Long-term outcome and prognostic predictors of medically treated acute type B aortic dissections. *Ann Thorac Surg* 2004; 78: 1268-1273.
6 Estrera AL, Miller CC, Goodrick J et al. Update on outcomes of acute type B aortic dissection. *Ann Thorac Surg* 2007; 83: S842-845.
7 Nienaber CA, Zannetti S, Barbieri B et al. INvestigation of STEnt grafts in patients with type B Aortic Dissection: design of the INSTEAD trial–a prospective, multicenter, European randomized trial. *Am Heart J* 2005; 149: 592-599.
8 Sueyoshi E, Sakamoto I, Hayashi K et al. Growth rate of aortic diameter in patients with type B aortic dissection during the chronic phase. *Circulation* 2004; 110 (11 Suppl 1): II256-261.
9 Song JM, Kim SD, Kim JH, et al. Long-term predictors of descending aorta aneurysmal change in patients with aortic dissection. *J Am Coll Cardiol* 2007; 50: 799-804.
10 Crawford ES, Crawford JL, Safi HJ et al. Thoracoabdominal aortic aneurysms: preoperative and intraoperative factors determining immediate and long-term results of operations in 605 patients. *J Vasc Surg* 1986; 3: 389-404.
11 Leurs LJ, Bell R, Degrieck Y et al. Endovascular treatment of thoracic aortic diseases: combined experience from the EUROSTAR and United Kingdom Thoracic Endograft registries. *J Vasc Surg* 2004; 40: 670-679.
12 Tespili M, Banfi C, Valsecchi O et al. Endovascular treatment of thoracic aortic disease: Mid-term follow-up. *Catheter Cardiovasc Interv* 2007; 70: 595-601.
13 Attia C, Villard J, Boussel L et al. Endovascular repair of localized pathological lesions of the descending thoracic aorta: midterm results. *Cardiovasc Intervent Radiol* 2007; 30: 628-637.
14 Livi U, Piccoli G, Ciccarese G et al. Stent-grafting of the thoracic aorta: feasibility and early results in acute and chronic lesions. *J Cardiovasc Med (Hagerstown)* 2007; 8: 504-510.
15 Chu MW, Forbes TL, Kirk Lawlor D et al. Endovascular repair of thoracic aortic disease: early and midterm experience. *Vasc Endovascular Surg* 2007; 41: 186-191.
16 Czerny M, Zimpfer D, Rodler S et al. Endovascular stent-graft placement of aneurysms involving the descending aorta originating from chronic type B dissections. *Ann Thorac Surg* 2007; 83: 1635-1639.
17 Yang J, Zuo J, Yang L et al. Endovascular stent-graft treatment of thoracic aortic dissection. *Interact Cardiovasc Thorac Surg* 2006; 5: 688-691.
18 Kiyotaka I, Shinichi S, Keiji U. Early and medium-term results of stent-graft treatment of DeBakey type III aortic dissection. *J Cardiovasc Surg (Torino)* 2006; 47: 651-657.
19 Piffaretti G, Tozzi M, Lomazzi C et al. Complications after endovascular stent-grafting of thoracic aortic diseases. *J Cardiothorac Surg* 2006; 1: 26.
20 Kaya A, Heijmen RH, Overtoom TT et al. Thoracic stent grafting for acute aortic pathology. *Ann Thorac Surg* 2006; 82: 560-565.
21 Chen S, Yei F, Zhou L et al. Endovascular stent-grafts treatment in acute aortic dissection (type B): clinical outcomes during early, late, or chronic phases. *Catheter Cardiovasc Interv* 2006; 68: 319-325.
22 Bockler D, Schumacher H, Ganten M et al. Complications after endovascular repair of acute symptomatic and chronic expanding Stanford type B aortic dissections. *J Thorac Cardiovasc Surg* 2006; 132: 361-368.
23 Gaxotte V, Thony F, Rousseau H et al. Midterm results of aortic diameter outcomes after thoracic stent-graft implantation for aortic dissection: a multicenter study. *J Endovasc Ther* 2006; 13: 127-138.
24 Suzuki S, Imoto K, Uchida K et al. Midterm results of transluminal endovascular grafting in patients with DeBakey type III dissecting aortic aneurysms. *Ann Thorac Cardiovasc Surg* 2006; 12: 42-49.
25 Dong Xu S, Zhong Li Z, Huang FJ et al. Treating aortic dissection and penetrating aortic ulcer with stent graft: thirty cases. *Ann Thorac Surg* 2005; 80: 864-868.
26 Guo W, Gai LY, Liu XP et al. The endovascular repair of aortic dissection: early clinical results of 178 cases. *Zhonghua Wai Ke Za Zhi* 2005; 43: 921-925.
27 Kusagawa H, Shimono T, Ishida M et al. Changes in false lumen after transluminal stent-graft placement in aortic dissections: six years' experience. *Circulation* 2005; 111: 2951-2957.
28 Kato M, Matsuda T, Kaneko M et al. Outcomes of stent-graft treatment of false lumen in aortic dissection. *Circulation* 1998; 98 (19 Suppl): II305-11.
29 Shimono T, Kato N, Hirano T et al. Early and mid-term results of endovascular stent grafting for aortic aneurysms. *Nippon Geka Gakkai Zasshi* 1999; 100: 500-505.
30 Fattori R, Napoli G, Parlapiano M et al. Endovascular treatment in diseases of the thoracic aorta. *Radiol Med (Torino)* 1999; 98: 379-385.
31 Fattori R, Napoli G, Lovato L et al. Descending thoracic aortic diseases: stent-graft repair. *Radiology* 2003; 229: 176-183.
32 Czermak BV, Waldenberger P, Fraedrich G et al. Treatment of Stanford type B aortic dissection with stent-grafts: preliminary results. *Radiology* 2000; 217: 544-550.
33 Won JY, Lee DY, Shim WH et al. Elective endovascular treatment of descending thoracic aortic aneurysms and chronic dissections with stent-grafts. *J Vasc Interv Radiol* 2001; 12: 575-582.

34. Kato N, Hirano T, Shimono T et al. Treatment of chronic type B aortic dissection with endovascular stent-graft placement. *Cardiovasc Intervent Radiol* 2000; 23: 60-62.
35. Kato N, Shimono T, Hirano T et al. Midterm results of stent-graft repair of acute and chronic aortic dissection with descending tear: the complication-specific approach. *J Thorac Cardiovasc Surg* 2002; 124: 306-312.
36. Duda SH, Pusich B, Raygrotzki S et al. Endovascular implantation of stent-grafts in the thoracic aorta -mid-term results of a prospective controlled study. *Rofo* 2002; 174: 485-489.
37. Nienaber CA, Fattori R, Lund G et al. Nonsurgical reconstruction of thoracic aortic dissection by stent-graft placement. *N Engl J Med* 1999; 340: 1539-1545.
38. Bortone AS, Schena S, D'Agostino D et al. Immediate versus delayed endovascular treatment of post-traumatic aortic pseudoaneurysms and type B dissections: retrospective analysis and premises to the upcoming European trial. *Circulation* 2002; 106 (12 Suppl 1): I234-240.
39. Shim WH, Koo BK, Yoon YS et al. Treatment of thoracic aortic dissection with stent-grafts: midterm results. *J Endovasc Ther* 2002 ; 9: 817-821.
40. Pamler RS, Kotsis T, Gorich J et al. Complications after endovascular repair of type B aortic dissection. *J Endovasc Ther* 2002; 9: 822-828.
41. Lopera J, Patino JH, Urbina C et al. Endovascular treatment of complicated type-B aortic dissection with stent-grafts: midterm results. *J Vasc Interv Radiol* 2003 ; 14: 195-203.
42. Lambrechts D, Casselman F, Schroeyers P et al. Endovascular treatment of the descending thoracic aorta. *Eur J Vasc Endovasc Surg* 2003; 26: 437-444.
43. Lonn L, Delle M, Falkenberg M et al. Endovascular treatment of type B thoracic aortic dissections. *J Card Surg* 2003; 18: 539-544
44. Bortone AS, De Cillis E, D'Agostino D et al. Stent graft treatment of thoracic aortic disease. *Surg Technol Int* 2004; 12: 189-193.
45. Destrieux-Garnier L, Haulon S, Willoteaux S et al. Midterm results of endoluminal stent grafting of the thoracic aorta. *Vascular* 2004; 12: 179-185.
46. Li XX, Wang SM, Chen W et al. Endovascular stent-graft repair of aortic dissection. *Asian Cardiovasc Thorac Ann* 2004 ; 12: 99-102.
47. Hansen CJ, Bui H, Donayre CE et al. Complications of endovascular repair of high-risk and emergent descending thoracic aortic aneurysms and dissections. *J Vasc Surg* 2004; 40: 228-234.
48. Lee KH, Won JY, Lee DY et al. Elective stent-graft treatment of aortic dissections. *J Endovasc Ther* 2004; 11: 667-675.
49. Nathanson DR, Rodriguez-Lopez JA, Ramaiah VG et al. Endoluminal stent-graft stabilization for thoracic aortic dissection. *J Endovasc Ther* 2005; 12: 354-359.
50. Eggebrecht H, Herold U, Kuhnt O et al. Endovascular stent-graft treatment of aortic dissection: determinants of post-interventional outcome. *Eur Heart J* 2005; 26: 489-497.
51. Thompson M, Ivaz S, Cheshire N et al. Early Results of Endovascular Treatment of the Thoracic Aorta Using the Valiant Endograft. *Cardiovasc Intervent Radiol* 2007; 30: 1130-1138.
52. Fattori R, Nienaber CA, Rousseau H et al. Results of endovascular repair of the thoracic aorta with the Talent Thoracic stent graft: the Talent Thoracic Retrospective Registry. *J Thorac Cardiovasc Surg* 2006; 132: 332-339.
53. Brooks M, Loftus I, Morgan R et al. The Valiant thoracic endograft. *J Cardiovasc Surg (Torino)* 2006; 47: 269-278.
54. Taylor JD, Dunckley M, Thompson M et al. Endovascular Management of Chronic Type B Dissecting Aortic Aneurysm Utilizing Aortic and Renal Stents. *Cardiovasc Intervent Radiol* 2007; [Epub ahead of print].

21

DAMAGE REPAIR AFTER THORACIC EVAR

STEPHAN LANGER, GOTTFRIED MOMMERTZ, THOMAS KOEPPEL
GEERT WILLEM SCHURINK, MICHAEL JACOBS

Since Dake et al. [1] published their first results with transluminally placed homemade nitinol-Dacron endografts for the repair of descending thoracic aneurysm (DTAA) in 1994, this therapeutic approach has achieved wide acceptance in the treatment of different thoracic aortic pathologies. The available experiences are promising, showing acceptable mortality and paraplegia rates [2]. But the question wether open or thoracic endovascular repair (TEVAR) is the favourable therapy of thoracic aortic pathologies still remains unanswered. For some indications like traumatic aortic rupture, TEVAR has rapidly become therapy of choice [3], but for thoracic aortic aneurysm (TAA) and dissection, the current discussion is controversly due to frequent complications. Series involving stent grafting of TAA have shown that endoleaks occur in 3%-29% [4,5]. Of these, about 50% are life threatening type I endoleaks with unchanged vascularized aneurysm sacks. The risk of retrograde type A dissection after TEVAR is approximately 6.8% with a procedure related mortality of 40% [6]. Incomplete deployed or total collapsed stentgrafts in the thoracic aorta have been published in case reports in the majority of cases [7,8]. In case of stent-graft failure, secondary interventional correction is feasible [9], but in a small percentage damage repair by means of open surgery is required due to inadequate landing zones not suitable for extension cuffs or inappropriate morphological vessel changes due to progressive aneurysmal disease. In contrast to endovascular abdominal aortic repair (EVAR), less is known about complications and conversions after TEVAR. However, it is apparent that thoracic endovascular aortic failure repair (TEFAR) by means of open surgery comprises a large surgical trauma. In this chapter, the spare published data concerning TEFAR will be reviewed and discussed with our own experience in managing eight conversions to open repair following failed thoracic endografting.

Personal experience

Patient population

In a six year period between 6 June 2001 and 6 June 2007 we performed altogether 316 thoracic and thoracoabdominal operations in the European Vascular Center Aachen-Maastricht. Of these, 210 were conventional open repairs and 106 endovascular procedures. In 50 endovascular patients (47.1%) the indication for acute thoracic aortic stentgrafting was given as shown in Table I. In 5 patients (4.7%) of the endovascular group plus 3 patients who were referred from other centers conversion to open repair was necessary. Thus we overview 8 TEFAR patients due to severe and endovascularly not rectifiable complications. The mean age of the 5 male and 3 female patients was 51.7 years (range 40-63 years). The initial aortic pathologies before TEVAR were various and included acute symptomatic type B dissection in 2 patients, expanding chronic type B dissection in 2, expanding chronic arch and descending dissection following previous Bentall procedure for type A dissection in 1, chronic false aneurysm in one and traumatic rupture in 2 patients (Table II).

The indications for open surgical correction included retrograde type A aortic dissection in two (patients 1 and 2 in Table II), type Ib endoleak with contained rupture in 1 patient (patient 3), false aneurysm rupture due to distal stent migration in 1 patient (patient 4) and type Ia endoleak in four (patients 5-8). Four patients underwent emergency procedures and 4 were elective conversions.

Emergency surgery

In 2 patients with retrograde type A dissection emergency surgery was necessary. The first patient initially suffered from acute type B dissection and developed critical mesenteric and leg ischemia. After uneventful stentgrafting he developed acute retrograde type A dissection 38 days later which was caused by an intimal tear induced by the proximal bare springs of a Talent endograft. During acute conversion, a supracoronary ascending aorta and arch replacement with elephant trunk procedure was performed. The supracoronary vessels were revascularized with a 12 mm prosthesis to the innominate artery and an 8 mm graft to the left common carotid artery and left subclavian artery. After excising the proximal bare stents, the remaining endograft in the descending aorta was hand sewed to the arch prosthesis as shown in the surgeon's draft (Fig. 1). In patient 2 a retrograde type A dissection occurred at the third post implantation day for acute expanding type B dissection, also caused by bare spring induced intimal injury. The operative procedure was analogue to the first patient.

The third patient also operated on in emergency setting was previously treated with an endograft for chronic expanding type B dissection and developed a contained rupture due to a distal type I endoleak and repressurized false lumen, not suitable for endovascular correction because of an inadequate distal landing zone. The endograft was totally removed during conversion and followed by descending aortic replacement. The fourth patient suffered from polytraumatic injuries including a severe thoracic blunt trauma induced contained aortic rupture. Initial successful endovascular repair was performed by placing a Talent endograft. Thirty-one days later he had to undergo emergency conversion because of delayed proximal descending rupture due distal device migration, as assessed by computed tomography (CT) scanning. Open repair included removal of the entire endograft and hemi arch and descending aortic replacement.

Table I	INDICATIONS FOR THORACIC STENT-GRAFTING IN OUR PERSONAL EXPERIENCE (N=106)
Aortic pathology	*N*
Acute (n=50)	
Dissection	19
Symptomatic TAA	3
Ruptured TAA	12
Traumatic rupture	9
Esophageal/bronchial fistula	7
Elective (n=52)	
TAA	46
Chronic dissection	6
TAAA	4
Total	106

Table II OVERVIEW OF THORACIC CONVERSION PROCEDURES

No.	Age	Gender	Aortic pathology	Indication for TEVAR	Failure	Ttc	Conversion	Outcome
1	52	M	Acute type B dissection	Mesenteric and peripheral ischemia	Retrograde type A dissection	38 d	Supracoronary arch replacement, elephant trunk	Discharged
2	63	F	Acute type B dissection	Progressive dilatation	Retrograde type A dissection	3 d	Supracoronary arch replacement, elephant trunk	Discharged
3	43	F	Chronic type B dissection	TAA repair	1. Endoleak Ib 2. contained rupture	10 d	Descending aortic replacement	Discharged
4	40	M	Traumatic rupture Polytrauma	False TAA repair	1. distal stent migration 2. rupture	31 d	Hemi-arch and descending aortic replacement	Died
5	53	F	Chronic type A dissection Bentall 2002	TAA repair	Endoleak Ia	7 d	Arch and prox. descending aortic replacement	Discharged
6	59	M	Chronic type B dissection	TAA repair	Endoleak Ia + II	10 m	Hemi-arch and descending aortic replacement	Discharged
7	47	M	Chronic false TAA	TAA repair	1. Endoleak Ia 2. aortobronchial fistula 3. TIA	37 m	Hemi-arch and descending aortic replacement	Discharged
8	49	M	Traumatic rupture	Sealing rupture	Endoleak Ia	23 d	Supracoronary arch replacement	Discharged

Ttc: time to conversion
d: day
m: month

ELECTIVE SURGERY

The main TEVAR failure in our 4 electively converted patients were type Ia endoleaks. Additionally we noticed 1 type II endoleak, 1 aortobronchial fistula and 1 device related transient ischemic events based on embolization. In 2 cases additional endovascular therapy was not feasible due to unfavourable anatomical situation; the remaining 2 young patients refused further endovascular hybrid procedures and decided for open repair.

Patient number 5 had developed a growing distal arch and proximal descending aortic aneurysm

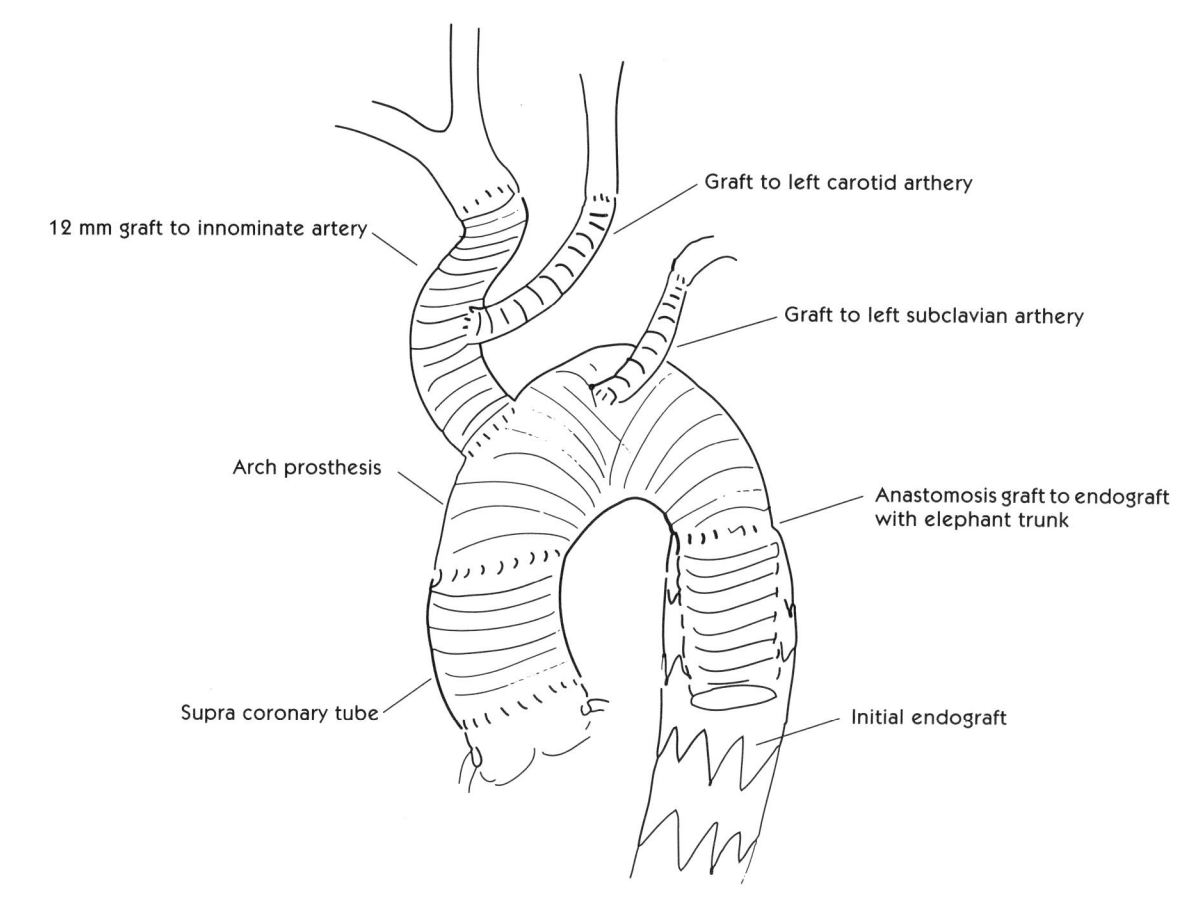

FIG. 1 Surgeons draft showing the operative details after conversion for retrograde type A dissection. Notice the anastomosis between the aortic arch graft and the endograft in an end-to-end fashion with "elephant trunk" technique.

as a consequence of a previous type A dissection, which was initially treated with a Bentall procedure in 2002. In 2006 she presented a large distal arch and descending aneurysm causing croakiness due to recurrent laryngeal nerve compression. To maximize the proximal landing zone, a carotid-carotid bypass was implanted prior to stentgrafting, but the fibrotic dissection membrane prevented complete deployment of the Valiant endograft, resulting in a large type Ia endoleak. Successful conversion to arch and proximal descending aortic replacement combined with complete endograft removal followed one week later.

The sixth patient developed a growing distal arch and descending thoracic aneurysm as a consequence of a type B dissection in 2002. In 2006 he received TEVAR (Talent). The proximal landing zone of the covered part of the device was deployed just distally to the left common carotid artery. During follow up, he presented with a small proximal type Ia and a large type II endoleak nine months later caused by retrograde left subclavian artery bleeding. Despite successful intervention by means of a transbrachially placed occluder device in the proximal sublavian artery (Figs. 2A, B), the aneurysm sack was still vascularized by the type Ia endoleak with subsequent enlarging of the arch and descending aneurysm. Repeat ballooning as an attempt to achieve apposition or endovascular extension after supra-aortic debranching were considered inappropriate in this relatively young patient and conversion to hemi-arch and descending aortic replacement was decided.

Patient number 7 had a history of more than 30 years. In 1971, at the age of 11 years, he underwent

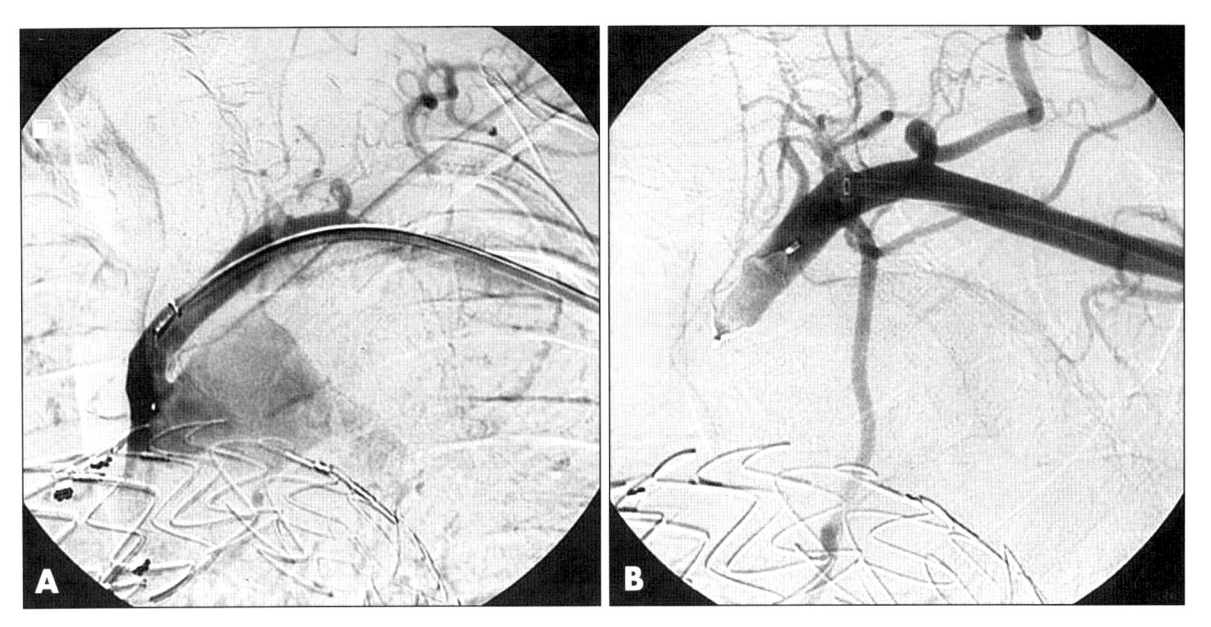

FIG. 2 Endovascular type II endoleak repair (A). The backbleeding left subclavian artery was closed by means of a transbrachially introduced occluder device (B).

left thoracotomy and aortic patch plasty for a false aneurysm after traumatic isthmus rupture. In 2004 he developed paralysis of the left recurrent laryngeal nerve caused by a large anastomotic aneurysm at the aortic patch (Fig. 3A) which was treated with a Talent thoracic endograft. Three uneventful years later he was referred to our department because of cerebral embolizations and hemoptysis. CT-scan confirmed a new type Ia endoleak and a proximal stent migration into the ostium of the left common carotid artery causing repeat cerebral embolization (Fig. 3B). The hemoptysis originated from an intraoperativly confirmed small aortobronchial fistula. Because further endovascular treatment would indicate sternotomy with debranching of the supra-aortic vessels and extension of the endograft, this otherwise healthy patient decided for open repair with hemi-arch and descending replacement after complete removal of the device.

The eigth patient was a morbid obese 49 year old man suffering from hypertension and a rupture of the proximal descending thoracic aorta induced by extreme blood pressure rise during tire changing. The chest x-ray at admission and the following CT-scan demonstrated an extended hematothorax (Figs. 4A, B). In a life saving procedure the leakage close to the left subclavian artery was covered successfully using a Zenith endograft and 3 000 mL blood was drained from the left chest. The control CT scan demonstrated a small type Ia endoleak due to steepness of the aortic arch causing mal-alignment of the device in the inner arch (Fig. 4C). Unfortunately the patient had ascending and arch dilatation with a diameter largen than 42 mm not allowing further endovascular extension as part of a hybrid procedure. After clinical improvement he underwent open supracoronary ascending and aortic arch replacement with preservation of the aortic valve. The graft was sewn to the descending endograft in an end-to-end fashion.

PREOPERATIVE DIAGNOSTIC EVALUATION

Morphologic and anatomic assessment of the thoracoabdominal aorta and iliac access vessels were performed by multi-slice CT and since 2006 dual source spiral CT. Cardiac evaluation included echocardiography and dipyridamole-thallium scanning. In case of detected ischemia, coronary angiography followed. The 4 emergency patients only had echocardiography prior to surgery. Coronary heart disease could be diagnosed in one case; no patient suffered from valve disorders. In all patients the renal function was normal (mean serum creatinine 88μmol/L). Further risk factors were hypertension in 5 and obesity in 2 patients.

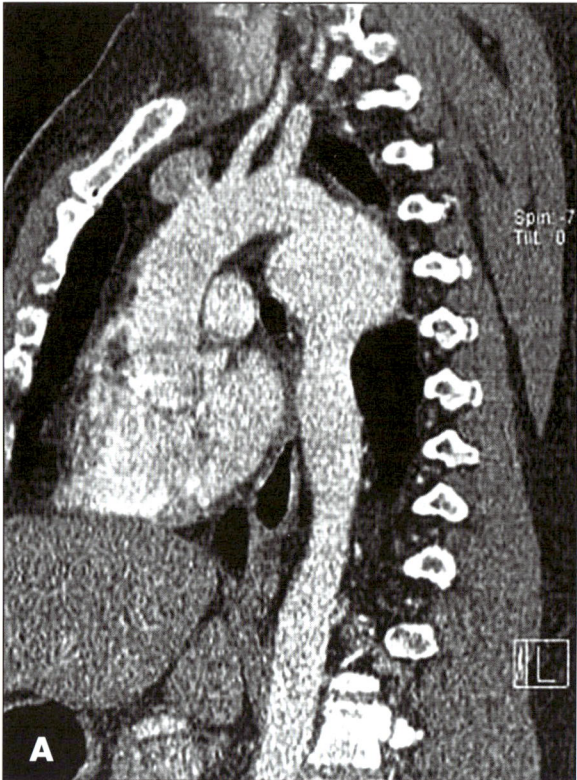

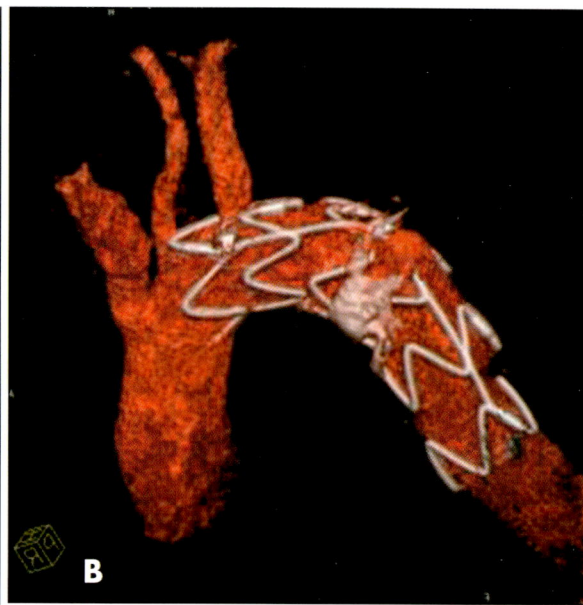

FIG. 3 A - Anastomotic aneurysm in the descending aorta after patch plasty 31 years ago. B - Device migration towards the ostium of the left common carotid artery causing recurrent cerebral embolization.

SURGICAL PROTOCOL

Surgical access was either by sternotomy or left thoracotomy, depending on the extension of the aortic pathology. If aortic valve or ascending replacement is necessary, a sternotomy is required. In case of arch or distal hemi-arch and simultaneous descending aortic replacement a left thoracotomy through the fourth or fifth intercostal space is recommendable. An open anastomosis under cardiac arrest until the level of the innominate artery can be performed using this approach.

In case of extended pathologies including the aortic arch, total extracorporeal circulation with cardiac arrest and selective antegrade brain perfusion is mandatory. If only a descending aortic problem exists, left heart bypass only can be sufficient, but limiting factors can be an inappropriate proximal clamp position and insufficient aortic quality to perform a solid anastomosis.

We recommend moderate hypothermia until 28° C, but profound hypothermia down to 18° can be necessary.

In case of left thoracotomy, cardiac arrest can be achieved by inserting and inflating a Foley catheter in the ascending aorta or ascending aortic graft for administering cardioplegia following opening of the aortic arch. If necessary, a vent should be inserted via the left pulmonary vein. Cerebral protection is established by means of selective antegrade perfusion through catheters with an inflatable balloon at the tip in the brachiocephalic and left carotid artery. These perfusion catheters are connected to the extra-corporeal system and are equipped with pressure channels allowing pressure controlled perfusion of the brain. Furthermore, in each catheter volume flow is assessed with ultrasound flow meters (Transonic, Ithaca, NY, USA). Total antegrade cerebral flow is approximately 10 ml/kg/min with a mean arterial pressure of 60 mmHg. Transcranial Doppler and electroencephalography is used to monitor cerebral perfusion continuously.

Spinal cord blood supply, visceral and renal perfusion is optimized by using continous retrograde aortic perfusion during cross clamping by cannulation of the left femoral artery. Additional spinal cord protection is provided by cerebrospinal fluid (CSF) drainage. Normally we leave the drainage

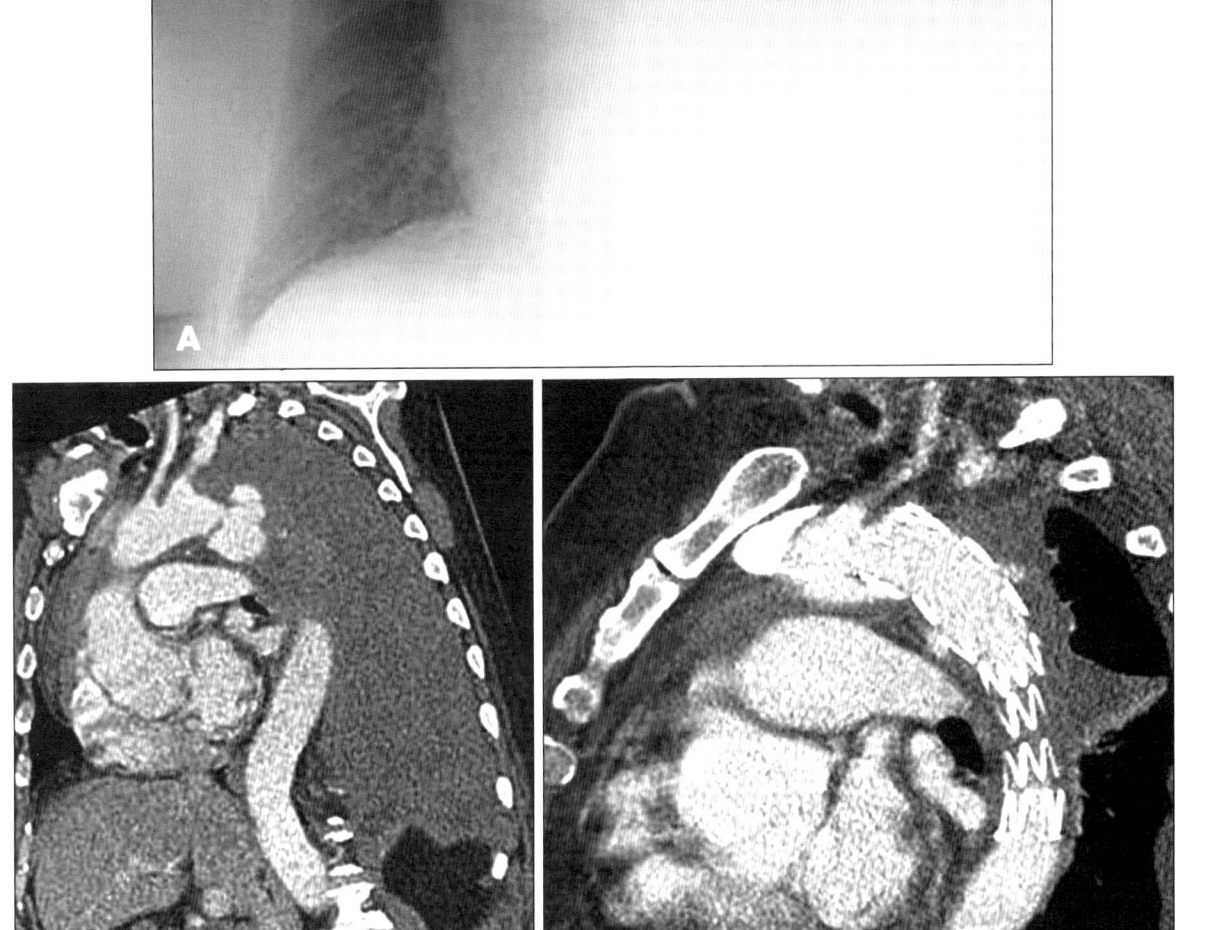

FIG. 4 A - Chest x-ray directly after admission demonstrating left thoracic fluid accumulation. B - CT-scan showing the level of the aortic rupture short distally of the left subclavian artery "loco typico" and the extended hematothorax. C - Small type 1a endoleak due to mal-alignement of the Zenith endograft at the inner curve of the aortic arch.

for 72 hours allowing spontaneous outflow and strive for pressures below 10 mmHg. In addition, motor evoked potential monitoring is carried out to assess spinal cord integrity, guiding intra-operative strategies to prevent neurological deficits. The details of this technique have been described before [10]. It might be a technical advantage to incorporate the endograft into the reconstruction, but it is always an individual decision, to remove or to leave the endograft. A short compendium of our surgical protocol is given in Table III.

In our series 3 patients underwent sternotomy; of these 2 had retrograde type A dissection and 1 with proximal type Ia endoleak in the arch. Total extra corporeal circulation was installed in the usual manner at a temperature of 28° centigrade in 6 patients. Two patients (number 4 and 8 in Table I) were operated under profound hypothermia (18°).

In 5 patients surgical access was performed via left thoracotomy because of distal arch and descending thoracic aortic pathology. However, in 4 of these patients cardiac arrest and antegrade cerebral perfusion was necessary because the aortic disease extended proximally until the brachiocephalic artery, not allowing proximal aortic clamping and therefore necessitating an open anastomosis. In 1 patient cardiac arrest was induced using only profound hypothermia only. Antegrade cerebral perfusion and vent insertion was provided in the same manner as decribed above. One patient was operated on with left heart bypass by means of cannulating the left femoral artery and left pulmonary vein (limited heparinization 0.5 mg/kg). CSF drainage and monitoring of MEP's was carried out in all 4 elective patients

Results

PERIOPERATIVE COURSE

All patients survived the surgical conversion. In both patients with retrograde type A dissection the intimal tear caused by the bare springs could be

Table III Surgical protocol for TEVAR

Extension of diseased aorta	Access	ECC	Neuromonitoring
Ascending aorta/ proximal arch/arch	Sternotomy	Total ECC Antegrade cerebral perfusion	TCD+EEG
Arch with proximal descending arch with DTAA/TAAA	Left thoracotomy Left thoracotomy/laparotomy	Total ECC Antegrade cerebral perfusion Distal aortic perfusion	TCD+EEG MEP
Distal arch with proximal descending Distal arch with DTAA/ TAAA	Left thoracotomy Left thoracotomy/laparotomy	Total ECC or LHB Distal arch perfusion	TCD+EEG MEP
DTAA/TAAA	Left thoracotomy Left thoracolaparotomy	LHB Distal aortic perfusion	MEP

ECC: extra corporeal circulation
DTAA: descending thoracic aortic aneurysm
TAAA: thoraco-abdominal aortic aneurysm
TCD: transcranial Doppler
EEG: Electroencephalography
LHB: left heart bypass
MEP: motor evoked potentials

identified intra-operatively. In both patients, as well as in patient 8 the ascending and arch prosthesis were sewn to the remaining endograft. In patient 1 and 2 an anastomosis between arch prosthesis and endograft was feasible after removal of the uncovered proximal bare metal stents of a Talent device. In patient 8 removal of proximal bare springs was not necessary because of a closed web design (Zenith). We could establish antegrade cerebral perfusion in these 3 patients and postoperative neurological outcome was uneventful.

In two of five left thoracotomies the operation was more difficult due to a redo procedure. Because of severe adherence of the left lung with the chest wall, surgical access was chosen one intercostal space higher and one lower than the previous approach. After complete dissection of severe left lung adherence, a temporary collapse using only right lung ventilation was appropriate to expose the entire arch and descending aorta. In 4 patients the proximal anastomosis was performed in an open end-to end-fashion under continuous antegrade cerebral perfusion. The level was in 1 patient proximal to the brachiocephalic artery and in three at the level of the left carotid artery. In one patient the clamp was positioned more distally between the left carotid and left subclavian artery. Distal clamp position was at mid-thoracic level in 2 at the diaphragm in 3 patients. In all patients retrograde distal aortic perfusion by cannulating the left femoral artery guaranteed lower body, renal and visceral perfusion. Urine output continued in all patients and motor evoked potentials were normal with a mean distal aortic pressure of 60 mmHg. In all 5 patients the endograft was removed completely. Operative data are shown in Table IV. The average cardiac arrest time was 50 min (range 35-121 min). Mean extra corporeal circulation time averaged 175 min (range 123-292 min) and surgical time 373 minutes (range 330-455 min).

POSTOPERATIVE COURSE

Seven patients were extubated within the first 48 postoperative hours. One patient with retrograde type A dissection developed postoperative sepsis due to necrotic cholecystitis and had to undergo open cholecystectomy. This patient was on ventilatory support during 4 days. One patient (patient 4, Table II) died 24 days after uneventful conversion in consequence of a rupture. Postmortem autopsy confirmed a graft infection and distal septic anastomotic leackage. We observed no renal failure, prolonged pulmonary insufficiency or myocardial infarction. We did not encountered any central or peripheral neurological deficits, especially no acute or delayed paraplegia. During a mean follow-up of

Table IV   PROCEDURAL CHARACTERISTICS IN OUR EXPERIENCE

N	Access	Cardiac arrest (min)	Cross clamp (min)	Extracorporal circulation (min)	Surgical time (min)
1	Sternotomy	35	135	292	455
2	Sternotomy	43	133	209	391
3	Left thoracotomy	No cardiac arrest	122	146	359
4	Left thoracotomy	121	120	215	350
5	Left thoracotomy	60	120	138	330
6	Left thoracotomy	45	NA	137	330
7	Left thoracotomy	49	NA	123	347
8	Sternotomy	60	112	147	420

NA: not available

14 months (range 4-71 months) all seven surviving patients are in good clinical condition and CT surveillance proved patent aortic side branches. Furthermore no technical complications like stenosis or anastomotic aneurysms were diagnosed.

LITERATURE SEARCH

Using the key words "TEVAR" or "thoracic stent" and "complication", "conversion" or "secondary intervention", a comprehensive search of the medical literature from 2000-2007 (Pubmed database) was performed. Articles including series or cases with surgical conversion to open repair after failed TEVAR were selected.

Comprehensive literature search identified altogether 38 patients in 12 publications including 1 meta analysis [11], 2 series from voluntary registries [12,13], 3 single center retrospective data [4,6,14] and 4 case reports [15-19]. Two reports evaluated causative anatomic or device factors that may increase the probability of stent graft collapse [7,8]. Table V demonstrates a compilation of the recently published studies or case reports dealing with thoracic conversions after TEVAR.

Discussion

This chapter describes the surgical treatment of failed thoracic endovascular aortic repair, demonstrating low morbidity, acceptable mortality and excellent late outcome in our own series. However, the analysis of the recently published studies shows on one hand a rapidly increasing and fascinating evolution of TEVAR techniques but, on the other hand only a small number of papers dealing with the consequences of severe complications. Consequently we have limited information on the incidence of secondary interventions or conversion to open repair.

Voluntary registries like the EUROSTAR registry or the United Kingdom thoracic endograft registry are certainly the largest compendium of endovascular thoracic procedures, but they only represent part of the entire implantation market. Considering these data, a high primary success rate of 87% in TAA and 89% in dissection can be obtained [2]. Further results including 213 TAA patients have shown a cumulative rate of freedom from intervention at 2 years of 83% [13]. Perhaps the most accepted indication for endovascular repair includes the emergency treatment of traumatic aortic rupture with verified reduced morbidity and mortality rates as compared to open repair [3]. Consequently an increasing use of TEVAR is documented in single center experience [14] or in a nationwide survey in Germany [20] and more procedures can be expected in the near future. Nevertheless, several complications like endoleaks [5], retrograde type A dissection [6], rupture [12,14], stent migration [17] and stent collapse [7,8] following this assumed "minimally invasive" therapy have been described. It can be expected that with increasing use of thoracic endografts the demand for open surgical repair after unsuccessful endovascular procedures will also increase.

RISK FACTORS FOR TEVAR FAILURE

According to the messages in literature and our own experience we identified acute and chronic dissections (5 of 8 cases) as possible risk factors for stent graft failure, particularly when devices with bare springs are used in acute type B dissection. Neuhauser et al. [21] described in 5 of 28 TEVAR (18%) for type B dissection serious complications. They identified as possible risk factors for retrograde type A dissection repeat balloon dilatation in a poor quality aortic wall and learned that endovascular stent-graft repair of thoracic aortic dissection is an alternative to surgical repair, but not without significant morbidity and mortality. We believe that endografts with uncovered bare springs should not be recommended for acute type B dissection. Additionally a stentgraft oversizing of more than 10% should be avoided to respect the vulnerable wall. Chronic dissections represent a different pathology. They often contain a strong fibrotic septum which may cause inadequate deployment of the devices with incomplete apposition. Particularly the inner curve of the distal aortic arch causing mal-alignment of current stentgrafts is an unsolved endovascular challenge, especially in younger patients with small diameters [8].

REASONS FOR CONVERSION

We found as main cause for conversion three early and two late type I endoleaks, 2 retrograde type A dissections and 1 rupture. Access failure did not occur. Comparable results in the few published series are present. Zipfel et al. [14] reported on 172 patients who underwent thoracic

Table V	THORACIC CONVERSIONS TO OPEN REPAIR IN LITERATURE				
First author [ref.]	Conversions	Failure	Device	Emergency/elective	Outcome
Grabenwoger [4]	4	3 endoleak Ia 1 retrograde type A dissection	NS	Elective	Uneventful
Böckler [16]	1	1 infection	Excluder	Elective	Uneventful
Eggebrecht [11]	7	NS	NS	NS	NS
Neuhauser [6]	3	3 retro A	Talent	1 emergency / 2 elective	1 died 2 uneventful
Flores [17]	1	1 endoleak Ia	NS	el	Uneventful
Iyer [19]	3	2 endoleak Ia 1 aortobronchial fistula	NS	2 emergency / 1 elective	Uneventful
Fattori [12]	3	NS	Talent	NS	NS
Zhang [18]	1	1 retrograde type A dissection	Excluder	emergency	Died
Muhs [7]	1	collapse	TAG	NS	Uneventful
Leurs [13]	6	1 endoleak III 1 stent kinking 1 infectious fistula 3 NS	NS	NS	NS
Zipfel [14]	6	3 access failure 1 bare spring penetration 1 retrograde type A dissection 1 endoleak Ia	3 Talent 1 TAG 1 Zenith 1 E-vita	4 emergency / 2 Elective	4 discharged 1 major complication 1 died
Bakaeen [15]	1	1 endoleak Ia+b	NS	Elective	Uneventful

NS: not specified

endografting of whom 15 suffered from endograft failure and six had conversion to open repair. Of these, 3 were converted immediately because of retrograde type A dissection, access failure and type Ia endoleak causing rupture after deployment. Reasons for conversions at a later date were access failure in 2 cases and aortic perforation by bare spring penetration. One death and one major complication occurred. Grabenwoger et al. [4] published 4 cases including three type Ia endoleaks and 1 retrograde type A dissection. All patients had an uneventful postoperative course. Both authors used extracorporeal circulation to perform open repair. Neuhauser et al. [6] described their experience focussed on 5 cases of retrograde type A dissection including three conversions. Causative reasons were tears in the aortic wall at the proximal landing zone in 3 cases, but in 2 cases the retrograde dissection was not related to the endografts.

Regarding the published cases and our experience, we can identify some factors that mandate open repair after failed TEVAR.
1) The most obvious constitutes retrograde type A dissection, requiring emergency repair.
2) Type I endoleaks, which can not be corrected by additional endovascular means (i.e. anatomic issues like ascending aortic disease, inadequate proximal area for hybrid bypass anastomosis, inappropriate distal landing zone).
3) Device related complications like migration, perforation, fistula, collapse, incomplete deployement or fracture which, for some reasons, can not be treated endovascularly.
4) Stent-graft infection with septicaemia.
5) In case of re-sternotomy after previous coronary artery bypass graft, as part of a hybrid procedure to maximize a landing zone in the arch a left thoracotomy might be less invasive.
6) Patients' wishes.

Time to conversion

In 6 patients we were confronted with immediate or short-term failure within the first 6 weeks, which represents a multifactorial event. Anatomical and technical factors including quality and length of the landing zones and appropriate devices are crucial. In addition, the anticoagulation status might be of importance, especially in polytraumatic injuries associated with increased transfusion requirements. In only 2 patients of our series a mid-term failure after 10 and 37 months was observed. Possible cause for mid- or long-term failure after initial successful endografting might be a continued aneurismal expansion at the level of the landing zones due to proximal or distal type I endoleaks as described by Bakaeen et al. [15]. This well known problem of time related morphological changes emphasizes the necessity of lifelong surveillance in TEVAR patients.

Conclusion

TEVAR seems to become the gold standard for many aortic pathologies. However, despite new and innovative improved devices and techniques, TEVAR failure represents a new aortic pathology, but fortunately, secondary endovascular treatment provides the solution in the majority of patients. For the remaining failures, in whom endovascular repair is not feasible, open surgery is the only alternative. The surgical outcome of these complex challenges is dependent on the infrastructure and multidisciplinary approach of the procedure comprising extracorporeal circulation, antegrade cerebral perfusion, distal aortic perfusion, cerebral and spinal cord monitoring. It would be recommendable to perform these procedures in centers with experience and the infrastructure offering these protective measures.

REFERENCES

1 Dake MD, Miller DC, Semba CP et al. Transluminal Placement of endovascular stent-grafts for the treatment of descending thoracic aortic aneurysms. *N Engl J Med* 1994; 331: 1729-1734.

2 Leurs LJ, Bell R, Degrieck Y et al. Endovascular Treatment of thoracic aortic diseases: combined experience from the EUROSTAR and United Kingdom thoracic endograft registries. *J Vasc Surg* 2004; 40: 670-679.

3 Lettinga-Van De PT, Schurink GW, De Haan MW et al. Endovascular treatment of traumatic rupture of the thoracic aorta. *Br J Surg* 2007; 94: 525-533.

4 Grabenwoger M, Fleck T, Ehrlich M et al. Secondary Surgical interventions after endovascular stent-grafting of the thoracic aorta. *Eur J Cardiothorac Surg* 2004; 26: 608-613.

5 Parmer SS, Carpenter JP, Stavropoulos SW et al. Endoleaks after endovascular repair of thoracic aortic aneurysms. *J Vasc Surg* 2006; 44: 447-452.

6 Neuhauser B, Czermak BV, Fish J et al. Type A dissection following endovascular thoracic aortic stent-graft repair. *J Endovasc Ther* 2005; 12: 74-81.

7 Muhs BE, Balm R, White GH et al. Anatomic Factors associated with acute endograft collapse after gore TAG Treatment of thoracic aortic dissection or traumatic rupture. *J Vasc Surg* 2007; 45: 655-661.

8 Hinchliffe RJ, Krasznai A, Schultzekool L et al. Observations on the failure of stent-grafts in the aortic arch. *Eur J Vasc Endovasc Surg* 2007; 34: 451-456.

9 Hobo R, Buth J. Secondary Interventions following endovascular abdominal aortic aneurysm repair using current endografts. A EUROSTAR Report. *J Vasc Surg* 2006; 43: 896-902.

10 Jacobs MJ, Mess W, Mochtar B et al. The value of motor evoked potentials in reducing paraplegia during thoracoabdominal aneurysm repair. *J Vasc Surg* 2006; 43: 239-246.

11. Eggebrecht H, Nienaber CA, Neuhauser M et al. Endovascular stent-graft placement in aortic dissection: a meta-analysis. *Eur Heart J* 2006; 27: 489-498.

12. Fattori R, Nienaber CA, Rousseau H et al. Results of endovascular repair of the thoracic aorta with the talent thoracic stent graft: the talent thoracic retrospective registry. *J Thorac Cardiovasc Surg* 2006; 132: 332-339.

13. Leurs LJ, Harris PL, Buth J. Secondary interventions after elective endovascular repair of degenerative thoracic aortic aneurysms: results of the European Collaborators Registry (EUROSTAR). *J Vasc Interv Radiol* 2007; 18: 491-495.

14. Zipfel B, Hammerschmidt R, Krabatsch T et al. Stent-grafting of the thoracic aorta by the cardiothoracic surgeon. *Ann Thorac Surg* 2007; 83: 441-448.

15. Bakaeen FG, Coselli JS, Lemaire SA, Huh J. Continued aortic aneurysmal expansion after thoracic endovascular stent-grafting. *Ann Thorac Surg* 2007; 84: 1007-1008.

16. Bockler D, Von Tengg-Kobligk H, Schumacher H et al. Late surgical conversion after thoracic endograft failure due to fracture of the longitudinal support wire. *J Endovasc Ther* 2005; 12: 98-102.

17. Flores J, Shiiya N, Kunihara T et al. Reoperations after failure of stent grafting for type b aortic dissection: report of two cases. *Surg Today* 2005; 35: 581-585.

18. Zhang R, Kofidis T, Baus S et al. Iatrogenic type A dissection after attempted stenting of a descending aortic aneurysm. *Ann Thorac Surg* 2006; 82: 1523-1525.

19. Iyer VS, Mackenzie KS, Tse LW et al. Early outcomes after elective and emergent endovascular repair of the thoracic aorta. *J Vasc Surg* 2006; 43: 677-683.

20. Eggebrecht H, Pamler R, Zipfel B et al. Stent-graft implantation in the thoracic aorta. results of an interdisciplinary survey in Germany. *Dtsch Med Wochenschr* 2006; 131: 730-734.

21. Neuhauser B, Greiner A, Jaschke W et al. Serious complications following endovascular thoracic aortic stent-graft repair for type b dissection. *Eur J Cardiothorac Surg* 2008; 33: 58-63.

22

SURVEILLANCE AFTER EVAR: INDICATIONS, COST AND MODALITIES

CLARK ZEEBREGTS, ERIC VERHOEVEN, IGNACE TIELLIU, WENDY BOS
TED PRINS, ROY DE JONG, JAN VAN DEN DUNGEN

Endovascular repair of abdominal aortic aneurysm (EVAR) has proven to be a viable alternative to open repair with superior early outcome. EVAR, however, is associated with late complications, such as the occurrence of endoleak(s), migration of the endograft, kinking of limb(s), component separation, and even rupture. Lifelong post-EVAR surveillance is therefore still advocated. Contrast-enhanced computerized tomography scanning (CTA) has been preferentially used as the imaging modality of choice and can be regarded as the gold standard. On the other hand, repeated exposure to radiation, intravenous contrast-induced nephropathy, inconvenience for the patient, and costs led several centers to adopt an alternative surveillance program, including plain X-ray and duplex ultrasound. In this chapter, we review our experience with a change of protocol that replaced standard CTA by plain X-ray + duplex ultrasound scanning (DUS), reserving additional imaging (i.e. CTA and/or angiography) on indication only. The new strategy gave significant economic advantages and the number of post-EVAR emergency cases due to missed complications did not increase. Possible missed endoleaks by DUS are only type II endoleaks without growth of the aneurysm and nowadays considered not to require intervention. We therefore plea a change of surveillance protocol as mentioned above in EVAR centers, provided that the results of both plain X-ray and duplex ultrasound are accurately assessed by trained personnel who understand graft design and position of radiopaque markers.

Outcome of the trials and the need for surveillance

Endovascular repair of abdominal aortic aneurysm (EVAR) has been well established and gained a firm position as a reliable alternative to open repair. Both the DREAM and EVAR-1 trial, comparing the two treatment options, found a lower 30-day mortality in those treated by EVAR (DREAM: 1.2% vs 4.6% (p=0.10), EVAR 1: 1.7% vs 4.7% (p<0.009) [1,2]. Secondary outcome measures, such as blood loss, hospital and ICU stay, recovery to normal daily live activities, all favored EVAR. The downside, however, included a higher number of mid- and long-term complications when compared to open repair. Kaplan-Meier re-intervention-free survival curves showed a clear advantage in favor for open repair. The DREAM trial showed a threefold higher re-intervention rate after EVAR, compared to open repair. Two-year outcomes reported a 12% re-intervention rate after EVAR against 6% in the open repair group [3]. EVAR-1 similarly described a reintervention rate of 15% after EVAR compared to 7% in the open repair group [4].

Mean hospital costs per patient up to 4 years in EVAR-1 mounted up to approximately € 20 000 for the EVAR group versus € 15 000 for the open repair group. Similar figures, with an almost equal difference between the groups, were found in the DREAM trial. With growing concerns in many European countries with regard to budgetary restrictions, an accurate and cheap follow-up imaging protocol is required.

As mentioned above, EVAR is related to a higher complication rate, of which a significant proportion does require treatment. Loss of fixation with migration, loss of sealing, and structural failure of the device all put the aneurysm at risk for rupture. With a growing aneurysm post-EVAR and a causative endoleak type 1 or 3, reintervention seems obvious, but with an endoleak type 2 (with or without aneurysm growth) further strategy is less clear. The natural history and clinical significance of these kinds of endoleaks is not yet completely known, and until more definitive data are available, ongoing life-long surveillance for detection and possible repair will be necessary in most cases.

The main goal of any follow-up strategy regardless the used imaging modality should include the detection of aneurysms remaining at risk for rupture after EVAR. Also, features that preclude limb occlusion or renal artery stenosis are noteworthy. In this chapter, the current diagnostic imaging tools to be used during follow-up after EVAR are listed focusing on their abilities to detect complications. We seek to find a rationale to the optimal follow-up imaging protocol and use own data and current literature. Challenges that need to be faced include patient compliance, reproducibility of imaging, sensitivity and specificity of the imaging modality, and cost-effectiveness of the technique.

Post-EVAR imaging

After EVAR, several features of the aneurysm, as well as the inserted endograft and their relation, can be measured. Most important among these parameters are the maximal diameter of the aneurysm, diameter of the aortic neck, occurrence of endoleak(s), migration of the endograft, kinking of limb(s), and component separation. A comparison of the various imaging modalities demonstrates that each provides useful information with some of the information being complementary to that acquired by other techniques, whereas other information is unique to a particular modality.

Imaging modalities

PLAIN X-RAY

Plain abdominal X-ray is probably the quickest, best manageable diagnostic imaging modality. Imaging in two to four directions provides information on stent-graft integrity and migration. Plain X-ray can, however, not be used as a stand-alone test, and has to be combined with other examinations. One of the features that can be accurately assessed with plain X-ray is the occurrence of kinking of endograft limbs. Kinking is the predominant factor of occlusion. In a recent series from Cochennec et al. [5] with 460 electively treated AAAs, 36 limbs in 33 patients (7.2%) occluded between day 0 and 71 months after EVAR. Limb kinking occurred in 14 limbs of 13 patients and was significantly associated with graft limb occlusion. Diagnosis of kinking was established on plain X-ray at the first month after operation in seven cases, and more than one year after the intervention in the other seven cases. In their series, none of the patient-related factors, such as gender, smoking habits, or dyslipidemia were predictive of occlusion. Specific anatomic features of iliac arteries, however, do correlate with early kinking, including angled aorto-iliac bifurcation, tortuosity and size of the iliac arteries, as well as distal extent of the graft. Obviously, the problem of early kinking, best detected on post-deployment control angiography without stiff guidewires inserted, can be solved by the insertion of one or more additional bare stents within the limb.

Late limb occlusion may occur during follow-up and may be preceded by aneurysm shrinkage, but migration of the graft as a distinct factor is clearly more important. Through migration, the whole body of the endograft may curl up within the aneurysm. As a consequence, kinking of the limbs may occur, but also proximal endoleaks. In the Eurostar registry [6], the presence of a kink was associated with increased incidences of proximal type 1 endoleak (HR 1.9), distal type 1 endoleak (HR 5.8), and midgraft type 3 endoleak (HR 3.3), all of which are in return associated with an increased risk for rupture of the aneurysm. As both migration and kinking of limbs can be clearly visualized with plain X-ray, it is clear that this imaging modality is a useful tool to detect post-EVAR complications early. Interpretation of the images, however, requires appropriate understanding of graft design and the position of radiopaque markers.

Duplex ultrasound scanning (DUS)

The assets and liabilities of DUS as a post-EVAR imaging tool seem clear. DUS is readily available and images can be provided at low cost, without radiation or use of nephrotoxic contrast agents. On the other hand, 10% to 15% of scans are inadequate due to obesity as a result of intervening skin and soft tissue, and the technique is largely operator dependent, which makes the technique less reproducible. Features that usually can be accurately assessed include the maximal diameter of the aneurysm, neck diameter and persistent flow within the aneurysm caused by an endoleak. (Figs. 1, 2) Approximately 25% of EVAR patients develop endoleaks. It is clear that type I and III endoleaks, both causing repressurization of the aneurysm, require treatment. The significance of type II side branch backflow endoleaks and their relation to post-EVAR aneurysm enlargement is still not well understood. The question remains whether those endoleaks that are possibly missed through DUS are really important and will ever lead to rupture of the aneurysm. As mentioned above, we usually advocate a CTA when the aneurysm is growing without evidence of endoleak on DUS.

CTA

Traditionally, contrast enhanced computerized tomography scanning (CTA) is considered the gold standard for post-EVAR surveillance. Images are relatively easy to interpret. Aneurysm diameter and volume can be measured accurately at all possible levels; endoleaks can be visualized with normal or delayed acquisition times. Characteristically, an endoleak on CTA is depicted as a collec-

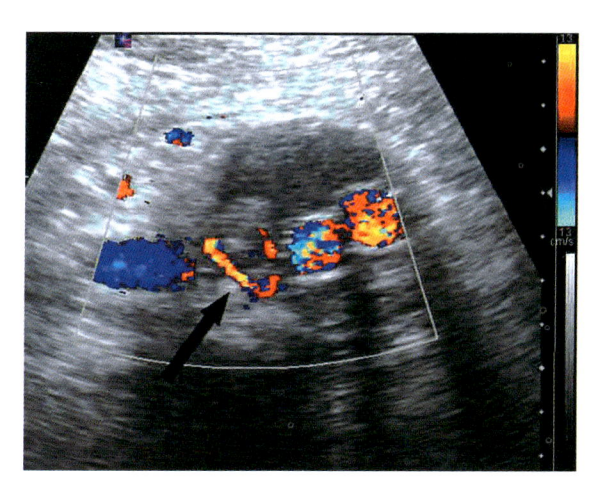

FIG. 1 A 65-year old male patient with a type 2 endoleak (arrow) two years after EVAR as detected with DUS. No further treatment has been initiated so far, as the maximal diameter of the aneurysm stays perfectly stable.

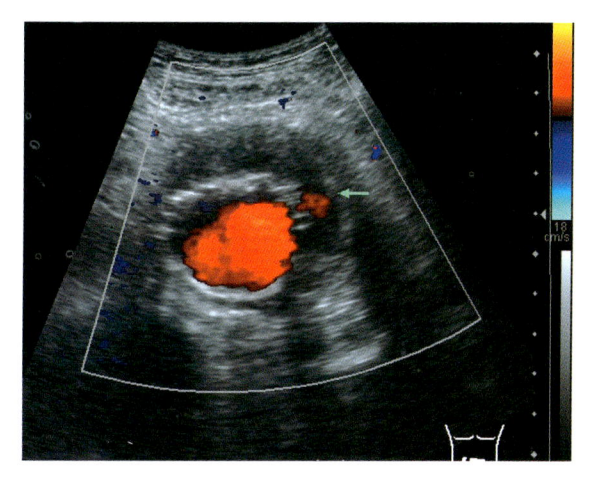

FIG. 2 Duplex ultrasound B-mode image of a type II endoleak 6 months after EVAR in an 85-year old male patient. Patent flow channel through the sarcral artery and inferior mesenteric artery.

tion of contrast within the aneurysm sac and outside the stent-graft (Fig. 3). Calcifications that may be interpreted as endoleaks must be identified by plain CT without contrast. Also, delayed CTA images can further add to the detection of endoleaks that occur due to back-flow from lumbar arteries and other side branches (type II endoleaks). Disadvantages of CTA are those related to radiation, contrast media, and cost.

OTHER IMAGING MODALITIES

Contrast enhanced magnetic imaging resonance (MRA) is another option for post-EVAR surveillance, especially for those patients that cannot have a CTA because of iodinated contrast allergy or severely deteriorated renal function. Endografts containing stainless steel do produce large MR artifacts and can not be followed by MRA. There are several reports of MRA used for endografts with nitinol (Gore Excluder) and elgiloy (Ancure) frames with satisfactory results comparable to CTA. Some even found MRA to be more sensitive than CTA in the detection endoleak and the determination of the type of endoleak during follow-up of mainly Ancure cases. [7]

Angiography is obviously used as a completion of all EVAR procedures, in order to detect intraoperative complications such as endoleaks or limb kinking and narrowing. As it is an invasive technique, with the use of contrast media and radiation, it seems less suitable for post-EVAR surveillance. Angiography can be a useful additional diagnostic and therapeutic tool especially in low flow type II endoleaks or diagnosis of prosthetic defects (type III endoleaks).

In experimental settings, the value of nuclear medicine techniques including positron emmision tomography scanning has been studied. So far, none of these imaging techniques can be used as a post-EVAR follow-up imaging tool.

Rationale for and results with our personal follow-up protocol

In our personal series of patients treated with endovascular repair, there have been two types of surveillance protocols. Before 1999 we used the Eurostar protocol, including CTA at discharge, one month, six months, one year, and yearly thereafter. Also, ankle-brachial index, plain abdominal X-ray and DUS were performed at the same intervals. From 1999 on, patients were discharged after plain abdominal X-ray only (completion angiogram not counted). DUS was only performed in selected cases (i.e. type II endoleak at completion angiogram). Follow-up started with CTA at one

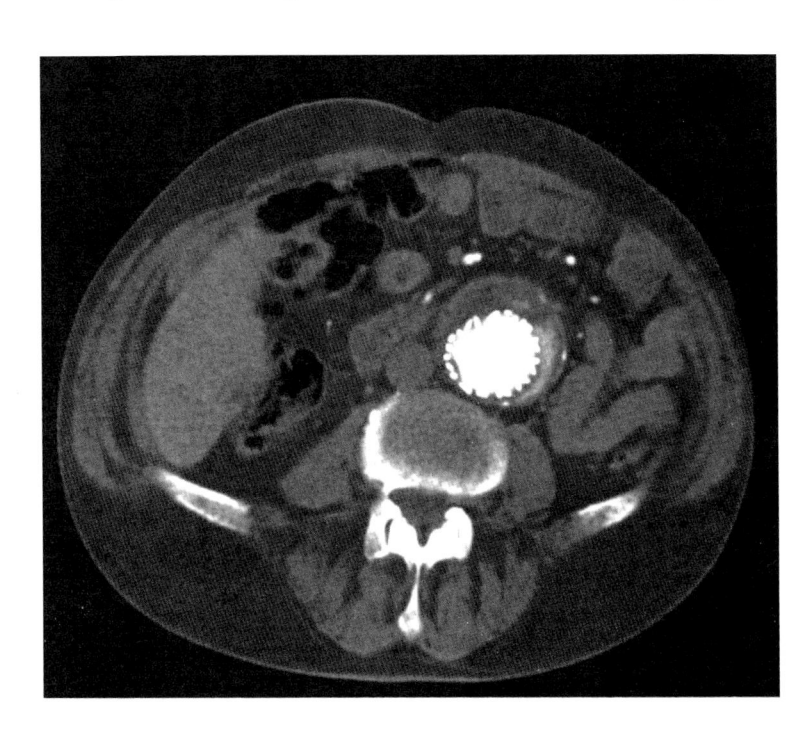

FIG. 3 Computerized tomography scan of a type 2 endoleak (same patient as in figure 2).

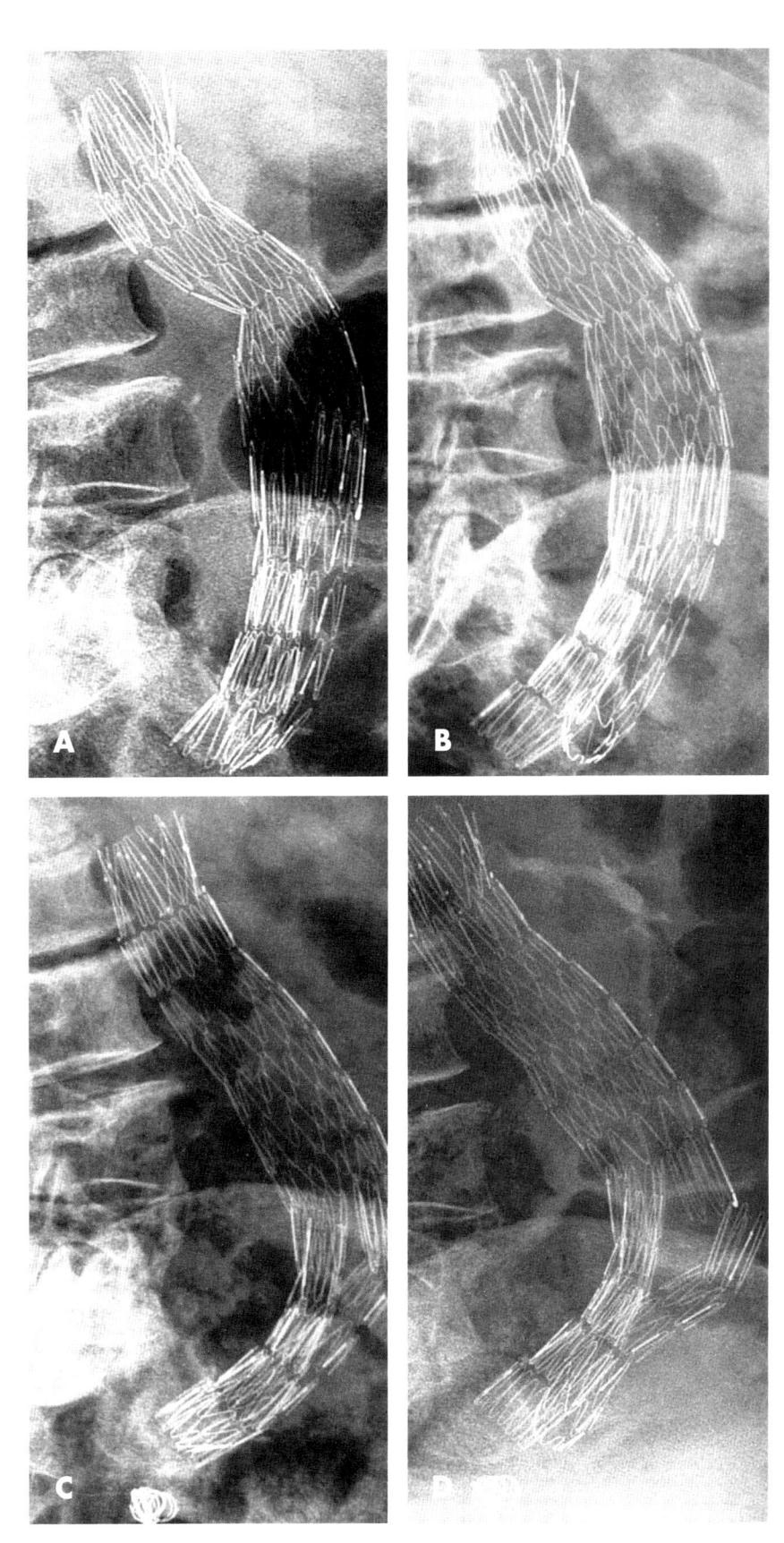

FIG. 4 Post-EVAR dislocation of the contralateral limb as shown on plain X-ray, eventually leading to a complete dislocation with an acute non-ruptured aneurysm as a consequence (views after 2 days [A], 6 months [B], one year [C] and 1.5 years [D]).

month, used as a reference for future examinations. Thereafter, patients were followed with abdominal X-ray and DUS at six months, one year, and yearly thereafter.

In an evaluation of 308 patients included between September 1996 and December 2003 with a mean follow-up of 36 (±22) months, one patient died of myocardial infarction the day after surgery, another required conversion to open repair because of technical reasons [8]. During this period of time a total of 126 late complications occurred in 102 patients. Different stent grafts had been used, and the Vanguard device was associated with the highest rate of complications. Also, 80% of all complications occurred in the first 100 stent grafts, suggesting that the learning curve might have played a role. Other devices, such as Gore Excluder and Cook Zenith, had three-year intervention free survival rates well above 90%. Re-interventions were performed electively in 31 patients (66%), and on an emergency basis in 16 (34%). The majority of elective re-interventions were needed because of a persistent endoleak, graft migration, or failure of the aneurismal sac to shrink. The majority of emergency re-interventions (88%) were required for acute leg ischemia depicting 14 limb occlusions. The other two acute re-interventions included one ruptured aneurysm treated by open repair, and one symptomatic aneurysm treated with a bridging stent graft. After the change of follow-up protocol we did not encounter an increase in emergency post-EVAR problems that required intervention.

With regard to kinking as found on plain X-ray, we encountered 14 primary limb occlusions as stated before and three occlusions after re-intervention for other reasons. Three of these 17 occlusions re-occluded after re-canalization. Nevertheless, we believe these results compare favorably with results from literature and may be explained by meticulous work-up, including accurate assessment of the landing zones. Small limb diameter and distal extent of the graft onto the external iliac artery have been identified as significant factors for limb occlusion [9]. Therefore, in our center we advocate the use of combined endografts (e.g. Cook Zenith body with Gore Excluder limbs) for those patients with short neck aneurysms that have angulated and/or narrow landing zones. Nevertheless, in our previous report we also encountered two patients that came in with acute aneurysms post-EVAR. Both aneurysms occurred due to limb disconnection and should have been detected. One of these patients was re-admitted with an acute non-ruptured aneurysm 21 months post-EVAR. In retrospect, plain abdominal X-ray had shown an initial migration of the contralateral limb (Fig. 4). At that stage a bridging stent-graft could have been easily inserted preventing the complete dislocation, which required a more complex procedure.

Analyzing the cost-effectiveness of this protocol in the same group of patients as referred to above, we determined a total saving of 897 CTs over a 3-year period (518 CTs in 204 patients without complications, 174 CTs in 55 patients with com-

Table I	COMPARISON OF VARIOUS POST-EVAR IMAGING STRATEGIES AND THEIR ABILITY TO VISUALIZE SPECIFIC EVAR-RELATED FEATURES (++ VERY GOOD; + GOOD; ± MODERATE; - POOR)				
EVAR related risk factors	CT	Duplex	Plain X-ray	Duplex + Plain X-ray
Presence of endoleak	+	++	-	++
Classification of endoleak	+	+	-	+
Aneurysm size/volume	++	+	-	+
Stentgraft integrity	±/+	-	+	+
Migration	+	-	++	++
Flow dynamics	-	+	-	+

plications not requiring re-intervention, and 205 CT's in 47 patients with complications requiring reintervention) [8].

Although EVAR outcome is to be regarded multifactorial as a result of various time eras, stent grafts, and ancillary products, we do feel that post-EVAR surveillance with plain X-ray and DUS only can identify problems requiring attention (i.e. additional imaging and re-intervention) at an early stage.

Comparison of DUS and CTA in literature

There are several studies that compared sensitivity and specificity of DUS to detect post-EVAR complications with CTA. The Table shows a summary of possible post-EVAR risk factors and the ability of various (combinations of) imaging modalities to visualize these features. A combination of DUS and plain X-ray seems very well capable of covering all the features to be measured.

Sun recently conducted a systemic review to identify the role of DUS in the detection of endoleaks and measurement of aneurysm diameter during post-EVAR follow-up [10]. The diagnostic accuracy of DUS was compared with that of CTA. A total of 21 studies published between 1991 and 2005 met the criteria and were included for analysis. The meta-analysis showed pooled estimates of sensitivity, specificity, positive predictive value (PPV), negative predictive value (NPV), and accuracy of color DUS compared with CTA (with 95% CIs) of 66% (52%-81%), 93% (89%-97%), 76% (65%-87%), 90% (86%-95%), and 91% (86%-97%), respectively, for unenhanced DUS. These figures were 81% (52%-100%), 82% (68%-97%), 58% (26%-90%), 95% (87%-100%), and 98% (91%-100%), respectively, for contrast-enhanced DUS. Clearly, the sensitivity in the detection of endoleak was improved with contrast-enhanced DUS versus unenhanced, but no significant differences were found with regard to specificity, PPV, NPV, and accuracy. Furthermore, the required dose of the ultrasound contrast agent for post-EVAR surveillance is still not well defined and the different published studies report the use of various doses. One of the advantages of DUS over CTA could be the additional hemodynamic information on blood flow and direction, in addition to morphological information,

enabling a more precise characterization of the type of endoleak. It is clear that DUS has it limitations and a lower sensitivity compared to CTA is the most important one. These limits are mainly due to echo reflection by the metallic part of the graft, extended calcifications, meteorism, obesity or an overly slow flow. [11] As stated previously, DUS depends to some extent on the personal experience of the physician and may not be reproducible in all centers. To this context, reviewing DUS examinations from different institutions over a 15-year period may be prone to severe bias. AbuRahma [12] therefore recently suggested to use a standardized DUS protocol, including (1) satisfactory use of duplex imaging without excessive overgain or undergain, (2) satisfactory B-mode imaging of the AAA sac and stent-graft, (3) a color DUS assessment of the entire AAA sac outside the graft in both longitudinal and transverse views to rule out endoleaks, and (4) the use of spectral Doppler scan waveform analysis within the AAA sac and outside the stent-graft to confirm or rule out potential endoleaks suggested by DUS assessment. These standardized duplex ultrasound protocols have been adopted by several centers resulting in excellent sensitivity and specificity of DUS in the detection of endoleaks. Some even reported a better sensitivity with DUS than with CTA [13].

Furthermore, it is clear from many studies that a large proportion of type 2 endoleaks resolve spontaneously. In addition, intervention will usually only be offered to those aneurysms associated with a post-EVAR increasing sac size. A follow-up strategy in which not every small endoleak will be detected, provided that the aneurysm shrinks or stays stable, seems well defendable. In a comparative study of DUS versus CTA, Sandford et al. [11] showed ratios of 81% likelihood of endoleak with a positive duplex ultrasound and a 96% likelihood of no endoleak with a negative duplex ultrasound. Importantly, there were no type 1 endoleaks, or endoleaks requiring intervention which were missed on duplex ultrasound.

With regard to cost-effectiveness, Bendick et al. [14] have evaluated the possible benefits of DUS surveillance with contrast agent compared to CTA. The charges for CTA in their institution averaged approximately € 2 000 per study with a 3-year total of € 16 000 per patient. The charges for DUS averaged € 369 per study with a 3-year total of € 3 000 per patient. Adding the costs of plain X-ray € 103 per study, brought the 3-year total of combined

DUS and plain X-ray to € 3 783 per patient, a savings of € 11 860 per patient. As a consequence, for every 100 EVAR patients a 3-year savings of more than € 1.1 million could be achieved.

Conclusion

Endovascular repair compares favorably to open AAA repair in terms of early mortality and morbidity, but requires an extensive post-EVAR surveillance programme to detect complications, such as persisting endoleaks (25%). CTA is more sensitive in the detection of endoleaks, but the leaks missed by DUS do not require intervention in most of cases. A combination of DUS and plain X-ray gives a wide range of information covering all EVAR related risk factors, is cheaper than CTA, with less radiation, and results in final EVAR outcome that is not worse than series that have CTA driven surveillance protocols. However, if DUS results are considered to be inadequate or an abnormality is detected, additional CTA is advocated.

REFERENCES

1. Prinssen M, Verhoeven EL, Buth J et al. Dutch Randomized Endovascular Aneurysm Management (DREAM)Trial Group. A randomized trial comparing conventional and endovascular repair of abdominal aortic aneurysms. *N Engl J Med* 2004; 351: 1607-1618.
2. Greenhalgh RM, Brown LC, Kwong GP et al. EVAR trial participants. Comparison of endovascular aneurysm repair with open repair in patients with abdominal aortic aneurysm (EVAR trial 1), 30-day operative mortality results: randomised controlled trial. *Lancet* 2004; 364: 843-848.
3. Blankensteijn JD, de Jong SE, Prinssen M et al. Dutch Randomized Endovascular Aneurysm Management (DREAM) Trial Group. Two-year outcomes after conventional or endovascular repair of abdominal aortic aneurysms. *N Engl J Med* 2005; 352: 2398-2405.
4. Anonymous. EVAR trial participants. Endovascular aneurysm repair versus open repair in patients with abdominal aortic aneurysm (EVAR trial 1): randomised controlled trial. *Lancet* 2005; 365: 2179-2186.
5. Cochennec F, Becquemin JP, Desgranges P et al. Limb graft occlusion following EVAR: clinical pattern, outcomes and predictive factors of occurrence. *Eur J Vasc Endovasc Surg* 2007; 34: 59-65.
6. Fransen GAJ, Desgranges P, Laheij RJF et al. EUROSTAR collaborators. Frequency, Predictive Factors, and Consequences of Stent-Graft Kink Following Endovascular AAA Repair. *J Endovasc Ther* 2003; 10: 913-918.
7. van der Laan MJ, Bartels LW, Viergever MA et al. Computed tomography versus magnetic resonance imaging of endoleaks after EVAR. *Eur J Vasc Endovasc Surg* 2006; 32: 361-5.
8. Verhoeven EL, Tielliu IF, Prins TR et al. Frequency and outcome of re-interventions after endovascular repair for abdominal aortic aneurysm: a prospective cohort study. *Eur J Vasc Endovasc Surg* 2004; 28: 357-364.
9. Erzurum VZ, Sampram ES, Sarac TP et al. Initial management and outcome of aortic endograft limb occlusion. *J Vasc Surg* 2004; 40: 419-423.
10. Sun Z. Diagnostic value of color duplex ultrasonography in the follow-up of endovascular repair of abdominal aortic aneurysm. *J Vasc Interv Radiol* 2006; 17: 759-764.
11. Sandford RM, Bown MJ, Fishwick G et al. Duplex ultrasound scanning is reliable in the detection of endoleak following endovascular aneurysm repair. *Eur J Vasc Endovasc Surg* 2006; 32: 537-541.
12. AbuRahma A. Fate of endoleaks detected by CT angiography and missed by color duplex ultrasound in endovascular grafts for abdominal aortic aneurysms. *J Endovasc Ther* 2006; 13: 490-495.
13. McLafferty RB, McCrary BS, Mattos MA et al. The use of color-flow duplex scan for the detection of endoleaks. *J Vasc Surg* 2002; 36: 100-104.
14. Bendick PJ, Zelenock GB, Bove PG et al. Duplex ultrasound imaging with an ultrasound contrast agent: the economic alternative to CT angiography for aortic stent graft surveillance. *Vasc Endovasc Surg* 2003; 37: 165-170.

23

SHORT-TERM MORBIDITY AND MORTALITY OF AAA ENDOGRAFTING

ZORAN RANCIC, DIETER MAYER, CHRISTIAN SCHMID
THOMAS PFAMMATTER, MARIO LACHAT

Sixteen years after its introduction, endovascular aneurysm repair (EVAR) of abdominal aortic aneurysm (AAA) still remains a matter of debate. Two main discussion points are: in which patients is EVAR a safer intervention than open repair, and does EVAR really offer life-long protection against AAA rupture. This chapter focuses on the short-term results (30-day mortality and morbidity) of AAA endografting and provides recommendations based on a review of the literature including randomized trials, registries, single or multicenter trials, meta-analyzes, reviews and collective series.

Thirty-day mortality

Vascular registries

In the Registry of Endovascular Treatment of Abdominal Aortic Aneurysm (RETA) overall 30-day mortality was 7% (Table I). It was significantly higher in unfit compared to fit patients (18% vs 4%) and in patients treated with an aorto-uni-iliac device and a crossover graft compared to tube and aorto-bi-iliac devices (12% vs 4%). Limitations of the registry are that 20% of the patients were considered unfit for open repair and that data were heterogeneous, reflecting a non-uniform group of patients and a wide range of devices used in the UK [1].

The EUROpean Collaborators on Stent/graft Techniques for aortic Aneurysm Repair (EUROSTAR) reports the results of endografts in current use only. In total 30-day mortality is 2.4%. However, the results differed among the various countries (i.e. Belgian cohort had slightly higher overall 30-day mortality of 3.1%). There were significant correlations between mortality rate and age, fitness of the patient, American Society of Anesthesiologists (ASA) class, and to a lesser extent with the aneurysm size [2,3]. In the EUROSTAR registry only 7% of the patients were considered unfit to justify an open AAA repair.

The first Vascunet Report on AAA surgery results from a pilot project to merge data from five national and one regional registry, with 33 780 aneurysm repairs collected from 1994 (Sweden), or 2005 (Switzerland) up to 2006 [4]; 15.3% (3 156) underwent EVAR with a 30-day mortality of 2%.

Lifeline registry contains data collected under four multicenter investigational device clinical trials that lead to Food and Drug Administration (FDA) approval in the USA. There was no difference in 30-day operative mortality between EVAR and open repair patients (1.7% vs 1.4%) [5].

Australian experience and safety profile of EVAR is presented within Australian Safety and Efficacy Register of New Interventional Procedure Surgery (ASERNIP-S) registry. Peri-operative mortality was 1.7%, mostly from cardiac causes, followed by neurological and intra-abdominal complications [6].

RANDOMIZED TRIALS

There are three prospective randomized controlled trials comparing EVAR with open repair. Two trials, UK EVAR 1 trial and the Dutch Randomized Endovascular Aneurysm Management (DREAM) trial, included patients who were considered fit enough for open surgical repair. The third trial, UK EVAR 2 trial, compared EVAR versus observation and medical treatment in patients unfit for surgery.

The EVAR 1 trial randomized 1 082 patients aged 60 years or older, with an aneurysm of at least 5.5 cm in diameter, anatomically suitable for EVAR and fit for open repair (543 assigned to EVAR, and 539 to open repair). Thirty-day mortality rate in the EVAR group was 1.7% and 4.7% in the open repair group (Table II). The most frequent cause of death was procedure related and cardiovascular [7].

The DREAM trial randomized 345 patients (174 patients in the open repair, and 171 in the EVAR

Table I   THIRTY-DAY MORTALITY IN VASCULAR REGISTRIES

Registry [ref.]	Type of study	Period	Number of patients	30-day mortality (%)
RETA [1]	Prospective	01. 1996 – 12.1998	611	7.0
EUROSTAR [2]	Prospective	07.1997 – 01. 2006	7 968	2.4
EUROSTAR – Belgian [3]	Prospective	01.2001 – 12.2005	2 068	3.1
VASCUNET [4]	Prospective	01.1994 – 12.2006	26 906	2.0
LIFELINE [5]	Collected data from randomized trials	01.1998 – 12.2005	2 664	1.7
ASERNIP-S [6]	Prospective	11.1999 – 05.2001	950	1.7

Table II   THIRTY-DAY MORTALITY IN RANDOMIZED TRIALS

Mortality	Trial [ref.]	EVAR	Open repair	No repair	P value
30-day	EVAR 1 [7]	1.7%	4.7%	-	0.009
	DREAM [8]	1.2%	4.6%	-	0.01
	EVAR 2 [9]	9%	-	-	-

group), with an aortic aneurysm of at least 5 cm in diameter. More than 80% of the patients in either groups were healthy or had only mild systemic disease. Thirty-day mortality rate was lower in the EVAR than in the open repair group (1.2% vs 4.6%) [8].

The EVAR 2 trial randomized 338 patients aged 60 or older, with an aneurysm of at least 5.5 cm in diameter, who were unfit for open repair (166 patients in EVAR group, 172 in no intervention group). Compared to EVAR 1, 30-day mortality for endografting was significantly higher (9% vs 1.7%). The mortality rate in the 47 patients who crossed over to receive EVAR was only 2% [9].

SINGLE-CENTER AND MULTI-CENTER RESULTS

Industry sponsored pre-FDA registration studies using one specific device generally show a lower short-term mortality compared to other single and multicenter studies (Tables III, IV) [10-15]. Reasons might be strict selection of patients, wider experience of institutions and tutors and a faster learning curve by using only one specific device.

Accordingly, there is a big difference among single center studies concerning 30-day mortality, ranging from 0% to 4.3% (Table IV) [16-18].

Thiry-day mortality of elective EVAR in a consecutive series of 650 EVAR procedures performed

Table III THIRTY-DAY MORTALITY IN SINGLE OR MULTI-CENTER TRIALS USING SPECIFIC DEVICES

First author [ref.]	Study comparing OR vs EVAR	Study type	Period	Type of device	Number of patients	30-day mortality (%)
Moore [10]	Yes	Prosp	11.1995 – 08.2002	AnCure	573	1.7
Zarins [11]	Yes	Prosp	06.1996 – 11.1999	AneuRx	1 192	1.0
Carpenter [12]	Yes	Prosp	NA	PowerLink	118	0.8
Matsumura [13]	Yes	Prosp	NA	Excluder	235	0
Qu [14]	No	Prosp	02.1999 – 09.2006	PowerLink	378	1.6
Van Herwaarden [15]	No	Prosp	12.1996 – 08.2003	AneuRx	212	2.4

Prosp: prospective; NA: not available

Table IV THIRTY-DAY MORTALITY IN SINGLE CENTER STUDIES

First author [ref.]	Study comparing OR and EVAR	Type of study	Period	Local anesthesia and analgo-sedation (%)	Number of patients	30-day mortality (%)
Biebl [16]	No	Retrospective	11.1999 – 12.2003	10.2%	167	0
Brewster [17]	No	Retrospective	01.1994 – 12.2005	1.8%	873	1.8
Du Toit [18]	No	Prospective	01.1998 – 12.2003	100% Epidural or propofol	163	4.2

since 1997 at University Hospital Zurich is 0.7%. With a few exceptions, all transfemoral implantations are performed under local anesthesia with slight systemic analgosedation. In patients with an appropriate infrarenal neck (neck diameter <30 mm and length >1.5 cm) and landing zone in the common iliac artery, 30-day mortality is 0%, high risk patients included.

META-ANALYSIS, SYSTEMATIC REVIEWS AND COLLECTIVE SERIES

The meta-analysis by Franks et al. [19] is the largest analysis of its kind in the published literature concerning EVAR for abdominal aorta aneurysms (Table V). The overall 30-day mortality rate after elective EVAR is low (3.3%), showing gradual reduction from 7.5% since it was first introduced (1991) to approximately 1.4% (2002). The apparent higher operative risk compared to randomized studies could be explained with the inclusion of results from the early experience in the analysis (when surgeons were not familiar with the "new equipment" or within learning curve). In this meta-analysis, 30-day mortality rate is 1.6% in the randomized controlled trials and 2.0% in non-randomized controlled trials, comparative studies and case series.

A major limitation of systematic reviews is the heterogeneity of inclusion criteria, and study population. There are many considerable variations among studies: fitness, primary technical success, operator experiences, different devices, so that the collective case mix is difficult to interpret [19-25].

THIRTY-DAY MORTALITY IN SUBGROUPS: HIGH RISK PATIENTS

There is no established consensus defining the "high risk patient". The determination of fitness in UK EVAR trial was left to the discretion of the surgeon participating in the trial. On the other hand there are several risk-scoring systems based on the patient's preoperative health status. For bedside use, the most applicable Scores are the Glasgow Aneurysm Score (GAS) and the Customized Probability Index [26].

EVAR 2 trial included patients at excessive surgical risk, medically unfit for open repair, that were randomized to either EVAR or no intervention. The 30-day mortality rate for EVAR was 9%. This high mortality rate could be explained with a significant proportion of EVAR-2 patients (8%) dying during the waiting time before EVAR, untreated comorbidities, and lack of preoperative medical treatment (statins, β-blockers) [9].

Table V THIRTY-DAY MORTALITY IN META-ANALYSES, SYSTEMATIC REVIEWS AND COLLECTIVE SERIES

First author [ref.]	Study comparing open repair and EVAR	Type of study	Period	Number of series	Number of patients	30-day mortality (%)
Franks [19]	No	Meta-analysis	1991 – 08.2003	161	28 862	3.3
Ho [20]	Yes	Systematic review	1991 – 11.2004	20	5 679	1.9
Drury [21]	Yes	Systematic review	01.2000 – 09.2004	61	18 316	1.9
Adriaensen [22]	Yes	Systematic review	06.1998 – 02.2001	9	687	2.4
Bush [23]	Yes	Collective series	05.2001 – 09.2003	123	717	3.1
Hua [24]	Yes	Collective series	01.2000 – 12.2003	14	460	2.8
Timaran [25]	No	Population based	01.2001 – 12.2004	1 000 hospitals/ 35 USA states	65 502	2.2

Table VI — Thirty-day mortality of high-risk patients

First author [ref.]	Cohort characteristics	30-day mortality EVAR N (%)	30-day mortality Open N (%)	Any complications EVAR N (%)	Any complications Open N (%)	1-year mortality EVAR N (%)	1-year mortality Open N (%)
Bush [27]	EVAR = 788 Open = 1 580	27 (3.4)	83 (5.2)	128 (16.2)	49 (31.0)	75 (9.5)	196 (12.4)
Napgal [28]	EVAR = 100	5 (5.0)	-	NA	-	NA	-
Jordan [29]	EVAR = 130 Open = 87	6 (4.6)	12 (13.8)	22 (16.9)	36 (41.3)	NA	NA
Sicard [30]	EVAR = 565 Open = 61	16 (2.9)	3 (5.1)	NA	NA	NA	NA

N: number of patients; NA: not available

Other studies (Table VI) report lower short-term mortality and morbidity rates in high-risk patients [27-30]. Influence of improvements in anesthetic options, surgical techniques, and intensive care management on the successful operations in high-risk individuals might not be neglected.

THIRTY-DAY MORTALITY IN SUBGROUPS: SMALL AAA

The threshold for differentiation of a small from a large aortic aneurysm is 5.5 cm. According to EUROSTAR registry patients with smaller aneurysms are younger than those with larger aneurysms, less frequently suffer from ASA class 3 or 4 disease, and less frequently had cardiac, renal and pulmonary comorbidity [31]. The same registry reports a 30-day mortality of 1.6% in patients with small aneurysms, compared to 4.1% in patients with large (≥6.5 cm), and 2.6% in patients with medium-sized aneurysms (5.5-6.4 cm). Cardiac complications occurred in 2.8%, pulmonary in 1.6%, with combined first-month systemic complications of 12% and statistically significant difference between small aneurysms and those larger than 6.5cm. On the other hand, there is no difference in early procedure related or device specific complications between small (<5.5 cm) and large aneurysms (≥6.5 cm). Operating time and rate of type I endoleaks at completion angiography was lower in the small aneurysm group of patients. These findings are associated with a lower frequency of significant angulations of the infrarenal neck, aneurysm and iliac arteries, and a narrower neck in patients with small aneurysms. Greater aortic neck lengths are additional characteristic of small aneurysms compared to larger ones [32]. In conclusion, considering the very good short time results, the statistically better survival in the early surgical group compared to surveillance group in UK Small Aneurysm Trial [33] after 9-years follow up, and the zero aneurysm ruptures and almost no aneurysm-related deaths in large series with aneurysm diameter <5 cm [32], endovascular repair of small aneurysms appears to be attractive in these patients and could result in more frequent use of this treatment modality in the future.

THIRTY-DAY MORTALITY IN SUBGROUPS: GENDER

Gender differences are well known in patients undergoing endovascular repair for AAA. Women are older than men [34] and the incidence of AAA is 5-6 times more frequent in men [35]. There are differences in aorto-iliac anatomy (in women common iliac arteries are smaller), as well the incidence of suitability for EVAR (more arterial kinking, narrower infrarenal aortic necks, more angulations between the proximal aneurysm neck and longitudinal axis of the aneurysm compared to men) [34,36]. It is worth to mention that the annual growth rate of AAA is significantly greater in women than in men (3.67 mm versus 2.03 mm) [37].

In earlier studies, the 30-day mortality rate after elective AAA endovascular repair was 12% for women and no death for men, and complication rates at 1 month of 41% for women, and 15% for men [38].

In Ouriel's study of 704 EVAR for AAA, the perioperative mortality was higher in females (3.1%) than in men (1.3%). However, this was not statistically significant. The only statistically gender specific difference seen in this study was the more frequent use of iliac conduits for introduction of the device in women (11%) than in men (2.8%) [35].

Zenith investigators encountered no difference between women and men with regard to short term mortality and morbidity. In the same study women experienced more type II endoleaks at 30 days (23.3% vs. 9.6%). This was explained with the aneurysmal thrombus load and the presence of circumferential neck thrombus (in women twice as much, 12% versus 6.5%) [36].

Thirty-day mortality in subgroups: octogenarians and nonagenarians

The frequency of AAA is rising up to 10% in octogenarians and nonagenarians with the ever increasing mean life expectancy in Western countries. Comorbid conditions often foreclose open surgical repair. Mortality rates in octogenarians and nonagenarians treated by EVAR are comparable with open repair. Furthermore, it even equalizes mortality rate with younger patients treated with EVAR [39-42].

In a small group of nonagenarians with a mean aneurysm diameter of 7.3 cm 30-day mortality rate was 12.5% [40]. Mid-term one-year survival rate was 83% whereas the one-year rupture incidence was 32.5% in patients refusing or unfit for elective repair with aneurysm diameter >7.0 cm [43], reflecting an advantageous outcome in interventionally treated nonagenarians.

Thirty-day mortality in subgroups: ruptured AAA

Since its introduction in 1994, a huge amount of literature about emergency-EVAR (e-EVAR) in ruptured abdominal aortic aneurysms has been published [44-50] showing overall evidence for the success of e-EVAR over open repair (absolute mortality reduction of >20% compared to open repair). Moreover, endovascular repair is, in all the studies, equally effective or better than open repair. However, because of a lack of reporting standards and standardized treatment algorithms no definite conclusions can be drawn and some authors/groups conclude that randomized controlled trials are needed to prove the efficacy and efficiency of emergency EVAR for ruptured abdominal aortic aneurysm. The authors are convinced that this evidence makes it an ethical issue to conduct randomized controlled studies comparing endovascular repair versus open repair for ruptured abdominal aortic aneurysm.

Predictors of 30-day mortality

The Glasgow Aneurysm Score (GAS) has been shown some years ago already to be a useful tool to predict immediate postoperative death after elective open repair of AAA [51-53]. This holds true for elective EVAR procedures [54]. Tertile 30-day mortality rates were 1.1% for patients with a GAS less than 74.4, 2.1% for those with a score between 74.4 and 83.6, and 5.3% for patients with a score over 83.6 ($p<0.001$). Multivariate analysis showed that GAS independently predicted postoperative

Table VII	Thirty-day mortality of octogenarians and nonagenarians				
First author [ref.]	Type of study (comparing studies or case series)	Period	Age (years)	Number of patients	30-day mortality (%)
Biebl [39]	Open vs EVAR	06.1999-09.2003	>80	49	0
Baril [40]	Case series	01.1997-01.2005	>90	16	12.5
Minor [41]	Case series	01.1997.-08.2002	>80	150	3.3
Lange [42]	EUROSTAR	01.1996-12.2004	>80	697	5.0

death (p<0.001). Other scoring systems such as the Modified Leiden Score (M-LS), and the Modified Comorbidity Severity Score (M-CSS) seem to be equivalent [55].

Similar predictions for open repair have been achieved by other scoring systems (E-PAS, WB-HOM) [56] which too accurately predicted the risk of mortality and morbidity in patients undergoing elective open AAA repair. Among these, E-PASS seemed to be the most accurate predictor in this patient population. Unfortunately up to now, these scoring systems have not been validated for EVAR.

Best treatment option can be assessed on risk stratification using simultaneously several scoring tools for open surgery (GAS, E-PASS) and EVAR (GAS, M-LS, M.CSS).

Thirty-day morbidity

INFLAMMATORY RESPONSE AND ACTIVATION OF COAGULATION FOLLOWING EVAR

The systemic inflammatory response syndrome following EVAR is a result of complex interactions between vascular endothelium, blood, thrombus within the aneurysm sac and the stent-graft [57] and ischemia-reperfusion injury caused by access artery clamping [58]. Clinically, post-implantation syndrome ranges from a milder form with increased inflammatory markers (CRP, leukocytosis) and fever to a huge systemic inflammatory response syndrome (SIRS) with (multiple) organ failure (cardiac, respiratory, renovisceral, cerebral) [59,60]. Increase of acute phase proteins (high-sensitivity CRP, alfa-1-antitripsin), pro-inflammatory cytokines (IL-6, IL-8, and TNF-alpha), and complement protein (C3a) are noted in up to 10% of the patients [59], which seems to be less than after open repair [61]. Potentially, peri-operative administration of anti-inflammatory drugs will additionally decrease peri-operative mortality.

Activation of coagulation is another physiologic response triggered by EVAR, and may contribute to hemorrhagic and thrombo-embolic complications. A study comparing activation of coagulation in asymptomatic patients treated with EVAR or open repair showed severe thrombin activation in the EVAR group [62]. In this small group of patients (N=30), one peri-operative myocardial infarct occurred in the EVAR group, and correlated with pronounced thrombin activity. Clinical impact ought to be defined, but all factors inducing thrombin activity should be minimized during the procedure (endovascular manipulation, volume of contrast media).

ISCHEMIC COMPLICATIONS

Ischemic complications following EVAR have been reported in up to 7% of the cases. Tissue ischemia occurs secondary to vessel occlusion (instable plaque with acute thrombosis, embolic occlusion, inadvertent occlusion of the vessel ostium by the stent-graft), low flow situation (low cardiac output syndrome, abdominal compartment syndrome) or insufficient tissue perfusion pressure (low systemic blood pressure combined with pre-existing arterial stenosis, or usage of vasoconstrictors).

The inferior mesenteric artery (IMA) is always sacrificed during EVAR but there are no clear data confirming its role in colon ischemia. Transient colon ischemia after EVAR has been reported in patients with previous segmental colon resection where IMA interruption may have impaired colonic collaterals [63]. Colonic ischemia is discussed to be usually a consequence of micro-embolization during catheter or sheath manipulation, and/or stent-graft deployment [63-66].

The role of unilateral or bilateral hypogastric artery interruption in pelvic ischemia is not completely defined. In a single center series among 88 patients with unilateral iliac artery coverage (without coil embolization) there is no incidence of ischemic colitis, spinal cord ischemia, or gluteal necrosis. Buttock claudication in 2 patients (9.5%) resolved after 4 months [63]. This is in accordance with results published by Mehta et al. [67]: out of 154 patients with aorto-iliac aneurysms where interruption of one (134 patients) or both internal iliac arteries (20 patients) did not result in severe colon ischemia or buttock necrosis. Persistent buttock claudication occurred in 12% of patients with unilateral and in 11% of patients with bilateral internal iliac artery interruption. They concluded that other factors such as distal embolization, failure to preserve collateral branches from the external iliac and femoral arteries may have contributed to ischemic complications. Overall, in patients with bilateral internal iliac artery interruption buttock claudication is reported to occur in 0%-57% cases. In another study, buttock claudication was the leading clinical symptom after bilateral internal iliac interruption (followed by erectile dysfunction), however, most patients show an improvement after one year [68]. There was no severe buttock necrosis at all.

On the other hand, Japanese surgeons, insist on preservation of the pelvic circulation through crossover bypass graft-to-ipsilateral internal iliac artery as an adjunct to aorto-uni-external iliac artery stent graft [69]. Other techniques are also referred including a fenestrated and branched revascularization of the internal iliac artery.

Remote access complications are the leading cause of limb ischemia after EVAR [70]. Stent-graft related causes are not well defined but the following are reported: 1. small limb diameter; 2. landing the graft limb in the external iliac artery [69]; 3. unsupported limb design of some devices [71]. With introduction of lower-profile devices with easier delivery systems and supported limb the frequency of ischemic complications after EVAR decreased. In a recent published study, Maldonado et al. [64] reported the incidence of overall ischemic events in the group of patients treated at same institution in two periods. In the second study period, over the last two years, Maldonado et al. [65] reported no ischemic events (Table VIII).

EVAR specific complications

The frequency of intra-operatively device related complications within the EUROSTAR registry (7 968 patients enrolled from July 1997 to August 2004) was 4.5%: among them, the most frequent were device migration, inability to advance the delivery sheath, and inability to deploy the device [2]. In-hospital local groin problems such as bleeding, hematoma, and false aneurysm (3.5%), arterial thrombosis (0.5%), emboli (0.3%) were observed. Thirty-day secondary repairs (transabdominal and extra-anatomic) were performed in 2.3% of patients.

In a systematic review of clinical trials comparing EVAR and open repair of AAA, seven studies were identified reporting the frequency of secondary procedures performed within 30 days post intervention. Secondary interventions were necessary in 8.4% (out of 1593 patients) in the EVAR groups, opposite to 4.4% (out of 1268 patients) in the open repair groups [20]. In another systematic review, three randomized controlled trials were identified with 759 EVAR procedures for elective AAA; in these randomized trials the overall frequency of graft thrombosis was 6.4%, of local wound infection 3.5% and of renal impairment 1.2%. In the 58 non-randomized trials, comparative studies and case series analyzed in the same review (17'377 EVAR procedures), the frequency of limb ischemia was 1.3%, local wound infection was reported in 6.8%, and renal impairment in 2.8% of the patients [21].

EVAR trial participants reported device specific results from the UK EVAR Trials. The frequency of secondary interventions in the EVAR 1 trial was 19.4% (Zenith group 17.6%, and Talent group 22.5%), and in the EVAR 2 Trial 21.7% (Zenith group 19.3%, Talent group 29.4%). The secondary intervention rate per 100 patient-years

Table VIII	Ischemic complications								
First author [ref.]	Study comparing EVAR and open repair	Study type	Period	Number of patients	Limb ischemia N(%)	Colon necrosis N(%)	Buttock Ischemia N(%)	Spinal Cord Ischemia N(%)	Total Ischemic events N(%)
Maldonado [63]	No	Retro	01.1994-12.2003	311	15 (4.8)	4 (1.3)	2 (0.6)	2 (0.6)	22 (7.1)
Maldonado [64]	No	Retro	01.1994-12.2005	430	15 (3.5)	4 (0.9)	2 (0.4)	2 (0.4)	22 (5.1)
Dadian [65]	No	Prosp	11.1992-4.2001	278	NA	8 (2.9)	NA	NA	NA

Retro=retrospective study; Prosp=prospective study

was 6.4% in the Zenith versus 8.6% in the Talent group in the EVAR 1 trial, and 9.6% for the Zenith versus 15.1% for the Talent group in the EVAR 2 trial. The most frequent complications in EVAR Trials were: type 1 endoleak (EVAR 1 and 2), graft thrombosis (EVAR 1), and technical deployment problems (EVAR 1). It is worth to mention that during both trial periods Medtronic corrected the delivery system. [72].

The suprarenal fixation resulted in unintentional graft covering or impinging of barbs on renal ostia, respectively. If not detected during the intervention (and not treated by renal angioplasty and stent placement) these complications mostly lead to increase in creatinine level, but patients requiring postoperative hemodialysis are those with pre-existing chronic renal function or other significant comorbid conditions. In a study undertaken to asses the effect on renal function of open repair versus EVAR with Zenith suprarenal fixation, renal dysfunction occurred regardless of the type of repair. There was a lower incidence of elevated serum creatinine in the Zenith compared with open repair group before discharge. However, after exclusion of the patients with suprarenal clamping from the open surgery group this difference disappeared. Initial dysfunction stabilizes or improves at 12 and 24 months follow up [73].

Cardiac complications

Coronary heart disease is the main cause of hospital mortality causing about 50% of deaths within 30 days in patients after open elective surgery for AAA [74]. Many authors report reduced incidence of peri-operative, and cardiac complications during endovascular repair. In a study of 175 patients treated either with open repair (126) or EVAR (49), myocardial ischemia occurred in 34%, cardiac arrhythmias in 25%, and cardiac events at 30 days in 6% of all patients. Endovascular repair compared to open repair was associated with significantly less myocardial ischemia (10.2% vs. 50.8%), lower 30-day mortality (0% vs 8.7%), and 30-day cardiac event rates (0% vs 7.9%) [75]. Endovascular repair is associated with a lower peri-operative heart rate [76]. Higher peri-operative heart rate in patients undergoing open repair is the result of increased surgical stress (intra-operatively, during longer period of aortic occlusion, postoperative pain), and increased sympathetic tone (interruption of beta blockers, or use of sympathicomimetic drugs). The use of beta-blockers and tight heart rate control are associated with reduced peri-operative cardiac events, and are recommended in all patients with AAA treated with open or endovascular repair [76]. Further decrease of cardiac complications should be expected with aggressive pre-operative assessment of coronary artery disease, liberal use of local/regional anesthesia, long-term postoperative use of beta-blockers, and eventually statins [77].

Respiratory complications

Respiratory complications after elective EVAR range between 0% and 5.2% according to the literature [78]. This is a significant reduction compared to respiratory complications after open repair that range between 8% and 16.5% [79]. Patients with the highest peri-operative mortality are those with limiting chronic obstructive pulmonary disease (COPD), dyspnoe at rest, oxygen dependency, or FEV-1 <1L/s [80]. Uses of local/regional anesthesia, early extubation after general anesthesia, intensive physiotherapy are the main elements for prevention of respiratory complications [81].

Type of anesthesia

Since the introduction of EVAR, the preferred type of anesthesia was general and still is accepted on a large scale in Europe as a traditional attitude. According to EUROSTAR registry general anesthesia has been used in 69% of 5 557 patients [82]. Other techniques: local (with additional intravenous medications, such as sedation and pain medication) and regional anesthesia (spinal and epidural) are used in remaining 31% of patients (25% in regional, and 6% in local). Potentially, contra-indications for local anesthesia might be insufficient cooperation (because of agitation) of the patient, severe obesity, or need for iliac access, as well as surgical learning curve. General anesthesia should be restricted to patients with contra-indications to epidural anesthesia necessitating access via iliac arteries [83]. Aforementioned EUROSTAR registry analysis comparing local (LA), regional (RA) and general anesthesia (GA) showed significantly reduced duration of operation in LA (115.7 min) and RA (127.6 min) compared to GA (133.3 min), as well as less admission to intensive care unit

(ICU, in LA 2%, RA 8.3%, and in GA group 16.2% patients required admission to ICU). Systemic complications were significantly lower both for LA (6.6%) and RA (9.5%) than for GA (13.0%) [84]. In high risk patients the advantages of LA and RA are more prominent: systemic complications are lower for LA (9.0%) and RA (10.7%), compared to GA (18.3%). Early death (within the 30-days) was reduced in EUROSTAR registries patients in RA (3.0%) compared to GA (4.3%) [82].

All these results emphasize the fact that LA and RA are safe, well tolerated, feasible in most of patients, so that widespread use of LA and RA, especially in high-risk patients, should be advised.

Learning curve

Mortality and adverse events leading to secondary intervention after endovascular AAA repair are significantly lower in patients who underwent endovascular AAA repair by a highly experienced specialist team of vascular surgeons and interventional radiologists than in those who underwent endovascular repair by a relatively inexperienced team [85]. Moreover, as an institution's experience with EVAR increases, an individual surgeon's learning curve shortens considerably [86].

Discussion

A review of the recent literature including randomized trials, registries, single or multicenter trials, meta-analyses, reviews and collective series, allows actually describing more specifically short term outcome of EVAR procedures.

Based on anatomical and/or device suitability, 20%-60% of the patients with AAA are suitable for EVAR. In elective patients, best results are achieved in low surgical risk males with AAA <6.4 cm in diameter and meeting the morphological criteria required for the specific device used. Acceptable results are achieved in females and/or patients with co-morbidities. In high risk patients or patients considered "unfit" for surgery, EVAR has highest mortality, but mortality rates as low as 2%-3% have been reported in various larger series. In ruptured AAA, EVAR achieves a relative risk reduction of 20% when compared to open surgery. There is no single published series reported showing mortality after EVAR to be higher than the mortality after open surgery.

Procedure-related morbidity has decreased during the last decade and is lowest in experienced teams, especially in those where surgeon and interventional radiologist are performing the procedure together. Devices, including delivery systems, have evolved and actually, technical complications in male patients with optimal anatomy for EVAR are <1%.

Morbidity related to patient comorbidities remains an issue. Underlying pathologies should be addressed with best medical treatment in all patients, irrespective the chosen treatment (EVAR or open repair). In patients unfit for surgery, it can be recommended first to make the patient fit for AAA repair, but AAA treatment should not be delayed for a too long time, especially in large AAA, as rupture risk increases dramatically with time. In patients with multifocal atherosclerosis, aspirin, lipid-lowering drugs and beta-blockers should be started at least 4 weeks before EVAR or open repair. Tight heart rate control during procedure (EVAR, open repair) increases not only early, but also late cardiac event free survival and is therefore recommended. Local anesthesia for transfemoral implantations seems to be best option: procedural volume load is minimized, catecholamine requirement exceptional, hepato- or nephrotoxic anesthetics are not required and complications related to intubation/extubation and artificial ventilation are completely avoided. Non-steroidal anti inflammatory or steroids might be necessary in rare patients suffering (high fever, discomfort) inflammatory response to EVAR. Clinical signification of the activation of the coagulation is unclear, but should be monitorized and eventually treated by aspirin and heparin administration, at least in patients with unstable coronary artery disease. In patients with prior colon surgery caution about the emergence of mesenteric ischemia is required. Thrombo-embolic complications are more prone to occur in patients with severe atherosclerotic disease of the descending or visceral aorta.

Open repair remains an effective therapy option in patients in whom EVAR is unsuitable. Even in high-risk old patients acceptable mortality rates of around 5% have been achieved. Risk scoring allows adequately predicts early and late mortality, representing a valuable tool to decide in which patient EVAR is the best option. Low-risk young patients with AAA >6.5 cm and with an expected survival of several decades (longer than the one of the stent-graft) are probably best treated by means of open repair.

Conclusion

Sixteen years after its clinical introduction, there is increasing evidence that EVAR offers substantial short-term advantage as compared to open repair for all types of patients (elective, emergent, low-risk and high-risk, small and large aneurysm, male and females). Unfortunately, there is still uncertainty concerning long-term outcome. Similarly, the results of EVAR for AAA in high risk patients seem to be far better than initially reported in a randomized study. As long-term outcome in these patients is not the major issue, EVAR should be, so far, "restricted" to patients with a high surgical risk (and maybe even patients unfit for surgery!) or those with a limited life expectancy presenting acceptable anatomical suitability for EVAR. However, the books are not closed, and several randomized trials are on the way to determine the value of treating high risk patients with EVAR. Moreover, EVAR for small aneurysms (<5.5 cm) may prove advantageous over large aneurysms and several randomized trials are under way. Early and late outcome can be assessed pre-operatively with for example the Glasgow Aneurysm Score (predicting 30-day and long-term mortality), helping to decide for which patient EVAR is best.

REFERENCES

1. Thomas SM, Gaines PA, Beard JD. Vascular Surgical Society of Great Britain and Ireland; British Society of Interventional Radiology. Short-term (30-day) outcome of endovascular treatment of abdominal aortic aneurism: results from prospective Registry of Endovascular Treatment of Abdominal Aortic Aneurism (RETA). *Eur J Vasc Endovasc Surg* 2001; 21: 57-64.
2. Anonymous. Eurostar Data Registry Centre - European Collaborators on stent-graft techniques for abdominal aortic aneurysm. *Progress Report – Endografts in current use only*, 2006.
3. Buth J, Harris, Leurs L et al. EUROSTAR report on Belgian endovascular abdominal aortic aneurysm elective repair between 2001 and 2005. *Rijksinstituut voor Ziekte- en Invaliditeitsverzekering* 2005
4. Anonymous. The European Society for Vascular Surgery. First vascular surgery database report. *DENDRITE Clinical Systems* 2007.
5. Anonymous. Lifeline Registry of EVAR Publications Committee. Lifeline registry of endovascular aneurysm repair: Long-term primary outcomes measures. *J Vasc Surg* 2005; 42: 1-10.
6. Boult M, Babidge W, Maddern G et al. Audit Reference Group. Endoluminal repair of abdominal aortic aneurysm-contemporary Australian experience. *Eur J Vasc Endovasc Surg* 2004; 28: 36-40.
7. Anonymous. EVAR trial participants. Endovascular aneurysm repair versus open repair in patients with abdominal aortic aneurysm (EVAR trial 1): randomised controlled trial. *Lancet* 2005; 365: 2179-2186.
8. Blankensteijn JD, de Jong SE, Prinssen M et al. Two-year outcomes after conventional or endovascular repair of abdominal aortic aneurysm. *N Eng J Med* 2005; 352: 2398-2405.
9. Anonymous. EVAR trial participants. Endovascular aneurysm repair and outcome in patients unfit for open repair of abdominal aortic aneurysm (EVAR trial 2): randomised controlled trial. *Lancet* 2005; 365: 2187-2192.
10. Moore WS, Matsumura JS, Makaroun MS et al. Five-year interim comparison of the Guidant bifurcated endogaft with open repair of abdominal aortic aneurysm. *J Vasc Surg* 2003; 38: 46-55.
11. Zarins CK, White RA, Moll FL et al. The AneuRx stent graft: four-year results and worldwide experience. *J Vasc Surg* 2001; 33(2 suppl): S135-145.
12. Carpenter JP; Endologix Investigators. Multicentre trial of the PowerLink bifurcated system for endvascular aortic aneurysm repair. *J Vasc Surg* 2002; 36: 1129-1137.
13. Matsumura JS, Brewster DC, Makaroun MS et al. A multicenter controlled trial of open versus endovascular treatment of abdominal aortic aneurysm. *J Vasc Surg* 2003; 37: 262-271.
14. Qu L, Hetzel G, Raithel D. Seven years' single center experience of Powerlink unibody bifurcated endograft for endovascular aortic aneurysm repair. *J Cardiovasc Surg* 2007; 48: 13-9.
15. van Herwaarden JA, van de Pavoordt ED, Waasdorp EJ et al. Long-term single-center results with aneurx endografts for endovascular abdominal aortic aneurysm repair. *J Endovasc Ther* 2007; 14: 307-317.
16. Biebl M, Hakaim AG, Oldenburg WA et al. Midterm results of a single-center experience with commercially available devices for endovascular aneurysm repair. *Mt Sinai J Med* 2005; 72: 127-135.
17. Brewster DC, Jones JE, Chung TK et al. Long-term outcomes after endovascular abdominal aortic aneurysm repair : the first decade. *Ann Surg* 2006; 244: 426-438.
18. Du Toit DF, Saaiman JA, Carpenter JP et al. Endovascular aortic aneurysm repair by a multidisciplinary team: lessons learned and six-year clinical update. *Cardiovasc J S Afr* 2005; 16: 36-47.
19. Franks SC, Sutton AJ, Bown MJ et al. Systematic review and meta-analysis of 12 years of endovascular abdominal aortic aneurysm repair. *Eur J Vasc Endovasc Surg* 2007; 33: 154-171.
20. Ho P, Yiu WK, Cheung GCY et al. Systematic review of clinical trials comparing open and endovascular treatment of abdominal aortic aneurysm. *Surgical Practice* 2006; 10: 24-37.
21. Drury D, Michaels JA, Jones L et al. Systematic review of recent evidence for the safety and efficacy of elective endovascular repair in the management of infrarenal abdominal aortic aneurysm. *Br J Surg* 2005; 92: 937-946.
22. Adriaensen ME, Bosch JL, Halpern EF et al. Elective endovascular versus open surgical repair of abdominal aortic aneurysms: systematic review of short-term results. *Radiology* 2002; 224: 79-747
23. Bush RL, Johnson ML, Collins TC et al. Open versus endovas-

cular abdominal aortic aneurysm repair in VA Hospitals. *J Am Coll Surg* 2006; 202: 577-587.

24. Hua HT, Cambria RP, Chuang SK et al. early outcomes of endovascular versus open abdominal aneurysm repair in the National Surgical Quality Improvement Program-Private sector (NSQIP-PS). *J Vasc Surg* 2005; 41: 382-389.

25. Timaran CH, Veith FJ, Rosero EB et al. Endovascular aortic aneurysm repair in patients with the highest risk and in hospital mortality in the United States. *Arch Surg* 2007; 142: 520-525.

26. Baas A, Blankensteijn J. Outcome of endovascular repair. In: Branchereau A, Jacobs M (eds). *Open Surgery versus Endovascular Procedures* 2007; pp 143-148.

27. Bush RL, Johnson ML, Hedayati N et al. Performance of endovascular aortic aneurysm repair in high-risk patients: Results from the Veterans Affair National Surgical Quality Improvement Program. *J Vasc Surg* 2007; 45: 227-234.

28. Napgal AD, Forbes TL, Novick TV et al. Midterm results of endovascular infrarenal abdominal aortic aneurysm in high-risk patients. *Vasc Endovasc Surg* 2007; 4: 301-309

29. Jordan WD, Alcocer F, Wirthlin DJ et al. Abdominal aortic aneurysms in "high-risk" surgical patients: comparison of open and endovascular repair. *Ann Surg* 2003; 237: 623-630.

30. Sicard GA, Zwolak RM, Sidaway AN et al. Endovascular abdominal aortic aneurysm repair: long-term outcome measures in patients at high-risk for open surgery. *J Vasc Surg* 2006; 44: 229-236.

31. Peppelbosch N, Buth J, Harris P et al. Diameter of abdominal aortic aneurysm and outcome of endovascular aneurysm repair: Does it matter? A report from EUROSTAR. *J Vasc Surg* 2004; 39: 288-297.

32. Zarins CK, Crabtree T, Bloch D et al. Endovascular aneurysm repair at 5 years: does aneurysm diameter predict outcome? *J Vasc Surg* 2006; 44: 920-930.

33. Anonymous. United Kingdom Small Aneurysm Trial Participants. Long-term outcomes of immediate repair compared with surveillance of small abdominal aortic aneurysms. *N Engl J Med* 2002; 346: 1445-1452.

34. Velasquez OC, Larson RA, Baum RA et al. gender-related differences in infrarenal aortic aneurysm morphologic features: issue relevant to Ancure and Talent endografts. *J Vasc Surg* 2001; 33(2 Suppl): S77-84.

35. Ouriel K, Greenberg RK, Clair DG et al. Endovascular aneurysm repair. Gender specific results. *J Vasc Surg* 2003; 38: 93-98.

36. Hugl B, Hakaim AG, Biebl M et al. Impact of gender on the outcome of endovascular aortic aneurysm repair using the Zenith stent graft: midterm results. *J Endovasc Ther* 2007; 14: 115-121.

37. Mofidi R, Goldie VJ, Kelman J et al. Influence of sex on expansion rate of abdominal aortic aneurysms. *B rJ Surg* 2007; 94:310-314.

38. Nordness PJ, Carter G, Tonnessen B et al. The effect of gender on early and intermediate results of endovascular aneurysm repair. *Ann Vasc Surg* 2003; 17: 615-621.

39. Biebl M, lau LL, Hakaim AG et al. Midterm outcome of endovascular abdominal aortic aneurysm repair in octogenarians. A single institutions' experience. *J Vasc Surg* 2004; 40: 435-442.

40. Barli DT, Palchik E, Carroccio A et al. Experience With Endovascular Abdominal Aortic Aneurysm Repair in Nonagenarians. *J Endovasc Ther* 2006; 13: 330-337.

41. Minor ME, Ellozy S, Carroccio A et al. Endovascular aortic aneurysm repair in the octogenarians. *Arch Surg* 2004; 139: 308-314.

42. Lange C, Leurs LJ, Buth J et al. Endovascular repair of abdominal aortic aneurysm in octagenerians: an analysis based on EUROSTAR data. *J Vasc Surg* 2005; 42: 624-630.

43. Lederle FA, Johnson GR, Wilson SE et al. Rupture rate of large abdominal aortic aneurysms in patients refusing or unfit for elective repair. *JAMA* 2002; 287: 2968-2972.

44. Acosta S, Lindblad B, Zdanovski Z. Predictors for outcome after open and endovascular repair of ruprured abdominal aneurysms. *Eur J Vasc Endovasc Surg* 2007; 33: 277-284.

45. Arya N, Makar RR, Lau LL et al. An intention to treat by endovascular repair policy may reduce overall mortality in ruptured abdominal aortic aneurysm. *J Vasc Surg* 2006; 44: 467-471.

46. Coppi G, Silingardi R, Gennai S et al. A single centre experience in open and endovascular treatment of hemodynamically unstable and stable patients with ruptured abdominal aortic aneurysms. *J Vasc Surg* 2006; 44: 1140-1147.

47. Franks S, Lloyd G, Fishwick G et al. Endovascular treatment of ruptured and symptomatic abdominal aortic aneurysms. *Eur J Vasc Endovasc Surg* 2006; 31: 345-350.

48. Hechelhammer L, Lachat ML, Wildermuth S et al. Midterm outcome of endovascular repair of ruptured abdominal aortic aneurysms. *J Vasc Surg* 2005; 41: 752-757.

49. Ockert S, Schumacher H, Böckler D et al. Early and midterm results after open and endovascular repair of ruptured abdominal aortic aneurysms in a comparative analysis. *J Endovasc Ther* 2007; 14: 324-332.

50. Greco G, Egorova N, Anderson PL et al. Outcomes of endovascular treatment of ruptured abdominal aortic aneurysms. *J Vasc Surg* 2006; 43: 453-459.

51. Biancari F, Leo E, Ylönen K et al. Value of the Glasgow Aneurysm Score in predicting the immediate and long-term outcome after elective open repair of infrarenal abdominal aortic aneurysm. *Br J Surg* 2003; 90: 838-844.

52. Biancari F, Heikkinen M, Lepäntalo M et al. Finnvasc Study Group. Glasgow Aneurysm Score in patients undergoing elective open repair of abdominal aortic aneurysm: a Finnvasc study. *Eur J Vasc Endovasc Surg* 2003; 26: 612-617.

53. Nesi F, Leo E, Biancari F et al. Preoperative risk stratification in patients undergoing elective infrarenal aortic aneurysm surgery: evaluation of five risk scoring methods. *Eur J Vasc Endovasc Surg* 2004; 28: 52-58.

54. Biancari F, Hobo R, Juvonen T. Glasgow Aneurysm Score predicts survival after endovascular stenting of abdominal aortic aneurysm in patients from the EUROSTAR registry. *Br J Surg* 2006; 93: 191-194.

55. Faizer R, DeRose G, Lawlor K et al. Objective scoring systems of medical risk: A clinical tool for selecting patients for open or endovascular abdominal aortic aneurysm repair. *J Vasc Surg* 2007; 45: 1102-1108.

56. Tang TY, Walsh SR, Fanshawe TR et al. Comparison of risk-scoring methods in predicting the immediate outcome after elective open abdominal aortic aneurysm surgery. *Eur J Vasc Endovasc Surg* 2007; 34: 505-513.

57. Gabriel EA, Locali RF, Romano CC et al. Analysis of the inflammatory response in endovascular treatment of aortic aneurysm. *Eur J Cardiothorac Surg* 2007; 31: 406-413.

58. Storck M, Scharrer-Pamler R, Kapfer X et al. Does a postimplantation syndrome following endovascular treatment of aortic aneurysm exist? *Vasc Surg* 2001; 35(1): 23-29.

59. Gerasimidis T, Sfyroeras G, Trellopoulos G et al. Impact of endograft material on the inflammatory response after elective endovascular abdominal aortic aneurysm repair. *Angiology* 2005; 56: 743-753.

60. Galle C, de Maertelaer V, Motte S et al. early inflammatory response after elective abdominal aneurysm repair: a comparison between endovascular procedure and conventional surgery. *J Vasc Surg* 2000; 32: 234-246.

61. Bölke E, Jehle PM, Storck M et al. Endovascular stent-graft placement versus conventional open surgery in infrarenal aortic aneurysm. A prospective study on acute phase response and clinical outcome. *Clinica Chimica Acta* 2001; 314: 203-207.

62. Englberger L, Savolainen H, Jandus P et al. Activated coagulation during open and endovascular abdominal aortic aneurysm repair. *J Vasc Surg* 2006; 43: 1124-1129.

63. Maldonado TS, Rockman CB, Riles E et al. Ischemic complications after endovascular abdominal aortic repair. *J Vasc Surg* 2004; 40: 703-710.

64. Maldonado TS, Ranson ME, Rockman CB et al. Decreased ischemic complications after endovascular aortic aneurysm repair with newer devices. *Vasc Endovasc Surg* 2007; 41: 192-199.

65. Dadian N, Ohki T, Veith FJ et al. Overt colon ischemia after endovascular aneurysm repair: The importance of microembolization as an etiology. *J Vasc Surg* 2001; 34: 986-996.

66. Mell M, Tefera G, Schwarze M et al. Absence of buttock claudication following stent-graft coverage of the hypogastric artery without coil embolization in endovascular aneurysm repair. *J Endovasc Ther* 2006; 13: 415-419.

67. Mehta M, Veith FJ, Ohki T et al. Unilateral and bilateral hypogastric artery interruption during aortoiliac aneurysm repair in 154 patients: a relative innocuous procedure. *J Vasc Surg* 2001; 33(2 Suppl): S27-32.

68. Zander T, Baldi S, Rabellino M et al. Bilateral hypogastric artery occlusion in endovascular repair of abdominal aortic aneurysms and its clinical significance. *J Vasc Interv Radiol* 2007; 18: 1481-1486

69. Unno N, Inuzuka K, Yammamoto N et al. Preservation of pelvic circulation with hypogastric artery bypass in endovascular repair of abdominal aortic aneurysm with bilateral iliac artery anueurysms. *J Vasc Surg* 2006; 44: 1170-1175.

70. Carroccio A, Faries PL, Morrissey NJ et al. Predicting iliac limb occlusions after bifurcated aortic stent grafting: anatomic and device-related causes. *J Vasc Surg* 2002; 36: 679-684.

71. Ouriel K, Clair DG, Greenberg RK et al. Endovascular repair of abdominal aortic aneurysms: device-specific outcome. *J Vasc Surg* 2003; 37: 991-998.

72. Anonymous. The EVAR Trial Participants. Secondary intervention and mortality following endovascular aortic aneurysm repair: device specific results from the UK EVAR Trials. *Eur J Endovasc Surg* 2007; 34: 281-290.

73. Greenberg RK, Chuter TA, Lawrence-Brown M et al. Analysis of renal function after aneurysm repair with a device using suprarenal fixation (Zenith AAA Endovascular Graft) in contrast to open surgical repair. *J Vasc Surg* 2004; 39: 1219-1228.

74. Norman PE, Semmenst JB, Lawrence-Brown MM. Long-term relative survival following surgery for abdominal aortic aneurysm. A review. *Cardiovasc Surgery* 2001; 9: 219-224.

75. Feringa HH, Karagiannis S, Vidakovic R et al. Comparison of the incidence of cardiac arrhythmias, myocardial ischemia, and cardiac events in patients treated with endovascular versus open surgical repair of abdominal aortic aneurysms. *Am J Cardiol* 2007;100: 1479-1484.

76. Feringa HH, Bax JJ, Boersma E, et al. High-dose beta-blockers and tight heart rate control reduce myocardial ischemia and troponin t release in vascular surgery patients. *Circulation* 2006;114(1suppl): I334-349.

77. Kertai MD, Boersma E, Westerhout CM et al. Association between long-term statin and use and mortality after successful abdominal aortic aneurysm surgery. *Am J Med* 2004; 116: 96-103.

78. Arko FR, Hill BB, Oclott C et al. Endovascular repair reduces early and late morbidity compared to open surgery for abdominal aortic aneurysm. *J Endovasc Ther* 2002; 9: 711-718.

79. Adriaensen ME, Bosch JL, Halpern EF et al. Elective endovascular versus open surgical repair of abdominal aortic aneurysms: systematic review of short-term results. *Radiology* 2002; 3: 739-747.

80. Brewster DC, Cronenwett JL, Hallett JW Jr et al. Guidelines for the treatment of abdominal aortic aneurysms. Report of a subcommittee of the Joint Council of the American Association for vascular Surgery and Society for Vascular Surgery. *J Vasc Surg* 2003; 37: 1106-1117.

81. Nevelsteen A, Lacroix H, Daenens K et al. Pulmonary complication after surgery for infrarenal aorta. In: Branchereau A, Jacobs M (eds). *Complications in vascular surgery, Part II*. Armonk, Futura Publishing Company 2002, pp 63-70.

82. Ruppert V, Leurs LJ, Rieger J et al. Risk-adapted outcome after endovascular aortic aneurysm repair: analysis of anesthesia types based on EUROSTAR Data. *J Endovasc Ther* 2007; 14: 12-22.

83. Bettex DA, Lachat M, Pfammatter T et al. To Compare general, epidural and local anaesthesia for endovascular aneurysm repair (EVAR). *Eur J Vasc Endovasc Surg* 2001; 21: 179-184.

84. Ruppert V, Leurs LJ, Stechmeier B et al. Influence of anesthesia type on outcome after endovascular aortic aneurysm repair. An analysis based on EUROSTAR data. *J Vasc Surg* 2006; 44: 16-21.

85. Laheij RJ, van Marrewijk CJ, Buth J et al. The influence of team experience on outcomes of endovascular stenting of abdominal aortic aneurysm. *Eur J Vasc Endovasc Surg* 2002; 24: 128-133.

86. Forbes TL, DeRose G, Lawlor DK et al. The association between a surgeon's learning curve with endovascular aortic aneurysm repair and previous institutional experience. *Vasc Endovascular Surg* 2007; 41: 14-18.

SHORT TERM MORTALITY AND MORBIDITY IN TAA ENDOGRAFTING

DAVID BECKETT, STEVEN THOMAS, SYED TANSHEET MUSTAFA
MATHEW KADUTHODIL

Endovascular treatment of thoracic aortic pathology has been used to treat degenerative disease, false aneurysms, both acute and chronic dissection, intramural hematoma, traumatic aortic injuries and infected aneurysms. These lesions are traditionally associated with a high surgical mortality and morbidity. Endovascular repair has proven to be a less invasive alternative and one that is particularly attractive for patients with severe co-morbidities. While over the past decade thoracic endovascular aortic repair (TEVAR) has shown encouraging results within the short term with growing data regarding its durability, it is still associated with significant morbidity and mortality both in the short term and on long-term follow-up. Within this chapter we focus solely on the short term (30-day) mortality and morbidity associated with TEVAR.

Mortality

Mortality is the most important criterion in appraising the results of thoracic aortic aneurysm (TAA) treatment. In open operation, the mortality rates differ substantially between 3% and 26% [1]. The avoidance of proximal aortic cross clamp, thoracotomy and surgical exposure of the mediastinum might play a major role in reducing the overall peri-operative complications and mortality [2].

Thirty-day mortality rates are reported as between 0% and 25%, with most centers reporting rates below 10% [3]. In general the results of TEVAR cannot be compared directly to the reported results for conventional surgical repair. This is because the results reported for TEVAR are often in patients with significant comorbidity such that they are not good candidates for open surgery [4].

Only one comparative study was identified that compared EVAR to open repair (OR) prospectively in a non-randomized cohort study [5]. Bavaria et al. conducted a study in which they compared 140 patients who underwent endovascular repair for descending thoracic aortic aneurysm with open surgical repair in 94 patients. There was no statically significant difference between the two groups in age, gender and peri-operative risk factors. Of 140 patients technical success was possible in 137 in the endovascular cohort (success rate: 97.8%). Peri-operative mortality, i.e. death within 30 days of procedure or within the first hospital admission, was 2.1% (n=3) in the EVAR group, while it was 11.7% (n=11) in the OR cohort (p=0.04). The incidence of spinal cord ischemia was 2.9% (4/140) in the EVAR group while the OR cohort showed a significantly increased incidence of 13.8% (13/94). The incidence of stroke was similar in endograft and surgical cohort (3.6% (n=5) vs 4.3% (n=4). The endovascular cohort had a lower incidence of respiratory and renal complications, but higher peripheral vascular complications when compared to the OR cohort in the study. However, there was no significant difference between the EVAR group and the OR group in terms of 2-year survival, which was 78% and 76%, respectively. Taking this into account it would appear that endovascular repair has a clear and significant advantage in terms of the early mortality of the procedure compared with open surgery.

Spinal cord ischemia and paraplegia

Paraplegia remains one of the most feared complications of surgical treatment for TAA. Fortunately, the results following TEVAR show very encouraging results with a reduced incidence of spinal cord ischemia with the most recent studies reporting rates below 5% [2]. The incidence of spinal cord ischemia and paraplegia appears to be consistently low even in patients in whom long aortic segments and the "danger zone" (T8-L1), that usually gives origin to the anterior spinal artery, has been covered by endograft [4].

This lower complication rate compared with open surgery can be explained by the shorter procedural time, the persistent blood circulation throughout the procedure, and the absence of aortic cross clamping, so the likelihood of a steal phenomenon in the perfusion of spinal cord is reduced. The stent-graft procedure is also associated with a lower incidence of postoperative respiratory failure and less prolonged hypotension, lowering the risk of delayed paraplegia [6]. However, since large numbers of intercostal arteries are acutely occluded even in endovascular repair especially when long stent-grafts are implanted, spinal cord ischemia can still occur [1].

Concomitant or previous abdominal aortic aneurysm repair and long thoracic aortic exclusion appear to be important risk factors for spinal cord ischemia, of both TEVAR and open repair. Using short segments and a step approach if long segments need to be covered may reduce paraplegic complications [6]. Spinal cord protective measures such as cerebrospinal fluid (CSF) drainage, use of steroids, and prevention of hypotension should be used for patient with aforementioned risk factors. Successful treatment of stent-graft induced paralysis by CSF drainage has been reported in some studies [6].

Stroke

Strokes can be caused by manipulation of wires, catheters and the device in the aortic arch, especially if there is atheromatous disease. The incidence of this complication is now lower with new endografts than the 7 +/- 3% rate previously reported [6]. Recent studies show the incidence of stroke to lie between 0%-4% [2].

The main modifications to device design that have been important to try to prevent stroke include keeping the tip of delivery system as short and flexible as possible and curved designs to aid passage of the device around the arch. In addition technical aspects of the procedure should ensure that there is little manipulation of the device within the arch, that the device has been completely flushed free of air and adequate peri-procedural anticoagulation is ensured.

Coverage of the LSA

To ensure successful exclusion of the treated thoracic pathology there must be adequate normal or relatively normal aorta within the proximal and distal landing zones to achieve good anchorage and an effective seal at these sites. The supra-aortic

vessels pose a limitation on the proximal landing zone with the majority of pathology located at or close to the origin of the left subclavian artery (LSA). Recent literature has shown that coverage of the LSA is acceptable with some exceptions [7,8,9]. Contraindications without revascularization include:
- aberrant left vertebral artery;
- dominant left vertebral artery;
- previous coronary artery bypass with a patent internal mammary artery;
- functioning A-V fistula.

With this in mind there is a role for carotid and vertebral duplex, computed tomography angiography (CTA), magnetic resonance angiography (MRA) and conventional angiography (DSA) to assess patency, size and location of the vertebral arteries. MRA also has a role in the assessment of the circle of Willis.

A recent study showed an incidence of left upper extremity symptoms of 21% in patients who had the subclavian artery occluded during TEVAR, though this is in keeping with observations elsewhere that after LSA coverage 63%-100% of patients remain asymptomatic [7,10]. Despite this apparent high rate of symptoms the majority of patients do not require intervention, as demonstrated by the fact that of the four symptomatic patients in the study by Reisenman et al. [10] only one patient required intervention for his upper extremity symptoms. Partial coverage of the LSA, however, was associated with an increased risk of type 1A endoleak.

Symptoms include those of vertebrobasilar insufficiency and left arm ischemia. Intervention may be warranted, but data now would support expectant management of left arm ischemia in the first instance, if the limb were not threatened.

Endoleak and aortic complications

The classification of endoleaks has been well documented and is illustrated in Table I. Endoleaks after thoracic endovascular therapy are a serious complication and have been reported in up to 14% of cases [11]. Data pertaining to the early 30-day outcome from the combined experience of the EUROSTAR and United Kingdom Thoracic Endograft Registries in relation to endoleaks suggests that the incidence is low (Table II) [4]. En-

Table I	Classification of endoleak
I	*Attachment site leaks*
A	Proximal
B	Distal
C	Iliac occluder
II	*Collateral vessel leaks*
A	Simple or to and from (from single vessel)
B	Complex (flow through 2 or more vessels)
III	*Graft failure*
A	Midgraft hole
B	Juctional leak or disconnect
C	Other causes of failure (suture holes, etc)
IV	*Graft wall porosity*
V	*Endotension*
A	Without endoleak
B	With sealed endoleak
C	With type I or III endoleak
D	With type II endoleak

doleak after stent-graft treatment of the descending TAA was usually graft fixation related type I endoleak. Type II endoleaks were relatively uncommon which is in accordance with the available literature. Type II endoleak may develop from the LSA. These may be successfully excluded by coil embolization at the origin of the LSA (Figs. 1-3). Type-I endoleak is amenable to further endovascular management in the form of additional endoluminal stent-grafting, stenting or angioplasty alone, embolization or open conversion. Rodriguez et al. [12] has recently evaluated their single center experience of endoluminal graft repair of various thoracic aortic pathologies. Early endoleaks included 18 (5.5%) type I, four (1.2%) type II, and two (0.6%) type III. No intervention was required in 15 (six of them type I) of 24 endoleaks. Re-intervention related to management of early endoleaks involved deployment of an additional endoluminal graft in 11 patients, stenting in three, and coil embolization in one patient. Of these, one had a large persistent proximal type I endoleak treated with open conversion.

A recent publication found no significant difference in the number of endoleaks between elective and emergent endovascular repair of the thoracic

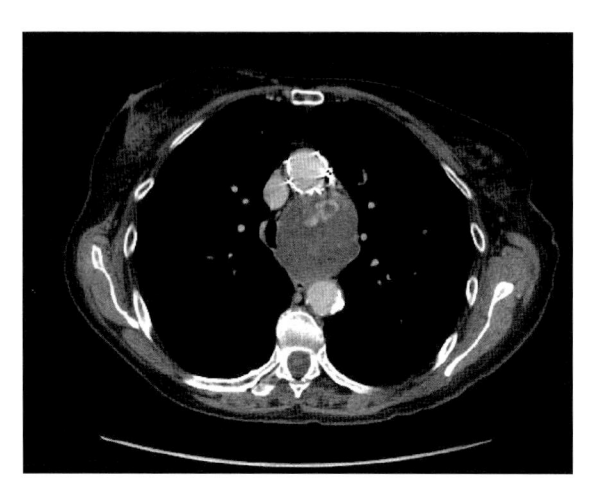

FIG. 1 Axial CT demonstrating contrast within the aneurysm sac following stent graft placement. (*Image provided courtesy of Prof. P Gaines*).

aorta [13]. This finding was later confirmed again by Rodriguez et al. [12] in which the urgency of the procedure was not a predictive factor for increased risk of endoleak (p=0.186). ANOVA analysis also showed that the type of pathology influenced the incidence of endoleak with TAA having absolute increased incidence of all endoleak types, type I, II, and III, though this was not statistically significant (p=0.49).

A potentially dangerous complication is that of a retrograde type A dissection after implantation of the stent-graft. The bare springs of the stent-graft may perforate the intimal and medial layer of the aortic wall. Uncontrolled movement at this point may cause forward and backward movements of the bare spring leading to perforation of the already damaged aortic wall. This complication has

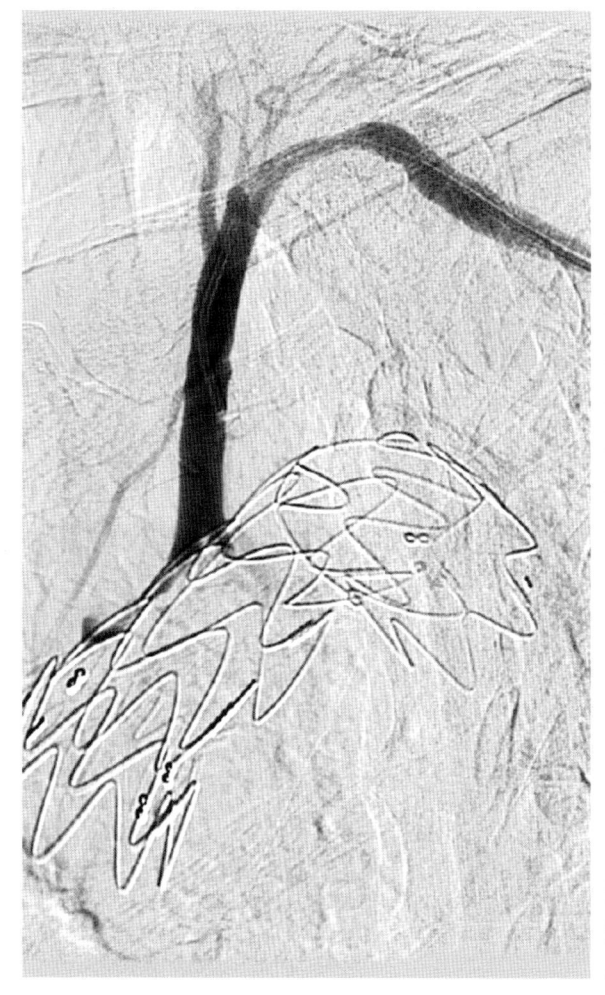

FIG. 2 Digital Subtraction angiogram demonstrating a type II endoleak from the left subclavian artery.

FIG. 3 Successful coil embolisation of the left subclavian artery. (*Image provided courtesy of Prof. P Gaines*).

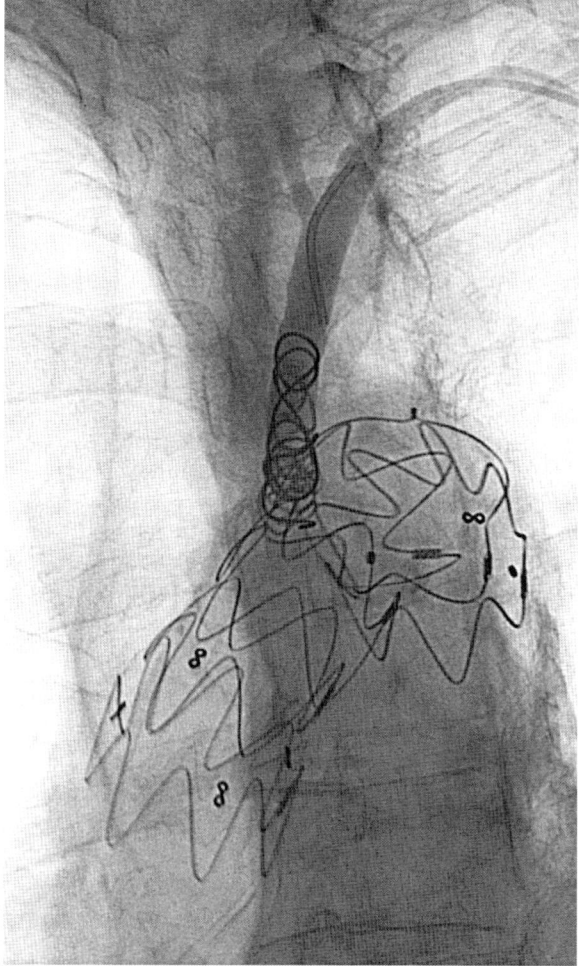

Table II	EARLY (30-DAY) OUTCOME. COMBINED EXPERIENCE FROM THE EUROSTAR AND UNITED KINGDOM THORACIC ENDOGRAFT REGISTRIES							
	Atherosclerotic aneurysm (N=249)		Aortic dissection (N=131)		False anastomotic aneurysm (N=13)		Traumatic rupture (N=50)	
	N	%	N	%	N	%	N	%
Endoleak								
Proximal	12	4.8	2	1.5	1	7.7	-	-
Midgraft	4	1.6	2	1.5	-	-	-	-
Distal	3	1.2	2	1.5	-	-	-	-
Perfusion from side branches	4	1.6	2	1.5	-	-		

been reported and has recently been described after using an Excluder stent-graft [14]. In a similar fashion there is the potential to transform a type-B intramural hematoma into a retrograde type-A thoracic dissection. Extreme care and appropriate device selection is paramount.

Stent-graft collapse

Collapse of the stent-graft is associated with considerable morbidity and mortality. In a recent series 2 of 7 patients presenting with stent-graft collapse died as a result of the collapse, with one other patient suffering significant morbidity [15]. Presentation may be the asymptomatic recognition of the problem at follow-up imaging or in the form of symptoms consistent with thoracic aortic occlusion including chest pain and distal ischemia. The true incidence is unknown.

A possible mechanism is that during systole high aortic flow, and the pressure drop this produces within the stent graft, causes stent-graft collapse, though this is usually followed by re-expansion during diastole. Such gross movements may occur commonly and are thought to be one of the causes of stent framework fatigue. If fracture of the supporting stent occurs this will potentially lead to collapse of the stent graft. Of note though is another potential cause with stent-graft collapse associated with poor apposition of the stent graft to the inner curve of the aortic wall with a >50% protrusion into the lumen of the arch. There is therefore the potential for blood to be forced behind the stent-graft at this site and this may also lead to stent-graft collapse. Deliberate placement across the origin of the left subclavian artery, may allow greater conformity to the thoracic arch, reducing the risk of this happening. In those patients in which stent-graft collapse is identified balloon angioplasty alone is usually futile due to the loss of any expansile force within the stent. Deployment of a large balloon mounted stent (Palmaz) is the preferred treatment. Presentation is varied but may occur from 3 days post implantation.

Puncture site complications

Most TEVAR procedures are performed using a surgical cut down, though there are a number of reports of the use of closure devices to allow percutaneous placement of the device.

Wound hematomas can develop with either percutaneous or open arterial access. The incidence was 2%-3% in one of the studies where the main approach was through surgical cut down [16], incomplete closure of the arteriotomy and abnormal clotting profile increases the risk of hematomas multifold.

Wound infection (1%-2%) is another potential complication at the puncture site, especially if a hematoma occurs. Such an outcome may be very problematic especially if there is vascular spread.

Damage to the access artery, may be caused at the time of implantation by a combination of the large caliber delivery system and pre-existing iliofemoral atheromatous disease, so it is important to assess the access vessels carefully when planning the approach. Access vessel damage may take the form of arterial dissections, pseudoaneurysms, distant embolization and rupture. Fortunately most of these complications are uncommon with access-related iliac artery rupture and thrombosis of the common femoral artery, reported as occurring in <1% of reported cases [16]. An alternative approach for vascular access include use of iliac or aortic conduits when the common femoral artery (CFA) or / and external iliac artery (EIA) are too unfavorable to permit safe device insertion.

Although only few studies are available, they show that percutaneous approaches for access have fewer complications compared to other forms of access approach. It should, however, be bore in mind that the outcome for a failed percutaneous approach may be catastrophic. Proper patient selection, exact puncture technique and accurate use of the device are important factors for success.

Systemic complications

Systemic complications when occurring mainly affect the renal, cardiac and respiratory systems. The incidence of long-term renal failure is poorly documented in the literature. The incidence of postoperative renal failure ranged between 4% to 8% in the different studies published. The most likely etiology is multifactorial. Chronically impaired renal function was found to be a major risk factor for acute post interventional renal failure. Other factors, including the type and total amount of contrast media, hemodynamic variables and atheroembolic causes can contribute to the occurrence of renal failure [17,18].

Respiratory complications occur in 4%-8%, with the main reported causes being pneumonia and respiratory failure. This may be explained due to a combination anesthetic factors, prolonged recovery and poor respiratory reserve prior to theatre.

Cardiac complications including myocardial infarction, arrhythmias and congestive cardiac failure occurred in 2%-5% of the patients, though when they occur are a major cause of morbidity and mortality [17].

REFERENCES

1. Scharrer-Pamler R, Kotsis T, Kapfer X et al. Complications after endovascular treatment of thoracic aortic aneurysms. *J Endovasc Ther* 2003; 10: 711-718.
2. Matsagas MI, Papakostas JC, Katsouras CS et al. Endovascular repair for thoracic aortic disease: tertiary single-centre experience in northwestern Greece. *Vascular* 2006; 14: 212-218.
3. Saratzis N, Saratzis A, Melas N et al. Endovascular treatment of descending thoracic aortic aneurysm with endofit stent-graft. *Cardiovascular and Interventional Radiology* 2007; 30: 177-181.
4. Leurs LJ, Bell R, Degrieck Y et al. Endovascular treatment of thoracic aortic diseases : combined experience from the EUROSTAR and United Kigdom Thoracic Endograft registries. *J Vasc Surg* 2004; 40: 670-679.
5. Bavaria JE, Appoo JJ, Makaroun MS et al. Endovascular stent grafting versus open surgical repair of descending thoracic aortic aneurysms in low-risk patients : a multicenter comparative trial. *J Thorac Cardiovasc Surg* 2007; 113: 369-377.
6. Rousseau H, Bolduc JP, Dambrin C et al. Stent-Graft repair of thoracic aortic aneurysms. *Tech Vasc Interv Radiol* 2005; 8: 61-72.
7. Görich J, Asquan Y, Seifarth H et al. Initial experience with intentional stent-graft coverage of the subclavian artery during endovascular thoracic aortic repairs. *J Endovasc Ther* 2002; 9 Suppl 2: II39-43.
8. Rehders TC, Petzsch M, Ince H et al. Intentional occlusion of the left subclavian artery during stent-graft implantation in the thoracic aorta: risk and relevance. *J Endovasc Ther* 2004; 11: 659-666.
9. Caronno R, Piffaretti G, Tozzi M et al. Intentional coverage of the left subclavian artery during endovascular stent graft repair for thoracic aortic disease. *Surg Endosc* 2006; 20: 915-918.
10. Reisenman PJ, Farber MA, Mendes RR et al. Coverage of the left subclavian artery during thoracic endovascular aortic repair. *J Vasc Surg* 2007; 45: 90-94.
11. Piffaretti G, Tozzi M, Lomazzi C et al. Complications after endovascular stent-grafting of thoracic aortic diseases. *J Cardiothorac Surg* 2006; 1: 26.
12. Rodriguez J, Olsen DM, Shtutman A et al. Application of Endograft to treat thoracic aortic pathologies : a single center experience. *J Vasc Surg* 2007; 46: 413-420.
13. Iyer VS, MacKenzie KS, Tse LW et al. Early outcomes after elective and emergent endovascular repair of the thoracic aorta. *J Vasc Surg* 2006; 43: 677-683.
14. Totaro M, Miraldi F, Fanelli F et al. Emergency surgery for retrograde extension of type B dissection after endovascular stent graft repair. *Eur J Cardiothorac Surg* 2001; 20: 1057-1058.
15. Hinchliffe RJ, Krasznai A, SchultzeKool L et al. Observations on the Failure of Stent-grafts in the Aortic Arch. *Eur J Vasc Endovasc Surg* 2007; 34: 451-456.
16. Ramaiah V, Rodriguez-Lopez J, Diethrich EB. Endografting of the thoracic aorta. *J Card Surg* 2003; 18: 444-454.
17. Wheatley GH 3rd, Gurbuz AT, Rodriguez-Lopez JA et al. Midterm Outcome in 158 Consecutive Gore TAG Thoracic Endoprostheses: single Center Experience. *Ann Thorac Surg* 2006; 81: 1570-1577.
18. Di Tommaso L, Monaco M, Mottola M et al. Major complications following endovascular surgery of descending thoracic aorta. *Interact CardioVasc Thorac Surg* 2006; 5: 705-708.

PRINTED BY
EDIZIONI MINERVA MEDICA
APRIL 2008
SALUZZO (ITALY)
CORSO IV NOVEMBRE, 29-31